*Clinical Guide to*

# PSYCHOTROPIC
# MEDICATIONS

*Clinical Guide*

—— TO ——

# PSYCHOTROPIC
# MEDICATIONS

Steven L. Dubovsky, M.D.

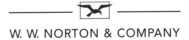

**W. W. NORTON & COMPANY**

*New York · London*

For information about permission to reproduce selections from this book, write to Permissions, W. W. Norton & Company, Inc., 500 Fifth Avenue, New York, NY 10110

Production Manager: Leeann Graham
Manufacturing by Quebecor World Fairfield Graphics

**Library of Congress Cataloging-in-Publication Data**

Dubovsky, Steven L.
    Clinical guide to psychotropic medications / Steven L. Dubovsky.
        p.      ; cm.
    "A Norton professional book."
    Includes bibliographical references and index.
    **ISBN 0-393-70419-X**
    1. Psychotropic drugs—Handbooks, manuals, etc.  I. Title.
    [DNLM: 1. Psychotropic Drugs—therapeutic use—Handbooks.
QV 39 D818 2004]

RM315.D877  2004
615'.788—dc22        2004058106

W. W. Norton & Company, Inc., 500 Fifth Avenue,
New York, N.Y. 10110
www.wwnorton.com

W. W. Norton & Company Ltd., Castle House, 75/76 Wells St.,
London W1T 3QT

1  3  5  7  9  0  8  6  4  2

# CONTENTS

# ABBREVIATIONS

| | |
|---|---|
| AA | arachidonic acid |
| AChE | acetylcholinesterase |
| ACTH | adrenocorticotrophic hormone |
| ADAS | Alzheimer's Disease Assessment Scale |
| ADCS-ADLsev | Alzheimer's Disease Cooperative study–Activities of Daily Living |
| ADD | attention deficit disorder |
| ADH | antidiuretic hormone |
| ADHD | attention deficit hyperactivity disorder |
| AED | antiepileptic drug |
| ALT | alanine aminotransferase |
| AMPA | $\alpha$-amino-3-hydroxy-5-methyl-4-isoxazole propionic acid |
| APUD | amine precursor uptake and decarboxylation |
| ASA | aminosalicylic acid (aspirin) |
| AUC | area under time-concentration curve |
| AV | atrioventricular |
| | |
| BAL | blood alcohol level |
| bcl-2 | b-cell lymphocyte-2 |
| BDNF | brain-derived neurotropic factor |
| BL | bilateral |
| BMI | Body Mass Index |
| BPH | benign prostatic hypertrophy |
| BPRS | Brief Psychiatric Rating Scale |
| BuChE | butylcholinesterase |
| BZD | benzodiazepine |
| | |
| CA | carbonic anhydrase |
| CAMP | cyclic adenosine monophosphate |
| CAST | Cardiac Arrhythmia Suppression Trial |
| CCB | calcium channel blocker |
| CDC | Centers for Disease Control, United States |

| CDRS | Childhood Depression Rating Scale |
|------|-----------------------------------|
| CDRS-R | Revised CDRS |
| CFS | chronic fatigue syndrome |
| CGI | Clinical Global Impressions |
| CGI-I | CGI for improvement |
| CI | cholinesterase inhibitor |
| CIBIC | Clinician's Interview-Based Impression |
| CNS | central nervous system |
| COPD | chronic obstructive pulmonary disease |
| CPK | creatine phosphokinase |
| CPT | Current Procedural Terminology or carnitine palmitoyltransferase |
| CR | controlled release |
| CSF | cerebrospinal fluid |

| D5S | 5% dextrose in saline |
|-----|------------------------|
| D5W | 5% dextrose in water |
| DA/ACH | dopamine/acetylcholine |
| DDAVP | arginine vasopressin |
| DL | deciliter |
| DHA | docosahexaenoic acid |
| DHEA | dehydroepiandrosterone |
| DHEA-S | dehydroepiandrosterone sulphate |
| DSM | *Diagnostic and Statistical Manual* |
| DST | dexamethasone suppression test |

| EAA | excitatory amino acid |
|-----|------------------------|
| ECT | electroconvulsive therapy |
| EFA | essential fatty acid |
| EKG | electrocardiogram |
| E-EPA | ethyl-eicosapentaenoic acid |
| EPA | eicosapentaenoic acid |
| ER | emergency room |

| FBS | fasting blood sugar |
|-----|----------------------|
| FDA | Food and Drug Administration, United States |
| FSH | follicle stimulating hormone |

| GAD | generalized anxiety disorder |
|-----|-------------------------------|
| G-CSF | granulocyte colony stimulating factor |
| GGT | gamma glutamyl transferase |
| GHB | gamma hydroxybutyrate |
| GI | gastrointestinal |

| | |
|---|---|
| GLU | glutamate |
| Gm | granulocyte-macrophage |
| GM-CSF | granulocyte-macrophage colony stimulating factor |
| GnRH | gonadotropin-releasing hormone |
| | |
| H1 | histamine-1 (receptor) |
| HAM-A | Hamilton Anxiety Rating Scale |
| HAM-D | Hamilton Depression Rating Scale |
| HCA | heterocyclic antidepressants |
| HDL | high density lipoprotein |
| HLA | human leukocyte antigen |
| HPA | hypothalamic-pituitary-adrenal cortical |
| HRSD | Hamilton Rating Scale for Depression |
| HRT | hormone replacement therapy |
| Hs | hour of sleep (bedtime) |
| Hz | Hertz (cycles per second) |
| | |
| IQ | intelligence quotient |
| IU | International Units |
| | |
| L | litre |
| LA | long acting |
| LAAM | L-alpha-acetylmethodol acetate |
| $LD_{50}$ | dose that will kill 50% of subjects |
| L-dopa | L-dihydroxyphenylalanine |
| LDL | low density lipoprotein |
| LFT | liver function test |
| LH | luteinizing hormone |
| LOCF | last observation carried forward |
| | |
| MADRS | Montgomery-Asberg Depression Rating Scale |
| MAO | monoamine oxidase |
| MAO-A | monoamine oxidase-A |
| MAO-B | monoamine oxidase-B |
| MB | muscle-brain component |
| MCPP | meta-chlorophenylpiperidine |
| MDD | major depressive disorder |
| $Mg^{2+}$ | magnesium |
| MHD | monohydroxy derivative |
| MHPG | methodoxy-4-hydroxyphenylglycol |
| MMSE | Mini Mental State Exam |
| MS | either mental status or morphine sulphate |

| | |
|---|---|
| n | number |
| Na-K | sodium-potassium |
| NCQA | National Committee on Quality Assurance, United States |
| NE | norepinephrine |
| NE-5HT | norepinephrine-serotonin |
| NMDA | N-methyl-D-asparate |
| nM | nanomolar |
| nmol | nanomol |
| NMS | neuroleptic malignant syndrome |
| NNT | number needed to treat |
| NOS | not otherwise specified |
| NPI | Neuropsychiatric Inventory |
| NT | neuroleptic threshold |
| | |
| OCD | obsessive compulsive disorder |
| OR | odds ratio |
| | |
| P50 | positive deflection at 50 msec |
| P450 | short for CYP450 |
| PABA | *p*-aminobenzoic acid |
| PANDAS | pediatric autoimmune disorder associated with streptococcal infection |
| PANSS | Positive and Negative Syndrome Scale |
| PCOS | polycystic ovary syndrome |
| PCP | phencyclidine |
| PDD | pervasive developmental disorders |
| PLMS | periodic limb movements of sleep |
| PSA | prostate specific antigen |
| PTH | parathyroid hormone |
| | |
| REM | rapid eye movement |
| RIMA | reversible inhibitor of MAO-A |
| RLS | restless legs syndrome |
| RR | relative risk |
| rTMS | repetitive transcranial magnetic stimulation |
| RUL | right-sided unilateral |
| | |
| SA | sinoatrial |
| SAMe | S-adenosylmethionine |
| SANS | Schedule for Assessment of Negative Symptoms |
| SD | standard deviation |
| SIADH | syndrome of inappropriate antidiuretic hormone secretion |

| SJW | St. John's Wort |
|---|---|
| SPECT | single photon emission tomography |
| SR | sustained release |
| SRI | serotonin reuptake inhibitor |
| | |
| $T_3$ | triiodothyronine |
| $T_4$ | thyroxine |
| TBI | traumatic brain injury |
| TIA | transient ischemic attack |
| TNF | tumor necrosis factor |
| TRH | thyrotropin releasing hormone |
| TSH | thyroid stimulating hormone |
| | |
| VNS | vagus nerve stimulation |
| | |
| WBC | white blood cell count |
| | |
| XR | extended release |
| | |
| Y-BOCS | Yale–Brown Obsessive–Compulsive Scale |
| YMRS | Young Mania Rating Scale |

# PREFACE

Modern psychopharmacology is progressing at a breakneck pace. Not only is new knowledge emerging every day, but practitioners ranging from psychiatrists, primary care physicians, and other medical specialists to nonphysician clinicians with prescribing authority are finding it necessary to use psychotropic medications in their daily practices.

There is no shortage of information about these medications. In fact, so many studies are being published that it seems impossible to keep up with them. The most that it seems possible to do is to glance at the abstract. More frequently, it is necessary to rely on summaries of recent research in lectures, newsletters, special issues of journals, and from manufacturers. Practitioners are inundated with material from pharmaceutical representatives that is difficult to interpret critically in the context of a busy practice.

This book is designed for busy clinicians who need rapid access to essential data about somatic therapies in psychiatry. Evaluating the clinical utility of the studies and opinions that flood the practitioner's office every day is a major challenge. Manufacturers obviously present research in a manner that favors their products. It is less obvious that, despite their best intentions, academicians cannot avoid evaluating their results in the light of their favorite theories and biases. In this volume, seminal studies that are frequently quoted to support a particular point of view are critically evaluated and placed in perspective.

Understanding the limitations of research in psychopharmacology is especially important; most of the "gold standard" (i.e., double-blind, placebo-controlled) studies are conducted with patients who resemble those seen in primary care practice rather than those seen by the psychiatrist. Most of these studies exclude patients with substance abuse and with comorbid psychiatric or medical conditions. Studies of antidepressants usually exclude patients with psychotic and bipolar depression and with significant suicide risk, and industry-sponsored studies of mood-stabilizing medications do not include the patients with complex forms of mood cycling who are common in specialty practice. The primary outcome variables are almost always changes in one, or at most a small number of, symptom rating scale scores, with little discussion of the clinical significance of statistically significant changes and no evaluation of changes in functioning.

The most important limitation of current psychopharmacological research is that the basic premise is usually that a single treatment is equivalent to, or better than, another treatment or is more effective than a placebo. This approach ignores the reality that psychiatric disorders, especially those treated by the specialist, are physiologically complex and often require combinations of treatments. In contrast, research in serious medical illnesses such as AIDS and cancer investigates which treatment combinations are most effective and in which order they should be sequenced for which patients. Psychiatric research has not yet taken this step, leaving decisions about treatment combinations to clinical experience and the consensus of experts who may or may not actually treat the conditions about which they make treatment recommendations.

The summaries in this book combine published research and clinical experience. I have cited and attempted to place in context important recent studies and reviews, but to avoid clutter I have not referenced every point. Much of the information the clinician needs for rational prescribing can be found in this volume, but no professional book is complete, and more detailed discussions of pathophysiology and pharmacology can be found in texts such as *The Pharmacological Basis of Therapeutics*, the *American Psychiatric Press Textbook of Psychopharmacology*, the *Comprehensive Textbook of Psychiatry*, and the *American Psychiatric Press Textbook of Psychiatry*. Most important, although the information presented here was up to date as of the time this book was written, today's facts are likely to become tomorrow's fantasies. The scientific clinician not only must keep up with new developments but must also conduct each patient encounter as if it were an experiment, testing hypotheses about the nature of the problem and the best treatment, and rejecting hypotheses that are not confirmed by the patient's improvement. I hope that this book will serve as a valuable partner in the never-ending experiment of clinical practice.

DENVER, COLORADO
NOVEMBER 2004

*Clinical Guide to*

# PSYCHOTROPIC
# MEDICATIONS

# CHAPTER ONE

# *Antipsychotics*

$A$ll antipsychotic medications treat psychosis of any cause; their action is not specific for any particular disorder.

Because most of the older antipsychotic drugs were sedating, they were incorrectly referred to as "major tranquilizers," in contrast to "minor tranquilizers," a term once used to describe antianxiety medications such as the benzodiazepines. However, in most cases, antipsychotics do not treat anxiety unless it is caused by psychosis or mental disorganization, whereas anxiolytic medications do not usually possess antipsychotic properties.

Neuroleptics (from the Greek for "to clasp the neuron") reduce psychosis and cause neurological side effects. The newer atypical antipsychotic drugs have fewer neurological side effects and appear to be as effective for psychosis; however, they may have other kinds of serious adverse effects. In this chapter, the term *neuroleptic* is used to refer to the older antipsychotic drugs, whereas clozapine, risperidone, olanzapine, quetiapine, ziprasidone, aripiprazole, and other newer medications with different pharmacological profiles are called *atypical antipsychotics* or simply *atypicals*.

This chapter covers the use of antipsychotic drugs in the treatment of

- Schizophrenia
- Delusional disorder
- Brief psychotic disorder
- Schizotypal and schizoid personality
- Borderline personality disorder
- HIV/AIDS-related psychotic symptoms
- Substance-induced psychosis
- Tourette's disorder
- Autism/pervasive developmental disorder

Other chapters address the use of antipsychotics for

- Mania (Chapter 5)
- Depression (Chapter 3)
- Aggression (Chapter 6)
- Delirium (Chapter 2)
- Agitation in dementia (Chapter 2)
- Anxiety (Chapter 7)

Table 1.1 provides a basic overview of the drugs addressed in this chapter.

## PHARMACOLOGY

All drugs that have antipsychotic properties block postsynaptic dopamine $D_2$ receptors. Although potency at $D_2$ receptor blockade parallels antipsychotic potency for the neuroleptics, this is not necessarily true of the atypical antipsychotics, which generally have less $D_2$ blockade than the neuroleptics. For all antipsychotic medications, $D_2$ receptor antagonism more precisely predicts acute neurological side effects and prolactinemia.

- $D_2$ occupancy around 60% is necessary for an antipsychotic effect.
- $D_2$ occupancy of 70% is associated with dysphoria and noncompliance.
- Prolactin elevation appears beyond 72% $D_2$ occupancy.
- As $D_2$ occupancy approaches 78%, extrapyramidal side effects (EPS) are more prominent.
- Observations that serum prolactin levels > 16 ng/mL predicted lower relapse risk in patients taking fluphenazine decanoate probably reflect more dopamine receptor blockade by the neuroleptic, indicating higher doses, more compliance, or greater $D_2$ receptor sensitivity.

Atypical antipsychotics have reduced $D_2$ occupancy and relatively higher $5HT_2$ occupancy, as well as possibly faster dissociation from the $D_2$ receptor.

- Clozapine produces significantly less $D_2$ occupancy than haloperidol and olanzapine (20–49% vs. 67–94% and 63–85%, respectively); risperidone $D_2$ occupancy ranges from 63 to 89%. The amount of $D_2$ occupancy predicts EPS.
- Clozapine moves on and off $D_2$ receptors 100 times faster than haloperidol.
  - This could permit less distortion of phasic dopamine signaling.
  - Transient receptor occupancy may result in less tolerance and receptor up-regulation and less EPS

## Table 1.1 Names, Classes, Dose Forms, Colors

| GENERIC NAMES | BRAND NAMES | DOSE FORMS (mg) | COLORS |
|---|---|---|---|
| | | **PHENOTHIAZINES** | |
| *Aliphatics* | | t:10/25/50/ | t: all orange |
| chlorpromazine | Thorazine | 100/200<br>sr: 30/75/150<br>200/300<br>o: 10/30/100<br>p: 25 mg/ml<br>s: 10 mg/5ml<br>sp: 25/100 mg/ml | |
| *Piperidines* | | t:10/25/50/ | t: all red |
| mesoridazine | Serentil | 100<br>o: 25 mg/ml<br>p: 25/mg/ml | |
| thioridazine | Mellaril | t: 10/15/25/50/<br>100/150/200<br>o: 30/100 mg/ml | t: chartreuse/<br>pink/tan/white<br>green/yellow/pink<br>o: straw yellows/<br>light yellow |
| | Mellaril-S | su: 25/100 mg/<br>5 ml | |
| *Piperazines* | | t:10/25/50/ | t: all red |
| fluphenazine | Permitil | t: 2.5/5/10<br>o: 5 mg/ml | t: light orange/<br>purple-pink/<br>light red |
| | Prolixin | t: 1/2.5/5/10<br>e: 0.5 mg/ml<br>o: 5 mg/ml<br>p: 2.5 mg/ml | t: pink/yellow<br>green/red |
| fluphenazine<br>decanoate | Prolixin<br>decanoate | p: 25 mg/ml | — |
| fluphenazine<br>enanthate | Prolixin<br>enanthate | p: 25 mg/ml | — |
| perphenazine | Trilafon | t: 2/4/8/16<br>o:3.2 mg/ml<br>p: 5 mg/ml | t: all gray |
| trifluoperazine | Stelazine | t: 1/2/5/10<br>o: 10 mg/ml<br>p: 2 mg/ml | t: all blue |
| | | **BUTYROPHENONES** | |
| haloperidol | Haldol | t: 0.5/1/2/5/<br>10/20<br>o: 2 mg/ml<br>p: 5 mg/ml | t: white/yellow<br>pink/green<br>aqua/salmon |
| haloperidol<br>decanoate | Haldol<br>decanoate | p: 50/100 mg/ml | — |

*(continues)*

**Table 1.1  Continued**

| GENERIC NAMES | BRAND NAMES | DOSE FORMS (mg) | COLORS |
|---|---|---|---|
| | | **THIOXANTHENES** | |
| thiothixene | Navane | c: 1/2/5/20<br>o: 5 mg/ml<br>p: 2/5 mg/ml | c: orange-yellow/<br>blue-yellow/<br>orange-white/<br>blue-white/dark<br>blue-light blue |
| | | **DIPHENYLBUTYLPIPERDINES** | |
| pimozide | Orap | t: 2 mg | t: white |
| | | **DIBENZAZEPINE** | |
| loxapine | Loxitane | c: 5/10/25/50 | t: dark green/<br>yellow-green/<br>light green-dark<br>green/blue-dark<br>green |
| | Loxitane-C<br>Loxitane-IM | o: 25 mg/ml<br>p: 50 mg/ml | —<br>— |
| | | **DIHYDROINDOLONE** | |
| molindone | Moban | t: 5/10/25/50/<br>100<br>o: 20 mg/ml | t: orange/lavender/<br>light green/blue/<br>tan<br>o: cherry |
| | | **THIENOBENZODIAZEPINE** | |
| olanzapine | Zyprexa | t: 2.5/5/7.5/<br>10/15<br>t: 5/10 | t: white (2.5–10 mg)/<br>/blue (15 mg)<br>t: yellow (orally<br>disintegrating) |
| | | **DIBENZODIAZEPINE** | |
| clozapine | Clozaril | t: 25/100 | t: all yellow |
| | | **DIBENZOTHIAZEPINE** | |
| quetiapine | Seroquel | t: 25/100/200/<br>300 | t: peach/yellow/<br>white<br>round/white<br>capsule |
| ziprasidone | Geodon | c: 20/40/60/80 | c: blue/white-<br>blue/blue-<br>white/white-<br>blue white |

(continues)

**Table 1.1 Continued**

| GENERIC NAMES | BRAND NAMES | DOSE FORMS (mg) | COLORS |
|---|---|---|---|
| | | BENZISOXAZOLE | |
| risperidone | Risperdal | t: 1/2/3/4 | t: white/orange/ |
| | Risperdal M-tab | t: 0.5/1/2 mg dissolves in mouth | t: coral |
| depot risperidone | Risperdal Consta | p: 25/37.5/50 mg per 2 mL | |
| | | QUINOLONE | |
| aripiprazole | Abilify | t: 5/10/15/ 20/30 | t: blue/pink/ yellow/white/ pink |

c = capsules; e = elixir; o = oral concentrate; p = parenteral concentrate; s = syrup; sp = suppository; sr = sustained-release spansules; su = suspension; t = tablets.

- Animal studies suggest that fast dissociation leads to less receptor up-regulation and reduced risk of tardive dyskinesia (TD).
- Quetiapine produces relatively high $D_2$ occupancy (58–64%) in 2–3 hours after a single dose, but this decreases to 0–27% within 12 hours. Rapid dissociation from the $D_2$ receptor may explain the low rate of EPS and prolactin elevation with quetiapine.
- Aripiprazole is a $D_2$ partial agonist.

Striatal $D_2$ occupancy was studied with single photon emission tomography (SPECT) in controls and in patients with schizophrenia treated with 7.5 mg olanzapine or 2.5 mg haloperidol (de Haan et al., 2003).

- Subjective well-being was greatest at $D_2$ occupancy between 60 and 70%.
- Olanzapine at 7.5 mg occupied 51% of $D_2$ receptors, vs. 66% with haloperidol 2.5 mg.
- There was substantial interindividual variability in $D_2$ occupancy.
- Based on these results, the dose of olanzapine probably must be > 7.5 mg for first-onset schizophrenia.
- The subjective response to 7.5 mg of olanzapine was not superior to haloperidol 2.5 mg.

Combined with reduced $D_2$ occupancy, the atypical antipsychotic drugs are as potent as the neuroleptics at antagonizing serotonin $5HT_2$ receptors. This feature has three important consequences:

- Because stimulation of $5HT_2$ receptors reduces dopamine release and increases $D_2$ receptor sensitivity, antagonizing $5HT_2$ receptors reduces acute motor side effects caused by dopamine antagonism and decreases the risk of TD caused by postsynaptic dopamine receptor supersensitivity.

- Because $5HT_2$ receptors mediate psychosis, blocking these receptors conveys an additional antipsychotic effect.
- $5HT_2$ antagonism contributes to antidepressant properties of many of the atypical antipsychotics.

Clozapine and probably other atypical antipsychotics also antagonize dopamine $D_1$ and $D_4$ receptors. Aripiprazole is a dopamine receptor partial agonist; it occupies receptors but has a less pronounced action than the parent neurotransmitter. If synaptic dopamine availability is low, the partial agonist binds to the receptor and acts like dopamine, although not quite as potently as the actual neurotransmitter, and net dopaminergic transmission increases. If synaptic dopamine concentrations are excessive, the partial agonist competes with dopamine for its receptor but has less of an effect on it, resulting in a net reduction of dopamine signaling. This dual action has been thought to be useful for the combination of psychosis and agitation, which may be related to increased dopamine signaling, as well as for lack of motivation and withdrawal, which could be related to reduced dopamine signaling in other regions. However, there is no actual evidence that this hypothesis is correct or that aripiprazole is more effective for negative symptoms than any other antipsychotic drug.

Receptor effects probably explain only a portion of the action of antipsychotics. For example, a study of the rat cortex found that clozapine and haloperidol modulate the expression of multiple genes involved in synaptic function and the regulation of intracellular calcium (Kontkanen, Toronen, Lakso, Wong, & Castren, 2002). Clozapine is also the only antipsychotic drug that has been shown to correct sensory gating abnormalities in schizophrenia, possibly through an action on the $\alpha7$ nicotinic receptor.

However, certain effects of atypical antipsychotic drugs can be predicted by their potency at blocking specific receptors. For example:

- Medications with the least $D_2$ blockade, such as clozapine and olanzapine, have the lowest incidence of acute EPS.
- Medications that are more potent as $D_2$ antagonists, such as risperidone, produce more EPS and prolactinemia (dopamine tonically inhibits prolactin release) and may be more rapidly effective against positive symptoms.
- Preparations that are potent histamine $H_1$ receptor antagonists, such as olanzapine and clozapine, produce more sedation and weight gain.
- Drugs that block noradrenergic $\alpha_1$ receptors, such as clozapine, produce more hypotension.

- Drugs that can enhance dopaminergic transmission, such as aripiprazole, are more likely to cause nausea and jitteriness.
- Ziprasidone, which has serotonin reuptake inhibitor properties, can cause jitteriness and sexual dysfunction.

In controlled studies, atypical antipsychotics have been found to be as effective as neuroleptics for positive symptoms (e.g., hallucinations, delusions, disorganization) and more effective for negative symptoms (e.g., social withdrawal, avolitional states). However, research suggests several modifications of these observations:

- The comparison antipsychotic drug in most studies was haloperidol, which has a therapeutic window; however, haloperidol levels were not measured in any studies of atypicals.
- The dose of olanzapine that was as effective as haloperidol in a direct comparison was 30 mg/day.
- Apparent preferential improvement of negative symptoms by atypicals compared to neuroleptics may be a function (to some extent) of less bradykinesia and "cognitive parkinsonism" with the atypicals.
- Improvement of cognition with the atypicals seems to be related more to reduced intrusive thinking and disorganization, mild improvement of some aspects of memory, and less of the interference with cognition by "cognitive parkinsonism" that occurs with the neuroleptics; no antipsychotic drug other than clozapine has been found to reduce the core cognitive dysfunction of schizophrenia, which involves deficient "gating" or filtering of irrelevant information. This deficit is corrected by inhaled (but not oral or intravenous) nicotine, which may be one reason why so many patients with schizophrenia smoke.
  - In a study of treatment-resistant schizophrenia, 24 patients taking fluphenazine and benztropine were randomized to olanzapine or haloperidol (plus benztropine) in doses of 10–30 mg/day (Arango, Summerfelt, & Buchanan, 2003).
    - There were no differences between the two groups in auditory sensory gating measured before and after 12 weeks of randomization by P50-evoked potentials.
  - Atypical antipsychotics have an anti-aggressive action separate from their antipsychotic effect, possibly related to $5HT_2$ antagonism, making these medications more useful for nonpsychotic agitation than the neuroleptics.

Atypical antipsychotics have a lower risk of parkinsonism and TD than the neuroleptics; however, these side effects have been reported with all of the newer medications. Clozapine may actually treat TD, as opposed to just temporarily suppressing it, as do the neuroleptics. Although the reported rate of TD (0.4–0.5%/year) is low for all the aypticals, further experience with these medications may be necessary to elucidate the true risk over time, compared with the 40% cumulative risk with the neuroleptics.

Each of the atypical antipsychotics has specific strengths and weaknesses:

- Risperidone
  - More potent $D_2$ antagonism
  - May be more effective for severe psychosis
  - Higher risk of prolactinemia
- Olanzapine
  - Less EPS and prolactinemia
  - Antidepressant properties
  - Greater risk of weight gain and diabetes mellitus
  - Chewable form useful for preventing "cheeking"
- Quetiapine
  - Extensive $H_1$ blockade results in high sedative property
  - Not as much weight gain as produced
  - Not reliable as antipsychotic at lower doses
  - Requires BID-TID dosing because of 6 hour half-life
  - Useful as sedative/hypnotic at dose of 25–100 mg
- Ziprasidone
  - No sedation or weight gain
  - Jitteriness common
  - Divided dose necessary
  - Prolongs QTc by mean of 9 msec, but no reports of adverse cardiac events
- Aripiprazole
  - No sedation or weight gain.
  - No cardiac effects
  - Can cause jitteriness or affective blunting
- Clozapine is the only atypical antipsychotic that is clearly effective in refractory schizophrenia (as opposed to treatment failure caused only by being unable to tolerate antipsychotics). Clozapine levels > 400 ng/mL seem to be more effective than lower levels. Relapse of schizophrenia has occurred when patients were switched from clozapine to olanzapine. In the treatment of schizophrenia, clozapine is given in divided dose.
  - A meta-regression analysis of heterogeneity of refractory schizophrenia studies (Moncrieff, 2003) suggested that clozapine was more likely to be found superior to other antipsychotics in the presence of
    - Shorter study duration
    - Higher baseline symptom severity

- Industry support of research
- Results suggested that meta-analyses combining data from different clozapine trials may overstate superiority of clozapine.
- In a small open study, 24 patients with refractory schizophrenia were treated with risperidone for 3 months (Cavallaro, Brambilla, & Smeraldi, 1998)
  - 8 patients had 20% improvement
  - Of the other 16 patients, 2 dropped out, 9 had at least 20% improvement with clozapine within the next month, and 5 patients had poorer response to clozapine.
  - At 37 months of follow-up, initial responses remained stable.
  - Clozapine therefore remained useful in a subset of patients unresponsive to risperidone.

With the exception of intravenous haloperidol for severe acute agitation, the higher rate of adverse neurological effects has made the neuroleptics second-line treatments for schizophrenia. Neuroleptics are generally divided into low-potency (i.e., more milligrams are necessary to produce the desired effect) and high-potency preparations; most of the low-potency medications are phenothiazines.

- Low-potency neuroleptics (e.g., chlorpromazine, thioridazine) have
  - Lower incidence of acute EPS
  - More anticholinergic side effects (e.g., dry mouth, blurred vision)
  - More antihistaminic effects causing sedation and weight gain
  - More alpha-adrenergic blockade and hypotension
  - More complex metabolic pathways with more active metabolites
- High-potency neuroleptics have
  - More acute EPS
  - Fewer anticholinergic and antihistaminic side effects
  - Fewer active metabolites

Because of long half-lives and accumulation in the brain, most neuroleptics can be administered in one daily dose. Although higher neuroleptic doses (e.g., 300–500 mg/day of chlorpromazine equivalent) are more rapidly effective for acute psychosis, long-term adherence is poor because of a high incidence of neuroleptic-induced dysphoria, bradykinesia, and motor side effects. Lower doses take longer to be acutely effective, but patients are more likely to continue them. Although there is little rationale for combining different neuroleptics, the combination of a neuroleptic and an atypical antipsychotic is sometimes effective for refractory schizophrenia.

Oral vs. parenteral neuroleptics:

- Peak concentration with oral form usually occurs in 2–4 hours.
  - 6–8 hours for pimozide
  - 15–30 minutes with IM preparations
  - Immediately with intravenous haloperidol
- Onset of anticholinergic effects with oral dosing occurs within 30–60 minutes.
- Acute EPS also can emerge rapidly.
  - More acute EPS with IM but not IV preparations
- Intramuscular doses are 2–4 times as potent as oral doses.

Several $D_2$ antagonist phenothiazines have neuroleptic side effects without much antipsychotic potency.

- Metoclopramide (Reglan) is used to enhance gastric motility.
- Triflupromazine (Vesprin), promazine (Sparine) and prochlorperazine (Compazine) are used as antiemetics.

## CLINICAL INDICATIONS AND USE

### Schizophrenia

Neuroleptics are more effective at relieving the positive than the negative symptoms of schizophrenia. The effectiveness of atypical antipsychotics in reducing positive symptoms is no greater than that of the neuroleptics, and they may be less effective for severe psychosis; however, because patients are more likely to tolerate and therefore continue atypicals, their efficacy is greater. Atypical antipsychotic drugs improve negative symptoms more than neuroleptics, although at least some of this apparent superiority comes from causing *less* bradykinesia, cognitive dulling, and other apparent negative symptoms.

- When the cognitive effects of neuroleptics and atypicals are compared, a significant portion of the superiority of atypicals may be related to less interference with cognition.
- Clozapine improved verbal fluency, psychomotor speed, and possibly preconscious information processing in six out of seven studies (Meltzer & McGurk, 1999).
- A 54-week randomized double-blind study included 20 patients treated with olanzapine (5–20 mg), 20 patients with risperidone (4–6 mg), and 15 patients with haloperidol (5–20 mg) (Purdon, Jones, & Stip, 2000). Independent of symptom improvement, olanzapine improved immediate recall and visual organization throughout the study; at 54 weeks, improvement with risperidone was similar to olanzapine;

haloperidol did not improve cognitve function. Olanzapine was the only medication to reduce parkinsonism, which could account for the early superiority in improvement of cognition. It cannot be concluded that olanzapine is superior to risperidone for cognition, because functions that risperidone seems to help most—namely, working and long-term memory—were not measured.

- 33 patients who were relatively stable following a first psychotic episode of schizophrenia, schizoaffective, or schizophreniform disorder were randomly assigned to olanzapine or risperidone for at least 7 weeks (Broerse, Crawford, & den Boer, 2002).
  - Patients were compared to 23 normal subjects.
  - Patients performed worse than controls on saccade tasks (a measure of visual information processing that is abnormal in schizophrenia).
    - Risperidone and olanzapine were not substantially different in impairment of saccadic measures.
- Atypical antipsychotics have been found to improve
  - Verbal memory
  - Executive function (ability to carry out tasks in sequence)
  - Visuospatial memory (remembering location of objects in space)
  - Reaction time
- Ability to gate irrelevant information—the core cognitive deficit in schizophrenia—is not improved as much by atypical antipsychotics as it is by clozapine.

## Choosing an Antipsychotic Drug

Because of better tolerability and possibly superior efficacy, atypical antipsychotics are generally preferable to neuroleptics as first-line therapies. However, some severely ill patients have a better response to neuroleptics, at least acutely. Since IM preparations of low-potency neuroleptics have a high risk of oversedation and hypotension, patients needing IM dosing are treated with IM haloperidol or ziprasidone. Patients who need extremely rapid control of dangerous psychosis and agitation can be treated with IV haloperidol.

The choice of a specific agent can be guided by the following factors.

- *Past response:* Patients who have previously had a good response to a particular medication might receive the same medication again, whereas patients who have had a poor response to, or have been unable to tolerate, a particular medication usually should not be treated with it again.
- *Initial response:* Patients who have severe side effects after one or two doses of an antipsychotic are not likely to continue it and should receive a different medication.

**Table 1.2  Choosing a Neuroleptic**

| PROBLEM | CHOICE |
|---|---|
| High dystonia risk (under 30-y.o. male; under 25-y.o. female) | High-potency atypical antipsychotics are a first choice, e.g., risperidone or olanzapine. Mid-potency neuroleptic somewhat decreases dystonia risk but may still need ACA. |
| Geriatric (high anticholinergic, orthostatic, sedation) risks, cognitive impairment, or delirium) | Risperidone or haloperidol; olanzapine acceptable if without sedation risk. |
| Predominant or severe negative symptoms | Risperidone, ziprasidone, olanzapine, or clozapine; quetiapine may be effective but optimal dosage can be difficult or impossible to find. |
| Treatment resistant | Risperidone, olanzapine, or clozapine (*see* augmentations on pp. 23–27) |
| TD or Parkinson's disease | Clozapine, olanzapine, or risperidone; first consider reducing L-dopa, which may be causing or exacerbating psychosis. Increased EPS with risperidone at doses of 5 mg or more and in geriatric patients at 2 mg or more. |
| Seizure risk | High-potency neuroleptics, risperidone, olanzapine, or quetiapine: low risks. Clozapine risks up to 5% seizures with 600+ mg qd. Molindone and fluphenazine have some increased risk but not as much as clozapine. |
| Obesity | Molindone; advise patient to lose weight. Avoid low-potency neuroleptics, e.g., clozapine (67% gain weight), chlorpromazine, chlorprothixine, thioridazine, or mesoridazine. Weight gain also with quetiapine and somewhat less for risperidone. Ziprasidone does not cause weight gain. |
| Cardiac arrhythmia | High potency (possibly medium potency). Avoid pimozide, thioridazine, and clozapine. |
| Extreme unresponsive agitation | Droperidol prn as adjunctive agent |
| Minimal compliance with medications | Haloperidol or prolixin decanoate, rarely pimozide orally. Haloperidol decanoate often only needs injection once a month. |
| Mental retardation | Haloperidol or an atypical antipsychotic that does not increase confusion and memory loss. However, an atypical antipsychotic drug that is effective for nonpsychotic agitation and does not impair cognition would be more appropriate for this group. |

- *Family history:* If a first-degree relative has done well with a particular medication, the patient may have a similar result.
- *Side-effect profile of the medication:*
  - Patients with severe insomnia might receive a sedating antipsychotic drug such as olanzapine, quetiapine, or chlorpromazine; initial choices for patients who cannot tolerate sedation include ziprasidone or aripiprazole, or possibly risperidone, fluphenazine, haloperidol, or trifluoperazine.
  - Patients who cannot tolerate weight gain or who have diabetes should not be treated with medications that can aggravate these problems (e.g., olanzapine, clozapine, and the low-potency neuroleptics). Ziprasidone, aripiprazole, and molindone are least likely to cause weight gain or metabolic changes.
  - Patients with heart block should not receive a neuroleptic (all are type Ia antiarrhythmics); olanzapine, risperidone, and aripiprazole do not have significant cardiac effects.
- Bedtime dosing of most antipsychotic medications improves compliance and reduces adverse effects because peak levels occur while the patient is asleep.
  - Activating antipsychotics such as ziprasidone and aripiprazole are more likely to interfere with sleep if they are given too late in the day.

### Atypical Antipsychotics versus Neuroleptics

- A comprehensive review of fixed-dose studies (Woods, 2003) of antipsychotic drugs found that 100 mg/day chlorpromazine was equivalent to
  - Haloperidol 2 mg
  - Risperidone 2 mg
  - Olanzapine 5 mg
  - Quetiapine 75 mg
  - Ziprasidone 60 mg
  - Aripiprazole 7.5 mg
- A multicenter industry-sponsored study randomized 309 chronically ill schizophrenia patients to haloperidol 5–20 mg with 1–4 mg prophylactic benztropine or 5–20 mg olanzapine plus benztropine placebo (Rosenheck, Davis, Evans, & Herz, 2003).
  - No significant differences were found in completion of the year-long trial (46% on olanzapine vs. 39% on haloperidol), final scores on Positive and Negative Syndrome Scale (PANSS), or quality of life.
  - Olanzapine patients had significantly less akathisia but not TD.
  - Weight gain was more common with olanzapine.

- No difference in cost of service was found.
- Cost of olanzapine was 4–5 times as high, increasing total annual health care costs by $3,000–9,000.

A meta-analysis of published trials of new antipsychotic drugs found the following (Davis, Chen, & Glick, 2003):
- Effect sizes (mean symptom score improvement/variance of results) > neuroleptics were
  - Clozapine: 0.49
  - Risperidone: 0.25
    - Corresponds to reduction of 4–6 points on the PANSS or 3–4 points on the Brief Psychiatric Rating Scale (BPRS)
  - Olanzapine: 0.21
- Haloperidol effect size compared to placebo: 0.60
  - Corresponds to decrease of 13 points on PANSS or 8 points on BPRS
- Effect size compared to placebo of aripiprazole, quetiapine, ziprasidone equivalent to neuroleptics.
- Therefore, clozapine, risperidone, and olanzapine were significantly more efficacious than neuroleptics, with superiority of clozapine over neuroleptics being twice as great as superiority of risperidone and olanzapine.
  - Risperidone and olanzapine had less than half the greater efficacy of haloperidol than haloperidol had over placebo; other atypicals were not more effective than neuroleptics, although they are better tolerated.
- Clozapine most effective at doses > 400 mg.
  - Most comparisons with clozapine used lower clozapine doses.
- Atypical antipsychotics > neuroleptics for negative symptoms, mood, thought disorder, and impulse control.

A meta-analysis of 30 controlled trials involving 2,500 patients found 5 that were 6 months–2 years in duration (Wahlbeck, Cheine, Essali, & Adams, 1999). Clozapine was more effective than other treatments, especially for refractory schizophrenia.

A public mental health system randomly assigned 108 patients with schizophrenia or schizoaffective disorder to risperidone, olanzapine, or neuroleptics (primarily haloperidol; Jerrell, 2002). Patients were followed every 3 months for 1 year.
- Compliance was greatest with olanzapine.

- Odds ratio for receiving supplemental neuroleptic or atypical was 2.7 for olanzapine and 4.13 for risperidone.
- All treatments produced equivalent improvements in both positive and negative symptoms and psychosocial functioning.
- Depression and mania symptoms increased significantly over time, with similar increases with all medications.
- No significant difference between medications in risk of rehospitalization.
- No significant differences in patient satisfaction.
- No difference between groups in cost of mental health care, except that olanzapine and risperidone were significantly more expensive than neuroleptics.

A consensus conference on the pharmacotherapy of schizophrenia made the following recommendations (Marder, Essock, Miller, et al., 2002):

- An atypical antipsychotic should be used before a neuroleptic for a first episode of schizophrenia or for patients whose history of past response to antipsychotics is unavailable.
  - The risks of neurological side effects with neuroleptics outweigh risks of weight gain with atypicals.
  - The risk of TD is definitely lower with atypicals.
- A neuroleptic can be first-line treatment for patients with a history of a better response to neuroleptics or to depot medications.
- Ziprasidone should be used only after patients have failed a trial of another atypical antipsychotic.
- There are no convincing differences between antipsychotic drugs in efficacy for positive symptoms.
- There are no conclusive data about whether greater improvement of negative symptoms with atypicals is a primary benefit of these medications or whether atypicals just produce fewer negative symptoms compared to neuroleptics.
- Some atypicals are more effective than neuroleptics for affective symptoms.
- Clozapine is the most effective antipsychotic for refractory patients.
  - At least one other atypical antipsychotic should be tried before clozapine.
  - Generic clozapine was equivalent to brand name clozapine in a prospective study of 20 schizophrenia patients (Makela, Cutlip, Stevenson, et al., 2003).
- Depot neuroleptics and atypical antipsychotics should be considered before oral neuroleptics for noncompliant patients.

INITIATING THERAPY WITH ATYPICAL ANTIPSYCHOTICS

Patients may differ substantially in their ability to tolerate or respond to one or another of the atypical antipsychotics.

- Unless the patient is severely agitated, starting with a low dose and increasing the dose slowly to stay below the threshold for intolerable side effects results in better long-term adherence.
- The optimal dose of risperidone for schizophrenia is around 2–4 mg/day.
  - Doses of 6 mg/day or less are as, or more, effective and better tolerated than higher doses; however, doses of 2 mg are 50% less effective than 6–16 mg doses (Davis et al., 2003)
  - A double-blind random assignment comparison of fixed doses of 2 and 4 mg of risperidone in 49 acutely psychotic patients led to similar degrees of improvement of positive and negative symptoms over 8 weeks, with each dose working at the same rate, but less fine motor dysfunction with the lower dose (Marco, Hofer, Gekle, et al., 2002)
- Although the recommended maximum dose of olanzapine is 20 mg/day, olanzapine was as effective as haloperidol and clozapine in a direct comparison only at doses of 30 mg/day.
  - Preliminary data suggest that the minimum effective level of olanzapine is around 9.3 ng/mL (Perry, 2001).
- The maximum recommended dose of quetiapine (800 mg) does not convey sufficient antipsychotic efficacy for some patients; higher doses (> 1200 mg) may be necessary.
  - A double-blind study found once-daily quetiapine to be as effective as twice-daily quetiapine in schizophrenia and schizoaffective disorder despite the short half-life of quetiapine (Chengappa, Parepally, Brar, & Goldstein, 2003).
- The recommended starting dose of aripiprazole is the same as the average therapeutic dose in early trials (15 mg); however, some patients require higher doses (20–30 mg/day).
- Clozapine and ziprasidone require bid dosing.
- Special issues with clozapine:
  - Clozapine is usually reserved for patients who have not responded to at least two other treatments.
  - A 2-year multicenter randomized trail with 980 patients with schizophrenia or schizoaffective disorder, who had had previous suicide attempts or current suicidal ideation, found that suicidal behavior (suicide attempts, hospitalization for suicide risk, or rescue interventions for suicidality) was 32% less with clozapine than with olanzapine (hazard ratio 0.76; $p = 0.03$; Meltzer, Alphs, Green, et al., 2003)
  - Start clozapine at a very low dose (e.g., ½ of a 25 mg tablet) and increase the dose slowly to allow time for tolerance to sedation.

**Table 1.3 Antipsychotic Drug Dosing**

| GENERIC NAMES | CHLORPROMAZINE EQUIVALENT DOSES (100 MG) | ACUTE DOSES (MG/DAY) | RANGES (MG/DAY) | P.R.N. (MG/PO) | P.R.N. (MG/IM) |
|---|---|---|---|---|---|
| aripiprazole | 15 | 15 | 10–30 | 5–15 | |
| chlorpromazine | 100 | 200–1600 | 25–2000 | 25–100 | 25–50 |
| clozapine | 75 | 150–500 | 75–700 | N/A | N/A |
| fluphenazine | 2 | 2.5–20 | 1–60 | 0.5–10 | 1–5 |
| haloperidol | 2 | 2–40 | 1–100 | 0.5–5 | 2–5 |
| loxapine | 15 | 60–100 | 30–250 | 10–60 | 12.5–50 |
| mesoridazine | 50 | 75–300 | 30–400 | 10–100 | 25 |
| molindone | 20 | 50–100 | 15–25 | 5–75 | N/A |
| olanzapine | 4 | 5–20 | 3–30 | N/A | N/A |
| perphenazine | 10 | 16–32 | 4–64 | 4–8 | 5–10 |
| pimozide | 0.5 | 10–12 | 1–20 | N/A | 1–3 |
| quetiapine | 100 | 200–800 | 100–1000 | N/A | N/A |
| risperidone | 1 | 2–8 | 1–16 | N/A | N/A |
| thioridazine | 100 | 200–600 | 40–800 | 20–200 | N/A |
| thiothixene | 0.5 | 6–30 | 6–60 | 2–20 | 2–4 |
| trifluoperazine | 5 | 6–50 | 2–80 | 5–10 | 1–2 |
| ziprasidone | 15 | 40–200 | 20–160 | 2–25 | N/A |

- Clozapine should be continued for at least 12 weeks before determining efficacy.
  - Evaluate patient for response at plateaus of 200–400 and 500–600 mg/day.
  - Increase > 600 mg only if adverse effects are not severe.
  - Improvement of schizophrenia may continue for 6–7 months.
  - Get plasma level if no response by 6 weeks.
- Optimal clozapine levels are around 350–504 ng/mL (Perry, 2001). Using these levels increases response rates in refractory schizophrenia from 30% to 55–80%. Some patients do better with levels > 504 ng/mL.
- Risk of seizures increases with dose.
  - Highest risk at doses of 600–900 mg/day.
  - Greater risk with more rapid dosage escalation.
- Risk of agranulocytosis is 1–2% (discussed on pp. 64–66).

**Table 1.4  Specific Neuroleptic Doses**

| GENERIC NAMES | FIRST ORAL DOSE (MG) | FIRST DAY TOTAL DOSE (MG/DAY) | THERAPEUTIC PLASMA LEVELS (MG/ML) |
|---|---|---|---|
| chlorpromazine | 50–100 | 300–400 | 30–100 |
| clozapine | 25 | 50 | 141–204* |
| fluphenazine | 1–2 | 2.5–10 | 0.2–3 |
| fluphenazine decanoate** | 12.5 | 12.5 | 0.15–2.7 |
| haloperidol | 1–5 | 3–20 | — |
| loxapine | 10–25 | 20–50 | — |
| mesoridazine | 50 | 150 | — |
| molindone | 10–25 | 50–75 | — |
| olanzapine | 5–10 | 10 | — |
| perphenazine | 4–8 | 16–32 | 0.8–12.0 |
| pimozide | 1–2 | 2 | — |
| quetiapine | 25 | 50 | — |
| risperidone | 0.5–1 | 1–2 | — |
| thioridazine | 50–100 | 150–300 | 1–1.5 |
| thiothixene | 5 | 4–13 | 2–20* |
| trifluoperazine | 2–5 | 4–20 | 1–2.3 |
| ziprasidone | 20 | 20–40 | — |

\* Women statistically higher than men.
\*\* Not given orally.

- Aripiprazole
  - Receptor actions
    - 5HT$_2$A antagonist
    - D$_2$ partial agonist
    - 5HT$_1$A partial agonist
    - Low affinity for alpha-adrenergic and H$_1$ receptors
    - No affinity for muscarinic cholinergic receptors
  - Metabolized by CYP
    - 3A4
    - 2D6
  - Does not alter levels of other P450 substrates
  - Elimination half-life 48–68 hours
    - 2 weeks to steady state

Table 1.5  Age-Related Antipsychotic Doses

| GENERIC NAMES | CHILDHOOD | | GERIATRIC DOSE RANGE (MG/DAY) |
| | WEIGHT ADJUSTED DOSE (MG/KG/DAY) | DOSE RANGE (MG/DAY)* | |
| --- | --- | --- | --- |
| aripiprazole | — | — | 10–25 |
| chlorpromazine | 3–6 | 45–430 (196) | 25–200 |
| clozapine | — | — | 100–400 |
| fluphenazine | 0.05–0.1 | 4.9–50 (10) | 2–10 |
| haloperidol | 0.05 | 1–4.5 | 0.5–6** |
| loxapine | 0.5–1 | 25–60 | 10–100 |
| mesoridazine | | | 75–200 |
| molindone | 0.5–1 | 25–50 | 50–150 |
| olanzapine | — | 4–10 (5) | 3–15 |
| perphenazine | 0.05–0.1 | 4–24 | 4–48 |
| pimozide | — | — | 10–50 |
| quetiapine | — | 50–150 | 50–300 |
| risperidone | — | — | 0.5–4 |
| thioridazine | 2–5 | 160–500 (282) | 25–200 |
| thiothixene | 0.5–1 | 2–24 (16) | 2–15 |
| trifluoperazine | 0.5 | 6–10 (0.5–15) | 2–15 |
| ziprasidone | — | — | 20–80 |

\* Mean in parentheses.
\*\* 0.03–0.05 mg/kg often enough.

- No prolactin elevation
- No changes in QTc
- 10, 15, 20, and 30 mg tablets
  - No dosage adjustment necessary for renal or hepatic impairment or for age.

## INITIATING THERAPY WITH NEUROLEPTICS

Acutely psychotic patients may need higher doses, but because adverse effects increase with higher doses, long-term adherence is reduced. Early neuroleptic side effects can be reduced by treating agitation with adjunctive benzodiazepines. The neuroleptic threshold (NT) is occasionally used to gauge initial neuroleptic dosing.

- The NT works best with high-potency neuroleptics because anticholinergic effects of low-potency preparations reduce acute EPS.
- The NT is the dose at which cogwheel rigidity first appears.
  - This is tested by flexing and extending the patient's elbow and wrist.
  - The patient can be distracted from the difficulty of relaxing the arm being tested by performing rapid alternating movements with the other arm.
  - Early appearance of parkinsonian side effects such as micrographia or decreased arm swing also can be used to assess the NT.
- Perform baseline testing 1–3 days before starting the neuroleptic.
- Initiate neuroleptic at 2 mg haloperidol equivalent.
- Increase dose by 2 mg every 1–2 days until early EPS appears.
- Lower neuroleptic doses are better tolerated, resulting in better long-term adherence; however, missing a few doses is more likely to result in rapid relapse.
- In multiple studies, the therapeutic plasma level of haloperidol is 5–18 ng/mL (Perry, 2001).
  - Higher levels do not appear to be more effective and may decrease the chance of response by inducing more dysphoria and EPS
- Trifluoperazine appears to have a therapeutic window of 1–2.25 ng/mL (Perry, 2001)

### TREATING AGITATED/COMBATIVE PATIENTS WITH SCHIZOPHRENIA

More sedating preparations may work better for some agitated patients. However, some paranoid patients become panicked when their hypervigilance is reduced by sedative effects, resulting in increased agitation.

- If possible, the patient should be offered an oral medication first to maintain some sense of control.
  - Elixirs have a faster onset of action and are preferable for noncompliant patients.
  - Because a goal of acute oral therapy for a combative patient is to maintain a therapeutic alliance, "snowing" the patient with a rapid dosage escalation may be counterproductive.
  - Give multiple daily doses to maintain optimal levels of sedation.
- The target dose is at the upper end of the therapeutic range (e.g., 15–20 mg/day of olanzapine); the dose can be reduced once the patient is calmer.

- If parenteral treatment is necessary, be sure that adequate personnel are available to control the patient while medication is being administered.
  - A belligerent patient may experience being approached by one or two people as a challenge, whereas a sufficient "show of force" may relieve the patient of the need to demonstrate prowess in standing up to persecutors.

Using IM antipsychotics:
- Initial dose of haloperidol: 2–5 mg
- Initial dose of IM ziprasidone: 10 mg
  - Subsequent doses 5–20 mg q 4–6 hours, maximum 80 mg/4 doses/ 24 hours
  - Peak concentration reached in 30 minutes.
  - A multicenter study randomized 132 patients with acute psychosis (*not* caused by substances or organic factors) to IM ziprasidone mesylate or IM haloperidol for 3 days, followed by the same drug in oral form for the next 4 days (Brook, Lucey, & Gunn, 2000).
    - Discontinuation rates were 9% from ziprasidone and 19% from haloperidol.
    - About 60% of patients in both groups received adjunctive lorazepam.
    - Ziprasidone produced significantly greater reductions in BPRS total and BPRS agitation scores, significantly more improvement in CGI scores, and fewer extrapyramidal side effects.
    - Mean increases in QTc intervals were 2.14 msec with ziprasidone and 2.22 msec with haloperidol.
  - A 1-day double-blind comparison of 2 mg and 10 mg of IM ziprasidone found that the 10 mg dose was significantly more effective in reducing agitation; patients were calmer but not sedated (Lesem, Zajecka, Swift, Reeves, & Harrigan, 2001).
- An experimental IM form of olanzapine reaches peak concentration two to five times that of oral preparation in 30 minutes.
  - Efficacy equal to IM haloperidol but with lower risk of dystonia.
  - Superior to lorazepam in reducing agitation in mania (Meehan, Zhang, David, et al., 2001).
- Reassess frequently.

"Rapid neuroleptization" (rapidly escalating doses of a neuroleptic such as haloperidol 2–5 mg IM q 1–2 hours until calm) is not more effective than slower-dosage escalation, and it produces more adverse effects.

Supplementation with a benzodiazepine can reduce the neuroleptic dose necessary to control behavior and can decrease akathisia.

- Lorazepam is the only benzodiazepine that is reliably absorbed with IM dosing.
  - Usual dose 1–2 mg, repeated as needed.
- Some patients may become disinhibited by a benzodiazepine.

For dangerous agitation, use IV haloperidol 1–5 mg as frequently as necessary, until patient is calm.
- This approach can produce tranquilization without excessive sedation.
- EPS less frequent than with IM dosing, but still may occur.
- Torsades de Pointes occasionally reported with IV haloperidol.
  - No reports of Torsades or significant QTc prolongation with IM ziprasidone.
- IV lorazepam 1–5 mg can be administered with haloperidol in the same syringe.

IV midazolam 1–2 mg repeated as necessary produces immediate sedation with brief duration of action.

When agitation or poor veins make it impossible to administer IV haloperidol and/or lorazepam, and IM ziprasidone or haloperidol is not appropriate, consider droperidol 2.5–15 mg IM.
- Onset of action usually within 3–10 minutes; peak effect in 20–30 minutes.
- Less sedating than most neuroleptics.
- QTc prolongation may occur; do not administer with other medications that slow cardiac conduction.

Avoid neuroleptics and droperidol for catatonic excitement.
- Some cases of catatonia are caused by severe EPS or neuroleptic malignant syndrome (NMS).
- Benzodiazepines are more effective and safer.
- Electroconvulsive therapy (ECT) is definitive treatment.

SCHIZOPHRENIA WITH COMORBID DEPRESSION

At least 50% of schizophrenia patients have one or more episodes of major depression.
- Half of depressive episodes occur during acute psychosis, making them difficult to identify.
  - When psychosis resolves and depressive symptoms persist, "postpsychotic depression" may be diagnosed.
- Persistent depression may inhibit functional recovery and lower the threshold for the recurrence of psychosis.
- Depressive symptoms should be distinguished from parkinsonian side effects such as bradykinesia.

- Grief over lost function can be difficult to differentiate from depression.
  - Symptoms are centered on what has been lost or not accomplished.
  - Insomnia present, but no other vegetative symptoms.
- Antidepressants are indicated for schizophrenia with depression.
  - No evidence that most antidepressants exacerbate psychosis.
  - Treating depression improves other schizophrenia symptoms.
  - Consider potential interactions when adding an antidepressant (see p. 198)
    - TCAs may have additive anticholinergic and cardiac side effects with neuroleptics.
    - Neuroleptics increase TCA levels.
    - SSRIs can elevate antipsychotic levels and have additive effect on prolactinemia and EPS.
    - Dopaminergic effect of bupropion could aggravate psychosis.

## TREATMENT-RESISTANT SCHIZOPHRENIA

Failure to respond as expected to antipsychotic medication may have many causes:

- Incorrect diagnosis
- Unrealistic expectations: Antipsychotic medications generally produce 30% improvement and are usually not curative.
- Noncompliance: Patients do not take antipsychotic medications as prescribed because of
  - Adverse effects, especially EPS, sedation, weight gain, and dysphoria
  - Medication cost
  - Belief that the medication unnecessary
    - Disagreement with the diagnosis
  - Paranoia (e.g., fears that medication is poisoned)
  - Reluctance to give up attachment to psychosis
  - Family members who encourage nonadherence
- Use of substances that exacerbate psychosis
- Dose too low or too high
  - Some medications (e.g., haloperidol) have therapeutic windows.
- Adverse effects may evoke more psychosis.
- Apparent negative symptoms may be antipsychotic side effects.
  - Seen with atypical antipsychotics as well as neuroleptics.
- The patient may need a different medication.
- High expressed emotion in the family.
  - Numerous studies show that unrealistic expectations of patient & excessive displays of negative emotions inhibit response to medications.

Approaches to treating inadequate response include the following:
- Address reasons for nonadherence.
- Reconsider the diagnosis.
  - Psychotic depression and chronic mixed psychotic bipolar illness can be mistaken for schizophrenia.
    - The content of psychosis and the presence of a formal thought disorder do not reliably distinguish between schizophrenia and bipolar disorder.
  - During regressed states (usually in the context of strong transference feelings), patients with personality disorders may develop schizophreniform conditions (i.e., brief psychotic disorder).
- Reassess substance use.
  - Prognosis is better in substance-abusing schizophrenia patients because treatment of substance use leads to improvement of psychosis.
- Check medication level.
  - Although only a few antipsychotics (e.g., haloperidol, clozapine) have established correlations between serum level and clinical effect, levels much lower than average suggest inadequate dose, rapid metabolism, or nonadherence. Very high levels may cause dysphoria that interferes with the therapeutic effect.
- Measure prolactin levels.
  - Neuroleptics and risperidone increase prolactin release because of reduction of tonic dopaminergic inhibition of prolactin-secreting neurons.
  - High prolactin levels do not cause psychosis, but they can aggravate depression, sexual dysfunction, and anergia, and they may increase the risk of endocrine-sensitive tumors such as breast cancer.
- Use liquid preparation (available for chlorpromazine, mesoridazine, thioridazine, fluphenazine, perphenazine, trifluoperazine, thiothixene, haloperidol, loxapine, molindone, ziprasidone) or chewable tablet (olanzapine).
- Consider depot antipsychotic (see pp. 29–31).
- Change medication.
  - Switch from one class of atypical antipsychotic to another.
  - For persistent psychosis on atypical antipsychotic, add or change to neuroleptic.
  - For failure to respond to other antipsychotics, try clozapine.

Augment the antipsychotic drug.
- Benzodiazepine mostly useful for agitation.
- Antidepressant useful for comorbid depression.
- Lithium may be useful for patients with prominent affective symptoms.

- Anticonvulsants may be helpful for patients with abnormal EEG or prominent negative symptoms.
  - Divalproex can reduce agitation.
    - Augmentation of haloperidol with valproate improved Clinical Global Impressions (CGI), BPRS, and Schedule for Affective and Negative Symptoms (SANS) scores more than haloperidol alone in one study but not in another (Conley & Kelly, 2001).
  - Lamotrigine 200 mg/day was added to clozapine in a 14-week placebo-controlled crossover trial in patients with clozapine-resistant schizophrenia (Tiihonen, Hallikainen, Ryynanen, et al., 2003).
    - Lamotrigine produced significantly greater reduction of positive but not negative symptoms.
- Omega-3 fatty acids
  - Evidence exists of a neuronal membrane dysfunction in schizophrenia.
  - Omega-3 fatty acid precursor (eicosapentaenoic acid) improved positive and negative symptoms by about 25% when added to a neuroleptic in a small study (Fenton, Dickerson, & Boronow, 2001).
- Serotonin $5HT_3$ receptor antagonists
  - The $5HT_3$ receptor promotes dopamine release in limbic and brainstem centers, contributing to nausea and possibly to psychosis.
    - $5HT_3$ antagonists (e.g., ondansetron) are used to treat cancer chemotherapy-induced nausea and may have antipsychotic properties.
    - Add ondansetron 4–8 mg tid to clozapine or other atypical.
- Cholinesterase inhibitors
  - Dysfunction of $\alpha7$ nicotinic cholinergic receptor has been demonstrated in schizophrenia (Freedman, 2003).
    - May be cause of social information-processing deficits in schizophrenia, which leads to secondary delusional explanations of maladaptive interactions.
    - Inhaled nicotine corrects information-processing deficits in schizophrenia; blocked by nicotinic receptor antagonist
  - Cholinergic agents may help to improve information processing in schizophrenia, with less need for pathological explanations of misunderstood social realities.

Some studies of cholinesterase inhibitors have been positive, some negative.

- Donepezil 5–10 mg added to 6 mg risperidone did not improve cognition or information processing in a 12-week study in schizophrenia, but heavy smoking in most patients may have reduced receptor sensitivity to increased acetylcholine availability (Friedman, Adler, Howanitz, et al., 2002).

- 24 patients with schizophrenia on 1–8 mg of risperidone assigned for 4 weeks to placebo or galantamine 16/24/32 mg (Allen, 2003).
  - Galantamine produced significantly more improvement on cognitive tests than placebo.
    - Verbal fluency
    - Continuous Performance Test (CPT) errors of commission
    - Delayed matching
  - More improvement of behavior with galantamine.
    - Dosing may have to be pulsatile, as it is with inhaled delivery systems, rather than consistent, to promote $\alpha7$ receptor function.
- Try antipsychotic combinations.
  - Neuroleptic often added to atypical antipsychotic.
  - Two atypicals may be combined.
    - Especially clozapine plus another atypical or a neuroleptic
    - Less rationale for other atypical combinations.
- NMDA receptor agonists
  - NMDA (N-methyl-D-aspartate) receptor antagonism by ketamine and PCP induces schizophrenia-like psychosis.
  - NMDA receptor hypofunction postulated in schizophrenia, with two results:
    - Decreased long-term potentiation impairs social learning.
    - Reduced input to NMDA receptors leads to compensatory increased glutamate release, resulting in downstream excitotoxicity and progression of neuronal loss.
  - Glycine site on NMDA receptor complex is glutamate co-agonist; stimulation of glycine receptor increases NMDA receptor activity.
  - Glycine agonists include glycine, serine, and D-cycloserine.
    - Glycine 60 gm/day improved negative symptoms, positive symptoms, and EPS in 19 patients.
    - Similar results seen with D-serine 30 mg/kg/day.
    - Improvement in some negative symptoms with 50 mg/day D-cycloserine.
- Cox-2 inhibitors
  - In a prospective double-blind study, 50 patients with an acute exacerbation of schizophrenia were randomly assigned to 5 weeks of risperidone (2–6 mg/day) plus placebo or 400 mg/day of the cyclo-oxygenase-2 inhibitor celecoxib (Muller, Riedel, Scheppach, et al., 2002).
    - The celecoxib add-on group had significantly greater improvement on the total PANSS score.

- The greatest difference was between weeks 2–4, suggesting an earlier response to treatment.
- ECT
  - 20% of schizophrenia patients improve with ECT.
    - Affective and acute symptoms predict better response.
  - ECT is highly effective for catatonia.
- Treatment of residual negative symptoms:
  - Add or change to atypical antipsychotic if patient is taking a neuroleptic.
    - Affective blunting and bradykinesia may be caused by neuroleptic.
    - Atypicals are at least somewhat more effective as primary treatment for negative symptoms.
    - More activating atypicals (e.g., aripiprazole, ziprasidone) may be preferable for patients with significant apathy.
  - Add antidepressant
    - TCAs (e.g., desipramine), SSRIs (e.g., fluoxetine), and MAOIs (e.g., seligiline) have been found to improve negative symptoms when added to neuroleptics.
    - Reduction of negative symptoms equivalent to that seen with atypical antipsychotics alone.
    - Depressive symptoms not necessary for antidepressant to be helpful.
    - Schizophrenia patients with negative symptoms may have family history of depression, even if they are not depressed themselves.
  - A double-blind placebo-controlled study of the neurosteroid dehydroepiandrosterone (DHEA) in 30 patients with chronic schizophrenia on stable antipsychotic doses (Strous, Maayan, Lapidus, et al., 2003) found:
    - In the 27 patients who completed at least half the study, those receiving DHEA had significantly greater reductions of negative symptoms (by about 30%), depression (by about 50%), and anxiety (by about 66%).
    - Reduction of negative symptoms was not a function of improvement of depression or anxiety.
    - Positive symptoms did not change significantly with either DHEA or placebo.

MAINTENANCE THERAPY

Resolution of an acute psychotic episode in schizophrenia may take up to a year. During this time, reduction of stress, especially expressed emotion in the family, promotes recovery. An antipsychotic drug is usually continued, although if higher doses were needed to control agitation and disorganization, the dose may be reduced gradually. The decision to continue the antipsychotic medication after psychosis has resolved depends on several factors:

- Patients with single schizophreniform episode (i.e., symptom duration < 6 months) who recover completely can probably withdraw antipsychotic medication slowly over 6–12 months, with close observation.
- Patients with good premorbid function, solid psychosocial supports, prominent affective symptoms or confusion, and complete recovery also may withdraw medication slowly over an extended period of time after a single psychotic episode.
- Maintenance antipsychotic medication should be considered in the presence of
    - Residual symptoms, including psychosocial dysfunction
    - Severe acute symptoms with important consequences, such as assault, legal charges, family dysfunction
    - More than one psychotic episode
    - Poor premorbid adjustment
    - Prominent family history of schizophrenia
    - Continued psychosocial or job stress

Approaches to maintenance medication include the following:
- Antipsychotic drugs are clearly superior to placebo in preventing relapse.
    - 15% per month relapse after discontinuing antipsychotic drug.
    - However, at least 30% will relapse over 2 years, despite maintenance treatment.
- Atypical antipsychotics are preferred maintenance treatments because of better tolerability and lower risk of TD.
- Lower doses are better tolerated but less potent at preventing relapse.
    - Aim for 20–50% of highest acute dose for maintenance.
- Intermittent treatment can be used if patient has supportive family and close observation is available: Patient takes no medication or very low antipsychotic doses, and medication is reinstituted or increased in dose immediately upon first sign of relapse.
    - Intermittent treatment with neuroleptics increases risk of TD more than continuous treatment.
        - May promote development of receptor supersensitivity.
- Single daily dose improves compliance and is pharmacologically appropriate for all antipsychotics except ziprasidone, quetiapine, and clozapine.
    - A long half-life (55 hours) could permit pimozide dosing every 2–3 days.

- Pimozide is used more frequently for Tourette's disorder and monosymptomatic hypochondriasis than schizophrenia.

Depot neuroleptics, the clinical effects of which last 2–4 weeks after each dose, are primarily indicated for patients with poor treatment adherence.

- Advantages of depot neuroleptics:
  - Patient does not have to remember medication each day.
  - Staff does not have to keep track of oral medications.
  - Dosing is more consistent, resulting in lower relapse rates than with oral medications.
- Disadvantages of depot neuroleptics:
  - Extrapyramidal and other side effects last longer than with shorter-acting oral medications.
  - The dose cannot be rapidly reduced or withheld in the event of severe adverse effects.
  - Limited efficacy found against negative symptoms.
- A review of six published randomized trials comparing depot fluphenazine to oral fluphenazine found no difference between the oral and the depot form for outcome and side effects (Adams & Eisenbruch, 2002).
  - Based on available data, the use of depot over oral fluphenazine is a matter of clinical judgment.

**Table 1.6  Use of Depot Antipsychotics**

| PREPARATION | FLUPHENAZINE DECANOATE | FLUPHENAZINE ENANTHATE | HALOPERIDOL DECANOATE | RISPERIDONE |
|---|---|---|---|---|
| Usual dose (mg) | 25 (6.25–100) | 25–75 (12.5–100) | 50–100 (50–300) | 25–50 |
| Usual frequency of injections (weeks) | 3 (2–6) | 2 (1–3) | 4 (2–5) | |
| Antipsychotic action begins (days) | 1–3 | 1–3 | 6–7 | |
| Peak plasma level (days) | 1–2 | 2–4 | 3–9 | |
| Protein binding | 80 | 80 | 92 | |
| Half-life (days) | 6.8–9.6 (one injection) 14.3 (many doses) | 3.5–4 (one injection) | 21 (one injection) 12 (many doses) | |
| Maximum dose recorded | 400 mg/week | 1250 mg/week | 1200 mg/injection | |

**Table 1.7  Approximate Equivalents of Oral and Depot Fluphenazine**

|  | PO | IM* |
|---|---|---|
| Low dose | 1–8 mg | 6.25–12.5 |
| Medium dose | 8–20 mg | 12.5–37.5 |
| High dose | 20–40 mg | 37.5–100 |

\* One study suggested 12.5 mg decanoate = 10 mg po.

- When all randomized trials in schizophrenia in which haloperidol decanoate, oral antipsychotics, or depot fluphenazine were evaluated, significantly fewer patients on depot preparations left a study early or did not improve compared with placebo, and patients on decanoate needed less additional antipsychotic medication (Quraishi & David, 2002).
  - In a single trial, there was no difference between oral and depot haloperidol.
  - There were no differences in outcome or side effects between depot haloperidol and other depot neuroleptics.
  - The choice of a depot neuroleptic therefore depends on individual preference rather than data favoring one over the other.
- Procedure for instituting depot neuroleptics:
  - Use fluphenazine or haloperidol decanoate.
    - Fluphenazine enanthate has more EPS and is usually not recommended.
  - Choose medication based on past response and family history.
  - Discuss preferred site of injection (thigh, shoulder, or buttock) with patient in advance.
    - Pain at injection site or embarrassment may lead to noncompliance.
  - Optimize dose of oral fluphenazine or haloperidol first.
    - Haloperidol dose can be adjusted by blood level.
  - Use test dose of 6.25 mg, administered in insulin syringe, to be sure that patient is not hypersensitive to vehicle (sesame oil) and can tolerate depot medication.
  - At equivalent dose of oral neuroleptic, gradually increase dose of depot medication and reduce oral dose.
    - For example, give full oral dose on first day of depot, then decrease oral dose by 10–20%/day, using additional supplemental oral doses as needed.
  - Equivalent doses
    - Fluphenazine decanoate: 1–10 times oral dose
    - Haloperidol decanoate: 10–20 times oral dose

- Fluphenazine decanoate administered every 2–6 weeks.
- Haloperidol decanoate given monthly (range 2–5 weeks).
- After stabilization, dose of depot medication can sometimes be reduced slowly to 5–10 mg fluphenazine or 20–50 mg haloperidol.
- Depot neuroleptics are not approved for children < 12 years old.
- Depot risperidone
  - Aqueous suspension of risperidone in a matrix of glycolic acid-lactate copolymer; after injection the copolymer is gradually hydrolyzed to produce slow release of risperidone.
  - Dose: 25, 50, or 75 mg q 2 weeks.
  - Of 400 chronic schizophrenia patients in a 12-week trial of IM long-acting risperidone 25, 50, or 75 mg or placebo every 2 weeks after a 1-week oral risperidone run-in, ≥ 20% reduction of PANSS scores was significantly greater with all risperidone groups (39–48% vs. 17% with placebo; Kane et al., 2003).
    - Weight gain was 0.5–1.9 kg with risperidone and −1.4 kg with placebo.
  - Must be refrigerated until use

### Delusional Disorder

Delusional disorder often has prodromal suspiciousness or eccentric behavior, with eventual development of recalcitrant symptoms and low (< 30%) response rate to antipsychotic medications. Patients with erotomania and paranoia may be chronically dangerous to others.

- Somatic type (monosymptomatic hypochondriasis), with a single delusion involving bodily function (e.g., being infested with parasites) may be difficult to distinguish from psychotic depression.
  - Older case reports suggest preferential response to pimozide; no controlled studies have been performed.
  - Some cases may represent overvalued body dysmorphic disorder and could respond to an SRI augmented with antipsychotic drug.
- Delusional jealousy also said to have a better response to pimozide.

### Brief Psychotic Disorder

Many patients with brief psychotic disorder experience transient regression in the context of an intense transference relationship (often with a therapist) and respond best to structure without medications.

- Low dose of antipsychotic medication (e.g., 0.25–2 mg risperidone) is preferable.
  - Higher doses may cause dysphoria and dissociated states, which worsen symptoms.

- Benzodiazepines can reduce agitation but also be disinhibiting.
- Lithium and anticonvulsants helpful for patients with marked affective symptoms or positive affective family history.
- Antidepressants useful for patients with comorbid depression.
- Improvement usually rapid, probably as result of high rate of spontaneous remission.

### Schizotypal and Schizoid Personality Disorders

Soft positive symptoms such as ideas of reference, "supernatural" experiences, and thought disorder may improve with antipsychotic drugs.
- Low doses are preferable.
    - 0.5–2 mg risperidol; 2–5 mg haloperidol
- Improvement occurs within a few weeks.
- More dropouts because of adverse effects (50%) than patients with schizophrenia.
- In a 9-week double-blind randomized placebo-controlled study, 25 patients with schizotypal personality disorder had significantly fewer negative symptoms, positive symptoms, and general symptoms with 0.25–2 mg of risperidone than with placebo (Koenigsberg, Reynolds, Goodman, et al., 2003).

### Borderline Personality Disorder

Brief psychotic episodes most frequently occur in patients with borderline and narcissistic personality disorders and can be treated as noted above. Transient disorganization with impulsive destructive or self-destructive behavior responds better to atypical antipsychotics than to neuroleptics because of probable anti-aggressive action of atypicals.
- Lower doses are better tolerated.
- Carbamazepine and lithium useful for affective dysregulation in personality disordered patients.
- Antidepressants indicated for comorbid major depression.
- Self-destructive behavior (e.g., cutting, burning) may be reduced with naltrexone.

### HIV/AIDS-Related Psychotic Disorders

Most HIV/AIDS patients develop neurological dysfunction prior to manifesting more obvious medical symptoms. Such patients are more vulnerable to the CNS side effects of all medications. Psychosis may occur early in course secondary to delirium, direct effects of HIV on the brain, substance use, or associated psychiatric disorders. Manic presentations are common.

- Atypical antipsychotics are first choice because of better tolerability.
  - Olanzapine desirable for patients with significant loss of appetite/weight.
- Low doses of all antipsychotics are preferable.
  - For example, risperidone 2–4 mg; olanzapine 2–10 mg
- Because olanzapine and clozapine are metabolized by CYP1A2, the HIV protease inhibitor ritonavir (which induces 1A2) can reduce half-life area under the time-concentration curve (AUC), and peak plasma concentration of these atypical antipsychotics.

### Autism/Asperger's

There is no specific treatment for pervasive developmental disorders. However, behavioral disturbances and lack of communication may be improved by some medications. Validated behavioral scales should be used to track clinical response.

- Neuroleptics
  - Haloperidol 0.5–4 mg/day can decrease uncooperative behavior, emotional lability, and irritability.
  - Low-potency neuroleptics are not as well tolerated.
- Atypical antipsychotic drugs
  - The most experience has been with risperidone (mean dose 3 mg) to reduce repetitive behavior, aggression, anxiety, depression, and irritability.
  - Less experience with newer atypicals, but all should be equally effective.
  - An 8-week multicenter trial in 82 boys and 19 girls, ages 5–17, with autism and severe aggression, angry outbursts, or self-injurious behavior found that risperidone 0.5–3.5 mg/day decreased behavioral dyscontrol 57% compared with 14% on placebo (McCracken, McGough, Shah, et al., 2002).
    - An overall response occurred in 69% of patients treated with risperidone but only 12% of those receiving placebo. There was no change in either group in social isolation or communication.
    - Benefit on risperidone was maintained at 6-month follow-up in 68% of responders at 8 weeks.
  - When previous antipsychotics were changed to ziprasidone 20–120 mg/day in 12 patients, 9 with autism and 3 with pervasive developmental disorder (PDD) NOS, 6 patients responded; 2 patients with comorbid bipolar disorder got "much worse" (McDougle, Kem, & Posey, 2002).

- In a 30-month open trial of olanzapine (mean dose 10.7 mg) in 25 children ages 6–16 with autism or PDD NOS, only 3 of 23 children who completed the study were responders (Kemner, Willemsen-Swinkels, de Jonge, Tuynman-Qua, & van Engeland, 2002).
- SSRIs and clomipramine
  - Reduce repetitive behaviors.
  - Decrease aggression.
  - Increase interactions and communicative use of language.
    - More initiation of, and response to, verbal communication
    - More appropriate speech
    - Less echolalia
- Anticonvulsants
  - Divalproex reduces mood swings, aggression, impulsivity.
    - Increased social awareness and relatedness
    - Decreased obsessive–compulsive behavior
    - May be more effective in patients with abnormal EEGs.

## SIDE EFFECTS

Neuroleptics can be categorized as low or high potency. Low-potency preparations (e.g., chlorpromazine, thioridazine, mesoridazine) require higher doses and have more sedative, hypotensive, and anticholinergic side effects but fewer acute extrapyramidal side effects (EPS); anticholinergic effects of these medications may reduce EPS. High-potency neuroleptics are more likely to cause EPS and prolactinemia, but they induce less sedation and fewer anticholinergic effects.

- Thioridazine (Mellaril) and mesoridazine (Serentil, a metabolite of thioridazine) produce more anticholinergic effects, inhibition of ejaculation, and EKG changes but are least likely to cause EPS.
  - Thioridazine can cause pigmentary retinopathy at doses > 800 mg/day.

### Anticholinergic Side Effects

Anticholinergic actions affect the heart, GI system, eyes, upper respiratory system autonomic regulation, and CNS, causing

- Dry mouth
- Blurred vision
- Dry eyes
- Precipitation of narrow angle glaucoma

- Photophobia
- Paralysis of accommodation/blurred near vision
- Constipation
- Paralytic ileus
- Urinary retention
- Fever
- Nasal congestion
- Tachycardia
- Hypotension
- Memory impairment
- Confusion
- Delirium

Combining medications that have prominent anticholinergic properties (e.g., thioridazine and benztropine) increases the risk of additive side effects. Anticholinergic side effects may become less noticeable over 1–4 weeks because patients stop paying attention to them, but side effects usually do not wear off completely. To reduce anticholinergic side effects:

- Switch to a less anticholinergic neuroleptic.
- Discontinue antiparkinsonian medication.
  - EPS often remits within a few months.
- Use a less anticholinergic antiparkinsonian drug (e.g., amantadine) if one is necessary.
- Add a cholinergic agent.
  - Bethanechol 10–50 mg tid–qid may reduce peripheral anticholinergic effects but is difficult to tolerate.
  - Cholinesterase inhibitors in usual doses (discussed in Chapter 2) are better tolerated and treat central anticholinergic side effects of other medications.
  - Physostigmine 1 mg IV can reduce acute central anticholinergic toxicity.
  - Cholinergic agents can counteract antiparkinsonian effect.

## Cardiovascular Side Effects

### EKG Changes and Dysrhythmias

All neuroleptics are type Ia antiarrhythmics like quinidine, procainamide, and disopyramide.

- These drugs act by blocking potassium channels, which slows cardiac repolarization and prolongs the refractory period, reducing the risk of reentry.

- Prolonged depolarization lengthens the QT interval.
- If depolarization is extended for too long, calcium currents are activated by accumulating intracellular potassium, creating a new depolarization (*afterdepolarization*) that may occur during the vulnerable period of the T-wave.
- Repeated afterdepolarizations may produce Torsades de Pointes.
  - Axis of depolarization rotates (or turns) around the isoelectric line.
  - A difficult to treat and potentially fatal ventricular arrhythmia results.
  - Hypokalemia (usually caused by diuretic use) increases the risk of Torsades.
- Prolongation of the QT interval corrected for heart rate (QTc interval) does not invariably lead to Torsades de Pointes.
  - Risk increases with QTc > 500 msec.
- QTc prolongation may occur with all neuroleptics, and with clozapine and ziprasidone. (Other medications commonly used by psychiatric patients that prolong the QTc interval are listed in Table 1.8.)
- QTc prolongation is most frequent with thioridazine and pimozide.
- Ziprasidone increased QTc intervals by a mean of 6–10 msec. at 160 mg/day in premarketing trials.

**Table 1.8  Commonly Used Medications That Prolong the QTc Interval**

| | |
|---|---|
| *Antiarrhythmic drugs* | *Atypical antipsychotics* |
| Type Ia: quinidine, disopyramide, procainamide<br>Type III: sotalol, amiodarone, ibutilide<br>Type IV: bepridil | Ziprasidone, risperidone, quetiapine<br>Olanzapine (isolated reports only; unclear association) |
| *Antihistamines* | *TCAs* |
| Terfenadine<br>Astemizole<br>Fexofenadine | *Serotonin receptor antagonists*<br>Ketanserin |
| *Antibiotics* | *SSRIs* |
| Erythromycin, clindamycin, trimethoprim-sulfametoxazole<br>Quinolones (e.g., levofloxacin)<br>Amantadine, pentamidine<br>Imidazoles (fluconazole)<br>Chloroquine, quinine | Fluoxetine, zimelidine (isolated reports only; uncertain relationship with Torsades) |
| *Triptans* | *Carbamazepine, vasopressin* (isolated reports only; QT prolongation mild) |
| *Neuroleptics* | *Diuretics* (hypokalemia increases likelihood of Torsades) |
| Thioridazine, mesoridazine, pimozide<br>Haloperidol | |

- No cases of Torsades have been reported with this medication.
- As of October 2001, 150,000 patient exposures to ziprasidone revealed no deaths attributable to the medication (Marder et al., 2002); this impression has not changed through 2004.
- In 1,733 patient-years of ziprasidone premarketing exposure, there were 0.56 sudden deaths per 100 patient years (vs. 2.5 during sertindole trials; Glassman & Bigger, 2001).
- QTc prolongation has not been a concern with the IM preparation.
- Torsades has been reported most frequently with thioridazine and with IV or oral haloperidol.
  - Sertindole was withdrawn because it was associated with syncope, arrhythmias, and sudden death.
    - 7.8% of QTc intervals were > 500 msec. in FDA New Drug Application for sertindole, vs. 0.06% with ziprasidone.
- Risk of Torsades and sudden death greatest with thioridazine but also associated with
  - Pimozide
  - Haloperidol
  - Droperidol
- In 97 schizophrenia patients starting clozapine at average age 37 (DC Henderson: Presentation at Society of Biological Psychiatry, May 2004:
  - Cardiovascular mortality 10% over next 10 years
  - Cardiac risk factors quadrupled over 5 years
  - No controls
- Monitoring recommendations:
  - Obtain baseline EKG in children, the elderly, and patients at risk of cardiac disease.
  - Baseline EKG not necessary in the absence of risk factors for significant QTc prolongation or cardiac disease, such as
    - History of heart disease, fainting, dizziness, or palpitations
    - Diuretic use or prolonged diarrhea
    - Family history of sudden cardiac death
    - Use of concomitant medications that prolong QTc interval
  - EKG monitoring recommended after dosage increases with pimozide and thioridazine.
  - If QTc increases by ≥ 20%
    - Check electrolytes.
    - Discontinue other medications that can cause QTc prolongation.

SUDDEN DEATH

QT prolongation may not predispose to sudden cardiac death with all medications.

- Records from 1993–1996 of outpatients in three U.S. Medicaid programs were reviewed for risk of sudden death with antipsychotic drugs (Hennessy, Bilker, Knauss, et al., 2002).
  - Compared with patients who had psoriasis or glaucoma (chronic illness controls), relative risk for patients with schizophrenia treated with antipsychotics was:
    - 1.7–3.2 for cardiac arrest and ventricular arrhythmia
    - 1.4–1.9 for sudden death
    - Risk with thioridazine increased beginning at 100 mg.
    - Risk with thioridazine dose at least 600 mg > haloperidol.
  - Risk with risperidone > thioridazine, but could reflect use of risperidone in medically ill patients
- Medical records of patients in five psychiatric hospitals who died suddenly during a 12-year period were compared with records of two controls matched for psychiatric illness and other relevant factors (Reilly, Ayis, Ferrier, Jones, & Thomas, 2002).
  - 1,350 patients died, 69 of them for unexplained reasons
  - Thioridazine was the only medication statistically associated with an increased risk of sudden death (OR 5.3, $p = 0.004$).
    - Higher doses had a greater risk.
  - The most likely cause of sudden death seemed to be Torsades de Pointes.
  - Preexisting ischemic heart disease and hypertension increased the risk of sudden death with thioridazine.
  - Not enough atypical antipsychotics were used during the study period to determine their risk of sudden death, but thioridazine had a greater risk than any other neuroleptic.
- Available data suggest that risk of sudden cardiac death is highest with thioridazine.
  - Risk is dose related.
  - Sudden death may not have been reported with other neuroleptics that cause QT prolongation (e.g., pimozide) because these medications are not used frequently.
  - Obtain EKG in patients who develop persistent tachycardia on antipsychotic drug.
- Risk of cardiac death may also be increased with clozapine

MYOCARDITIS

Reported with clozapine.

### Orthostatic Hypotension

Orthostatic hypotension is caused by blockade of postsynaptic alpha-adrenergic receptors, most frequently by low-potency neuroleptics and clozapine, but also with other neuroleptics and atypical antipsychotics.

- Failure of accommodation of blood pressure on standing up causes lightheadedness, dizziness, fainting.
  - Postural dizziness sometimes occurs without significant blood pressure changes.
  - Greatest risk is when patient gets up in middle of the night.
- Aggravated by low-salt or fluid intake, use of antihypertensives, hypothyroidism, or stimulant withdrawal.
- Management:
  - Use atypical antipsychotic agent other than clozapine first in patients with risk of postural hypotension.
  - Tell patient to stand up slowly over about 60 seconds.
    - If rising from a lying position, put feet on floor first, sit up for about 30 seconds, then stand up.
    - If patient develops severe symptoms of hypotension on standing, advise lying down and elevating legs above head until symptoms abate.
  - Suggest that patient wear support hose (including at night).
  - Ensure adequate salt intake, unless medically contraindicated.
- Medications that may be helpful:
  - Fludrocortisone 0.1–0.2 mg/day
    - Mineralocorticoid
    - Requires monitoring of electrolytes and blood pressure.
  - Dihydroergotamine
  - Tyramine
  - Acute treatment with volume expanders and alpha-adrenergic pressor agents if hypotension is medically dangerous.
    - Metaraminol
    - Phenylephrine
    - Norepinephrine
    - Do *not* use agonists for both alpha and beta receptors such as epinephrine or isoproterenol.
    - Beta-adrenergic agonism in the presence of continued alpha-adrenergic blockade causes vasodilation and aggravates hypotension.

### Stroke

The manufacturer reported in April 2003 that in four placebo-controlled trials in 1,230 patients, cerebrovascular events such as stroke and TIA, including fatalities, were significantly more frequent in elderly patients with psychosis and dementia treated with risperidone than placebo.

- Cerebrovascular events occurred in 3.8% or risperidone patients vs. 1.5% of those on placebo.
- Similar mortality seen with risperidone and placebo.

### Tachycardia

Antipsychotic drugs can elevate heart rate $> 100$ via anticholinergic (vagolytic) effect or as a compensatory response to hypotension.

- Most common with low-potency neuroleptics and clozapine
- Management:
  - Change the antipsychotic medication.
  - Use a beta-blocker that is not too lipophilic and has fewer central side effects (e.g., atenolol 25–100 mg/day).
  - Cholinesterase inhibitors may be useful.

### Thromboembolism

A case control study found that the risk of venous thromboembolism was increased seven times in patients taking neuroleptics (Zornberg & Jick, 2000).

- Risk was greatest with low-potency neuroleptics.
- Clozapine also had increased risk.
- No data on newer atypicals.
- Risk could be due to weight gain, sedation, or antiphospholipid antibodies interacting with risk factors such as smoking.

## Central Nervous System Side Effects

### Extrapyramidal Syndromes (EPS)

These syndromes may be acute or chronic, and there is some overlap between them (e.g., parkinsonism and neuroleptic malignant syndrome). All extrapyramidal syndromes are more common with neuroleptics than with atypical antipsychotics, but all of the atypicals have been associated with EPS. Among the atypicals, clozapine produces EPS least and risperidone most frequently.

Akathisia
- Most common type of EPS
- Begins within a few hours to 2 weeks of starting antipsychotic drug.
- Symptoms include
  - Inner restlessness
  - Jitteriness

- Fidgeting
- Rapid foot tapping
- Rocking back and forth
- Myoclonus
- Intense discomfort
- Some patients only experience subjective symptoms without outward change in activity.
- Akathisa may be confused with
  - Agitation
  - Anxiety
  - Mania
  - Restless legs syndrome (RLS)
- To differentiate between agitation and akathisia, ask if discomfort feels as if it is starting in muscles or in mind.
- In contrast with akathisia, RLS is characterized by:
  - Symptoms restricted to legs.
  - Unpleasant sensation in calves
  - Worse in, or restricted to, nighttime
  - Insomnia
  - Worse on lying down
  - Improves with walking
- Treatment of akathisia
  - Propranolol
  - Benzodiazepine
    - Only two valid randomized controlled trials (total N = 27) of benzodiazepines for akathisia have been published. An analysis found that clonazepam was significantly more effective than placebo for acute akathisia, with side effects equal to placebo (Lima, Soares-Weiser, Bacaltchuk, & Barnes, 2002a).
  - Amantadine
  - Anticholinergic drugs not reliably effective.
    - An attempt to perform a meta-analysis of all published randomized trials of anticholinergics to treat akathisia found no randomized controlled trials that could either support or refute use of anticholinergics to treat neuroleptic-induced akathisia (Lima, Weiser, Bacaltchuk, & Barnes, 2002b).

Parkinsonism
- Slow, rhythmic, pill-rolling tremor involving fingers, hand, and wrist moving as a unit.
  - Anxiety-related tremor is distinguished by fine, rapid, side-to-side movements.

- Micrographia
- Decreased arm swing
- Stiffness
- Stooped posture
- Impaired gait
- Masked facies
- Bradykinesia
- Cogwheel rigidity
- Drooling, seborrhea
- May be confused with negative symptoms, withdrawal, exacerbation of schizophrenia, depression
- Management:
  - Reduce dose.
  - Use atypical antipsychotic.
  - Use anticholinergic agent.
  - Try amantadine.

Dystonia
- Sustained abnormal involuntary muscle contraction causing repetitive movements or abnormal posture
- Affects tongue, face, neck, jaw, back.
- Spasms of tongue, jaw, and neck
- May present with blepharospasm.
- Stiff or thick tongue
- Retrocollis, torticollis
- Opisthotonos (titanic tightening of entire body, with torso and head extended)
- Oculogyric crisis (eyes locked upward)
- Laryngospasm
  - May compromise respiration.
- Torticollis (twisting of cervical muscles with unnatural head position)
- Very common (> 70%) with high-potency neuroleptics in younger patients
- Usually self-limited, lasting about 2 weeks
- Management:
  - Use atypical antipsychotic first, then
  - Anticholinergic agent
  - Diphenydramine
  - Benzodiazepine
  - Reserpine
  - Baclofen or other muscle relaxants

### Akinesia

- Paucity of spontaneous movement and emotional expression
- Apathy
- Rigid posture
- Reduced conversation
- Decreased arm swing
- May or may not be associated with parkinsonism
- Management:
  - Reduce dose.
  - Add antiparkinsonian drug.
  - Consider dopaminergic agent; but could aggravate psychosis.

### Paresthesias

- Burning dysesthesia occasionally reported with risperidone
  - Usually in hands and feet
  - Dose related

### Rabbit syndrome (perioral tremor)

- Occurs with long-term treatment.
- Rapid (5 Hz) tremor or lip and masticatory movements of mouth that mimic a rabbit.
- In contrast to TD
  - Continues during sleep.
  - Does not involve tongue.
  - Remits when neuroleptic is stopped.
- Responds to anticholinergics.

### Neuroleptic malignant syndrome (NMS)

- Incidence usually estimated at around 0.5% of neuroleptic-treated patients, but milder forms may be more common.
- Usually begins within 72 hours of starting neuroleptic, but onset may be after months of treatment.
- More common with neuroleptics but has been reported with all antipsychotic drugs, including clozapine.
- Signs and symptoms involve severe EPS, muscle breakdown, fever and autonomic instability; for example,
  - Muscle rigidity, rhabdomyolisis, myoglobinuria, elevated MB isoform of creatinine, hyperpyrexia, unstable pulse and blood pressure
- DSM-IV-TR research criteria for NMS include the following:
  - Both A Criteria must be associated with neuroleptic use:
    - Severe muscle rigidity
    - Elevated temperature

- Two or more B Criteria, not explained by another illness or substance use; must be associated with neuroleptic use:
  - Severe parkinsonism (catatonic appearance; tremors, dyskinesias; lead pipe muscle rigidity, akinesia; flexor-extensor posturing; festinating gait)
  - Altered consciousness (agitated, confused, obtunded, comatose; incontinence; patient may be alert)
  - Autonomic dysfunction (tachycardia, labile or increased blood pressure, diaphoresis, sialorrhea, tachypnea, pallor, dysphagia)
  - Laboratory abnormalities: (1) evidence of muscle damage (elevated creatine kinase MB isoform; myoglobinuria), (2) renal failure, (3) elevated white blood count, (4) elevated liver function tests (LFTs)
- Differential diagnosis of NMS includes
  - Anticholinergic toxicity
    - Similarities: fever, confusion, hyperreflexia, mydriasis, tachycardia
    - Differences: muscle relaxation, no parkinsonism, no muscle damage
  - Drug-induced hyperthermia (e.g., lidocaine, meperidine, stimulants, NSAIDs)
    - Similarities: fever, tachycardia, hyperreflexia with stimulants
    - Differences: no muscle changes, no parkinsonism
- Risk of NMS is increased by
  - Past history of NMS
    - Rechallenge with any neuroleptic has 33% risk of NMS recurrence.
  - High neuroleptic dose
  - Rapid neuroleptization
  - High-potency neuroleptics
    - May reflect greater use of high-potency neuroleptics.
    - If NMS does occur with a low-potency neuroleptic, it tends to be more severe.
  - Treatment with two or more neuroleptics
  - High ambient temperature
  - Dehydration
  - Developmental disability
  - Preexisting CNS disease
  - History of receiving ECT
  - Severe agitation
  - More time in restraint or seclusion
  - Low serum iron
    - Not clear if this finding is primary or secondary to NMS.

- Risk of fatal outcome
  - Age < 20 or > 60
  - Substance abuse
  - CNS disease
  - Developmental disability

Management of NMS:
- Stop neuroleptics and anticholinergic drugs.
- Maintain hydration
- Correct electrolyte disturbances
- Reduce fever
  - Antipyretics
  - Body cooling
- Treat associated pneumonia or pulmonary embolus.
- Supportive care has same duration of illness with and without addition of specific treatments.
  - Some reports suggest longer duration of NMS with specific treatments, but this may reflect greater severity of illness when these agents are used.
  - No controlled studies conducted of NMS treatment.
- Add specific treatment.
  - Bromocriptine
    - Reverses antidopaminergic effect of neuroleptic.
  - Amantadine
    - Alternative to bromocriptine
  - Other dopaminergic agent
    - Levodopa, levodopa-carbidopa
  - Dantrolene
    - Effective for malignant hyperthermia
    - Decreases muscle spasm by reducing calcium release from intracellular stores.
    - Hepatotoxicity at doses > 10 mg/kg/day
  - Calcium channel-blocker
    - Less experience but is sometimes effective.
    - Can reduce hypertension as well as other features.
  - Benzodiazepine
    - Most experience with lorazepam
  - Carbamazepine
    - Start with 1200 mg/day.
    - Follow with 500 mg/day.
  - ECT sometimes reduces NMS and does not increase it.

**Table 1.9 Drugs Used to Treat NMS**

| GENERIC NAME | DOSE |
|---|---|
| anticholinergic agents | — |
| bromocriptine | 7.5–60 mg/day po |
| dantrolene | 0.8–10 mg/kg/IV; 50 mg qd-qid po |
| levodopa | 100 mg bid po |
| carbidopa-levodopa | 25 mg tid-200 qid po |
| amantadine | 100 mg bid or tid po |
| lorazepam | 1.5–2 mg IV, then po |

- Plasmapharesis
  - May be necessary for NMS with depot preparation.
- Is it safe to restart antipsychotic medications after an episode of NMS?
  - As many as 80% of patients are able to reintroduce medication successfully.
  - Wait at least 2 weeks after NMS has remitted completely.
    - Benzodiazepines might be used temporarily as needed
  - Ensure adequate hydration.
  - Advise patient not to stay in overly heated environment.
  - Check temperature, WBC, and CPK regularly.
  - Use atypical antipsychotic agent first.
  - If neuroleptic is needed, try low-potency agent first.

SEIZURES

Seizures are uncommon with use of antipsychotic drugs; they occur most frequently with clozapine.
- More likely when antipsychotic dose is raised or lowered rapidly.
- There is a higher risk with low-potency neuroleptics than with high-potency agents.
  - Low risk with molindone, fluphenazine
- Lower risk with more frequent dosing and lower peak blood levels
  - Increased risk with higher blood levels
- Risk of clozapine-induced seizures is dose-related.
  - < 300 mg/day: 1–2%
  - 300–600 mg/day: 3–4%
  - > 600 mg/day: 5%
  - Abnormal EEG without seizures reported in 65% taking clozapine

- To reduce risk of seizures:
  - Increase dose slowly (e.g., 12.5 mg/week of clozapine).
  - Give divided dose.
  - Check blood level in patients at risk of seizures.
    - Past history of seizure
    - CNS disease predisposing to seizures
    - Traumatic brain injury
- Management of seizures:
  - Reduce antipsychotic dose.
  - Use an antipsychotic with a lower risk of seizures.
  - Obtain EEG.
  - Add anticonvulsant.
    - *Do not* combine carbamazepine and clozapine.
  - Once anticonvulsant level is maximized, increase antipsychotic dose gradually.
  - Consult with a neurologist about when to attempt to wean anticonvulsant.

## SEDATION

Comparative sedative side effects are summarized in Table 1.2.
- Sedation usually appears within first few weeks of treatment.
- Tolerance often develops to mild sedation.
  - Tolerance may not develop if sedation is substantial initially.
- Management:
  - Give entire dose at bedtime.
  - Reduce daytime doses.
  - Increase dose slowly.
  - Switch to less sedating neuroleptic.
  - Modafinil may be helpful, without increasing psychosis.
  - Nicotine transdermal patch or cholinesterase inhibitor may help associated cognitive impairment.

## TARDIVE DYSKINESIA

- TD involves involuntary choreoathetoid movements of limbs, face, trunk, or respiratory muscles.
  - Signs often are worse during stress and disappear during sleep.
  - Voluntary effort may temporarily suppress movements.
- Signs may be grouped into three categories:
  - Facial–lingual–oral

- Chewing, lip smacking, tongue protrusion and rolling ("fly catcher's tongue"), frowning, blinking, grimacing, pouting, licking, chewing
  - Limb choreoathetoid movements
    - Rapid, irregular choreiform movements
    - Slower, irregular athetoid movements
    - Rhythmic tremors
    - Lateral knee movements
    - Foot tapping, squirming, inversion, eversion
  - Truncal dyskinesia
    - Movements of neck, shoulders, hip
    - Pelvic gyrations and thrusts
    - Erratic respiration
- Spontaneous dyskinesias
  - Common in elderly
    - 1–5% of all elderly
    - Some apparent cases of TD are actually loose fitting dentures.
  - Reported in 15–20% of never-treated schizophrenia patients and 24% of patients with schizotypal personality.
    - Risk factors for spontaneous dyskinesia in these patients: prominent negative symptoms, lower IQ, hebephrenia
- Drug-induced TD
  - All antipsychotic medications can cause TD.
    - Risk is lowest with clozapine, but TD has been reported.
  - Risk factors:
    - Intermittent treatment with antipsychotic ("drug holidays" increase risk of TD, possibly by sensitizing postsynaptic dopamine receptors).
    - Longer use and higher doses of antipsychotic
    - Older female
    - Younger male
    - African ethnicity
    - Mood disorder (may reflect intermittent antipsychotic use in these patients).
    - Preexisting CNS disease
    - Diabetes mellitus
    - History of severe EPS
  - Usually begins after 6–36 months.
  - Risk is proportional to total antipsychotic dose.

- However, TD may develop after a few weeks with low doses in vulnerable patients.
- Anticholinergic drugs may increase TD risk, or at least lower threshold for expression of TD.
- Neuroleptics have 5–10%/year TD risk.
  - Lifetime risk around 40%
  - Prevalence figures vary substantially, but probably around 15% above spontaneous dyskinesia rate after 2 years.
- Atypical antipsychotic drugs have lower risk.
  - Estimated at around 0.5%/year.
  - However, sufficient long-term data have not yet accumulated to be sure that risk is as low as it appears.
- TD often appears with withdrawal or decrease in antipsychotic dose.
  - Increasing dose initially masks TD because of increased $D_2$ blockade, but TD eventually rebounds.
- Other medications that can cause TD:
  - Amoxapine (metabolite of loxapine with neuroleptic properties)
  - Other dopamine blockers not used as antipsychotics: metoclopramide (Reglan), prochlorperazine (Compazine), promethazine (Phenergan), trimethobenzamide (Tigan), thiethylperazine (Torecan), triflupromazine (Vesprin)
- TD is severe in 2–5% of patients.
- TD remits with medication discontinuation in about 50% of cases.
  - Total remission may take 3 years.
- TD often does not progress once it appears.
- Risk reduction:
  - Monitor all patients taking antipsychotics with a standardized scale, such as the Abnormal Involuntary Movement Scale (AIMS).
  - Reassess need for continued antipsychotic use regularly.
    - It is often necessary to continue an antipsychotic medication at some dose to prevent relapse of schizophrenia.
    - Mood disorder patients may not need continued treatment, and long-term neuroleptic use sometimes contributes to depressive relapse.
    - Consider reducing dose gradually if medication cannot be discontinued.
- Management of TD
  - If TD appears as antipsychotic is withdrawn, wait at least 6 months for symptoms to remit spontaneously before treating.
    - Remission rate is around 50% within 6 months.
    - Remission rate over the next 10 years is about 2.5–5%/year.

- Vitamin E 1200–1600 units/day
  - Clinically significant improvement in 50% of patients with TD, duration < 5 years.
  - In eight studies, vitamin E produced "clinically relevant improvement" (NNT = 5), with more deterioration of TD in patients not using vitamin E (Soares & McGrath, 2001). However, most studies were limited methodologically.
  - A large VA cooperative study was negative.
  - Not effective for TD of longer duration.
  - Not curative
- Acetazolamide 1.5–2 gm/day (tid dosing)
  - About 45% improvement of TD in one 2-month placebo-controlled study.
  - Add thiamine 500 mg tid to reduce risk of kidney stones.
  - Add daily orange juice 8 oz. or other potassium supplement.
  - May be helpful for longstanding TD.
- Ondansetron 4–8 mg/day in tid schedule
  - Short-term treatment reduces TD.
  - May be result of masking syndrome rather than true treatment.
- Clozapine sometimes reverses TD; improvement persists after clozapine withdrawn.
- Cholinergic agents
  - May restore DA/ACh balance
  - Choline 2–8 gm/day produced disappointing results.
  - Preliminary experience with cholinesterase inhibitors (e.g., donepezil 5–10 mg/day) encouraging but there have not been any large studies, and a review of published trials could draw no conclusions (Tammenmaa, McGrath, Sailas, & Soares-Weiser, 2002).
- Dopaminergic agents
  - May stimulate presynaptic receptors and decrease dopamine release or eventually desensitize $D_2$ receptors and reduce TD.
  - Amantadine 100 mg bid–tid
  - Levodopa 100–200 mg/day
  - Bromocriptine 2.5 mg/day
- Calcium channel-blockers (CCBs)
  - In schizophrenia trials, CCBs do not improve positive or negative symptoms but reliably decrease TD.
  - Verapamil 40–120 mg tid–qid

- Reserpine 1–6 mg/day
  - Older reports suggest benefit, but no studies reported.
- Anticonvulsants
  - Carbamazepine 100–800 mg/day
  - Valproate 1000–1500 mg/day: a review of five randomized controlled trials in which valproate was added to antipsychotics found no benefit of adding the anticonvulsant (Basan & Leucht, 2004).
- In 41 patients on stable antipsychotic dose, assigned to placebo or high doses (222 mg/kg) of a branched chain amino acid preparation (valine:isoleucine:leucine ratio 3:3:4) for at least 1 week of a 3-week trial, TD decreased significantly more in the amino acid group, with 37% decrease on amino acids vs. a 3.4% increase on placebo (Richardson, Bevans, Read, et al., 2003)
  - One-third of amino acid subjects had a reduction of 60% or more in TD movements, vs. none in the placebo group.
- Decrease in TD was correlated with decreased total aromatic amino acid levels but not with changes in antipsychotic drug levels.
- Rolipram, a selective cyclic AMP phosphodiesterase inhibitor, reduced both dyskinetic movements and excessive $D_2$ receptor density in rats in which TD was induced by chronic treatment with haloperidol (Sasaki, Hashimoto, Inada, Fukui, & Iyo, 1995).
  - Up-regulation of $D_2$ receptors, which is thought to be a mechanism of TD, decreases cAMP levels by inhibiting adenylate cyclase.
  - Rolipram reduces breakdown of cAMP.
- A review of six thorough randomized trials found significant improvement in TD with low-dose insulin compared with placebo but not with botulinin toxin, endorphin, estrogen, essential fatty acid, ganglioside, lithium, naloxone, cyproheptadine, phenylalanine, piracetam, tryptophan, or ECT (McGrath & Soares-Weiser, 2002).
- A review of published studies found that benzodiazepines were not more effective than placebo for TD (McGrath & Soares, 2002).

## Tardive Dystonia

Like TD, tardive dystonia develops after long-term antipsychotic use, either while continuing the medication or after medication withdrawal or dosage reduction.

- Tardive dystonia involves sustained involuntary muscle contractions that cause twisting, repetitive movements, or abnormal posture.
- Temporary voluntary control of movements may be possible.
- May occur spontaneously after traumatic brain injury in 7–48% of patients.

- Differences from TD:
  - More distressing and disabling
  - More frequent in men
  - Occurs after shorter exposure
    - Average $< 2.5$ years
  - Rarely remits
  - May be partially responsive to anticholinergics
- Risk factors:
  - Mania $>$ schizophrenia
  - High-potency neuroleptics
  - Young age
- Management:
  - Anticholinergic medication
  - Benzodiazepine
  - Clozapine
  - Reserpine
    - Depletes dopamine.
  - Tetrabenazine
    - Depletes and blocks dopamine.
  - Botulinum toxin type A injected into affected muscles
    - Average duration of improvement after injection about 12 weeks

OTHER TARDIVE SYNDROMES

- Tardive akathisia
  - Persistent restlessness
  - Treatment as for acute akathisia
- Tardive tics
- Tardive psychosis
  - A small number of patients treated long-term with neuroleptics develops new psychotic symptoms or exacerbation of previous psychosis upon withdrawal or reduction of neuroleptic dose.
  - Theoretically, postsynaptic $D_2$ receptors in limbic circuits have developed supersensitivity analogous to TD.
  - Often remits gradually after neuroleptic withdrawn.
  - Not yet reported with atypical antipsychotics.
  - Could be responsible for development of psychosis in nonpsychotic patients receiving chronic neuroleptic therapy.
  - No specific treatments have been studied.
    - Atypical antipsychotic, especially clozapine, would probably be first choice.

## Endocrine and Sexual Side Effects

Multiple systems may be affected.

PROLACTINEMIA

- Prolactin release is tonically inhibited by dopamine released from tuberoinfundibular neurons; dopamine-blocking agents such as the neuroleptics can elevate prolactin levels, sometimes substantially.
- Among the atypical antipsychotics, risperidone is most likely and clozapine lease likely to cause prolactinemia.
    - Olanzapine, quetiapine, and ziprasidone have little effect on serum prolactin.
    - Clozapine reduces prolactin release 16–80%.
    - Aripiprazole may reduce prolactin release slightly.
- Because SSRIs reduce dopamine release, they can exacerbate neuroleptic-induced prolactinemia as well as occasionally causing prolactinemia by themselves.
- Symptoms and signs of elevated prolactin:
    - Amenorrhea and menstrual irregulatities
    - Anovulation
    - Breast enlargement
    - Galactorrhea
        - Usually but not always with elevated prolactin
        - More common in women who have been pregnant in the past.
    - Promotion of growth of breast cancer
        - Primarily in cancers with prolactin receptors
    - Decreased libido and anorgasmia
        - Erectile as well as ejaculatory dysfunction may occur in men.
    - Osteoporosis
        - Risk correlated with amount and duration of prolactin elevation.
        - Cigarette smoking exacerbates osteoporosis caused by prolactinemia by interfering with protective effect of estrogen.
    - Depression
        - Psychosis is not increased by prolactin.
    - Sexual dysfunction
- Management of prolactinemia:
    - Dopaminergic agents inhibit prolactin release.
    - Bromocriptine
        - Available in 2.5 and 5 mg tablets.
        - Start with 1.25 mg/day and increase, as necessary, to 2.5–15 mg/day.

- Amantadine, pergolide, pramipexole, or bupropion also could be used.
- Dopaminergic agents may exacerbate psychosis.

## Hyperglycemia (Abnormal Glucose Tolerance Test)

- Untreated schizophrenia patients have a higher prevalence of diabetes mellitus than the general population.
  - A comparison of 26 patients with untreated first-episode schizophrenia and 26 controls matched for body mass index (Ryan, Collins, & Thakore, 2003) found that
    - No controls but 15% of patients had impaired fasting glucose (> 110 and < 126 µg/dL).
    - Patients had significantly higher mean fasting plasma glucose, insulin, and cortisol and more insulin resistance.
    - Patients had significantly lower fasting cholesterol.
    - No differences were found in serum triglycerides.

## Diabetes Mellitus

- Hyperinsulinemia occurs in as many as 71% of patients taking olanzapine.
  - Suggests dysfunction of insulin receptor.
- Could be caused by binding to insulin-sensitive glucose transporter.
  - More likely to occur with drugs with high intracellular concentration (e.g., clozapine, olanzapine).
  - More likely to occur in schizophrenia, probably because of increased incidence of diabetes mellitus and poor diet in these patients.
- Development of diabetes reported most consistently with clozapine and olanzapine
- Survey of a database in two large health plans of 7,933 patients with some form of psychosis (Gianfrancesco, Grogg, Mahmoud, Wang, & Nasrallah, 2002):
  - Compared with untreated patients, the risk of developing type 2 diabetes was increased
    - 7.4 times with clozapine
    - 3.5 times with low-potency neuroleptics
    - 3.1 times with olanzapine
    - 2.1 times with high-potency neuroleptics
    - Not at all with risperidone
  - The risk of diabetes with olanzapine increased with increasing doses.
  - Not yet reported with risperidone, ziprasidone, aripiprazole.

- Not always associated with weight gain.
- Glucose tolerance may return to normal with drug discontinuation.
- A British study examined data from 400 general practices with 3.5 million patients in England and Wales (Koro, Fedder, L'Italien, et al., 2002a):
  - All cases of schizophrenia (19,637 patients) who did not already have diabetes included
    - 451 patients who were identified as having developed diabetes within 3 months of starting an antipsychotic drug
    - Each schizophrenia patient who developed diabetes was matched with six schizophrenia patients who never developed diabetes.
  - Compared with no use of antipsychotics in schizophrenia.
    - Olanzapine increased risk of diabetes 5.8 times.
    - Risperidone increased risk of diabetes 2.2 times.
    - Neuroleptics increased risk of diabetes 1.4 times.
    - Olanzapine but not risperidone was significantly more likely than neuroleptics to be associated with development of diabetes.
  - Diet and severity of schizophrenia were not controlled in this study.
- A review of charts of 215 patients taking clozapine, olanzapine, risperidone, quetiapine, haloperidol, or fluphenazine found that glucose levels increased significantly on clozapine and olanzapine, and five patients taking clozapine required addition of a glucose-lowering agent (Wirshing et al., 2002).
- A Canadian study sponsored by the manufacturer of risperidone examined health care claims of 34,692 patients who received at least one prescription for risperidone or olanzapine from 1997–1999 (Caro, Ward, Levinton, & Robinson, 2002).
  - Relative risk of developing diabetes over the study period was 20% greater with olanzapine than risperidone.
    - Risk of developing diabetes was greatest during first 3 months of treatment with olanzapine.
- Review of 237 cases of diabetes or hyperglycemia in patients taking olanzapine (Koller & Doraiswamy 2002):
  - 188 were new-onset cases, 44 were exacerbations of preexisting diabetes, and 5 could not be classified.
  - The majority (73%) of all cases of hyperglycemia appeared within 6 months of starting olanzapine.
  - Metabolic acidosis or ketosis developed in 80 patients.
    - 41 patients had glucose levels > 1000 mg/dL, and 15 patients died.
  - When olanzapine was discontinued or reduced in dose, 78% had improvement of hyperglycemia.

- A retrospective analysis of a VA database reviewed 5,837 patients treated with olanzapine, risperidone, haloperidol, or fluphenazine from 1997–2000, who either received a diagnosis of diabetes mellitus or were treated with an oral hypoglycemic agent while taking the antipsychotic (Fuller, Shermock, Secic, & Grogg, 2003).
  - Overall risk of diabetes was 6.3%.
  - Olanzapine was 37% more likely than risperidone to be associated with developing diabetes (controlled for race, age, diagnosis, substance abuse, lithium, valproic acid, and other atypicals).
  - There was no difference between risperidone, fluphenazine, and haloperidol in the risk of developing diabetes.
- A randomized double-blind trial in refractory schizophrenia and schizoaffective disorder followed patients for 8 weeks on a fixed dose and for another 6 weeks on variable doses (depending on response) of olanzapine (mean dose 20–31 mg), clozapine (mean dose 444–477 mg), risperidone (mean dose 9–12 mg), and haloperidol (mean dose 20–26 mg; Lindenmayer, Czobor, Volkan, et al., 2003):
  - After 14 weeks, glucose levels increased significantly only with olanzapine (from 91.7–105.5 mg/dL).
  - However, glucose levels with all medications were still within the normal range.
  - Over the 14 weeks, cholesterol increased significantly only with olanzapine (from 179.8–197.6 mg/dL).
  - Weight gain over the study was
    - 7.3 kg with olanzapine ($p < 0.0001$)
    - 4.8 kg with clozapine ($p < 0.0003$)
    - 2.4 kg with risperidone ($p = NS$)
    - 0.9 kg with haloperidol ($p = NS$)
  - Weight gain significantly correlated with increased cholesterol on olanzapine or clozapine.
- A 31-year-old male patient with schizophrenia was treated with 10 mg olanzapine for 1 week, when his fasting blood glucose increased to 203 mg/dL; the dose was raised to 20 mg, and his fasting glucose went up to 284 mg (Meatherall & Younes, 2002). He developed weakness, polydipsia, and polyuria and died with a postmortem blood glucose of 954 mg/dL and unremarkable blood olanzapine concentrations.
  - Could have been coincidental, or precipitation of severe diabetes in a vulnerable patient
- Diabetes not always associated with weight gain.
- 50% of cases of diabetes that occurs with antipsychotic drugs remits when the drug is discontinued, and hyperglycemia returns when the drug is reinstituted (Ananth, Venkatesh, Burgoyne, & Gunatilake, 2002).

### HYPERLIPIDEMIA

- Not always correlated with weight gain or abnormal glucose tolerance.
- Can predispose to pancreatitis.
- A review of charts of 215 patients taking clozapine, olanzapine, risperidone, quetiapine, haloperidol, or fluphenazine (Wirshing et al., 2002) revealed:
  - Cholesterol levels decreased with risperidone and fluphenazine and increased on clozapine.
    - Six patients required addition of a cholesterol-lowering agent.
  - Triglyceride levels increased significantly with clozapine and olanzapine.
  - Patients taking clozapine, olanzapine, risperidone, and quetiapine had decreases in LDL levels, but any benefit from this was offset by decreased HDL levels on clozapine and olanzapine.
- Review of records from a medical database involving 400 general medical practices with 3.5 million patients (Koro, Fedder, L'Italien, et al., 2002b) revealed:
  - 18,309 patients in the database treated with an antipsychotic drug other than clozapine for at least 3 months for a diagnosis of schizophrenia and followed for an average of over 4 years.
  - 1,269 (7%) were diagnosed and/or treated for hyperlipidemia within 3 months of starting the antipsychotic medication.
  - Each hyperlipidemia subject was compared with six matched schizophrenia controls who did not develop hyperlipidemia.
  - Patients taking olanzapine were 4.65 times as likely to develop hyperlipidemia as schizophrenia controls taking no antipsychotics, and 3.36 times as likely to develop hyperlipidemia as those taking neuroleptics.
  - Small but statistically significantly increased risk of hyperlipidemia (1.38-fold) in patients taking neuroleptics compared to no medication.
  - No increased risk of hyperlipidemia with risperidone.

Monitoring recommendations for medications with risk of weight gain or diabetes:
- Check weight at baseline and then every 3 months. If weight increases, obtain fasting blood sugar (FBS), 2-hour postprandial glucose, cholesterol, and triglycerides.
- Screen for
  - Family history of diabetes
  - Hypertension
  - History of gestational diabetes or baby > 9 pounds

- Consider changing medication if weight increases >5% or FBS is elevated

## ALTERED THYROID FUNCTION TESTS

- Reported occasionally with neuroleptics
- Slight decrease of $T_3$, total $T_4$, and free $T_4$, without elevation of TSH.

## PRIAPISM

- Occasionally occurs with medications that block alpha-1 postsynaptic adrenergic receptors.
    - Primarily low-potency neuroleptics
    - Also reported with clozapine, risperidone, olanzapine, ziprasidone.

## SEXUAL DYSFUNCTION

- Erectile dysfunction/retrograde ejaculation
    - Reported with all neuroleptics.
    - Most common with thioridazine
        - 35–49%
- Other forms of sexual dysfunction
    - 25% of patients taking neuroleptics
        - 60% of patients taking thioridazine
    - Check prolactin levels.
    - Treatment:
        - Cyproheptadine 2–8 mg 2 hours before sex or up to tid.
        - Yohimbine 5.75 mg as needed or tid, *but* may aggravate anxiety and psychosis.
        - Amantadine 100–400 mg/day, *but* dopaminergic effect may aggravate psychosis.
        - Trazodone 50–300 mg at bedtime or in divided dose
        - Bupropion (75–300 mg) or stimulant (5–20 mg), *but* may aggravate psychosis.

### Eyes, Ears, Nose, and Throat Side Effects

## BLURRED VISION

Anticholinergic effect of neuroleptics, especially low-potency agents, frequently causes this problem.

- Affects near > far vision.
- Management usually with cholinergic agent.
    - Cholinesterase inhibitor
        - Not much published experience but often helpful.
    - Pilocarpine 1% eye drops

- Bethanechol 5–30 mg
  - Not as well tolerated as cholinesterase inhibitors.

## Dry Eyes

Anticholinergic effect of low-potency neuroleptics may cause this problem.

- More common in patients wearing contact lenses, and in the elderly.
- Management:
  - Artificial tears
    - Use cautiously with contact lenses.
  - Cholinesterase inhibitor

## Photophobia

Pupillary dilation caused by anticholinergic effects.

## Narrow Angle Glaucoma

Anticholinergic neuroleptics (especially low-potency ones) may precipitate narrow angle glaucoma.

- Get ophthalmological consultation for patients with history of eye or facial pain or halos around lights.

## Eye Pigmentation

Long-term use of neuroleptics, especially chlorpromazine, may increase pigmentation of parts of the eye.

- Probably dose dependent
- Granular deposits in back of cornea and front of lens
  - Star-shaped opacities in front of lens, if pigmentation advanced
- Vision usually unaffected.
  - If pupil is opaque, consultation with an ophthalmologist is necessary.
- Pigmentation of eye associated with photophobia or skin pigmentation.
- Pigmentary retinopathy:
  - Most frequently occurs with chronic use of > 800 mg/day of thioridazine.
    - Such doses are never justified.
  - May cause decreased visual acuity/blindness.
  - May remit with drug withdrawal, if retinopathy has not been present for too long.

## Cataracts

Reported with quetiapine in a single breed of beagle that is spontaneously prone to cataracts.

- No reports of cataracts in primates, including humans.

- Recommendation by manufacturer for ophthalmological examination every 6 months probably not justified.

## Gastrointestinal Side Effects

### Allergic Hepatitis

Cholestatic jaundice was reported soon after the release of chlorpromazine.

- A reaction to excipients in the pills, not to the active drug.
- Allergic hepatitis did not lead to permanent liver damage.
- Reversible when medication was discontinued.
- No cases reported after change of manufacturing process.
- No need for routine liver function tests.

### Elevated Liver Function Tests

Mild–moderate elevations of transaminases frequently occur with antipsychotics and other medications metabolized by the liver.

- Manifestation of enzyme induction by medication
- Often transient
- Usually not clinically important

### Constipation

Anticholinergic effects of low-potency neuroleptics can cause severe constipation and occasionally paralytic ileus.

- Management:
  - Increase bulk and fluids.
  - Add stool softener (e.g., docusate) and fiber (e.g., psyllium).
  - Cholinesterase inhibitor (see pp. 94–97)

### Dry Mouth

Anticholinergic effects of low-potency neuroleptics frequently cause this problem, which may cause difficulty speaking. Drinking a lot of fluid does not produce sustained release.

- Management:
  - Sugar-free gum or candy
  - Frequent brushing of teeth
  - Pilocarpine 1% mouthwash
  - Cholinesterase inhibitor

### Siallorhea

Occurs most frequently with clozapine.

- Management:
  - Anticholinergic agent
  - Clonidine patch
  - Pirenzepine 25–100 mg/day

## WEIGHT GAIN

Definitions
- Overweight: BMI (Body-Mass Index) 25–29.9 kg/m$^2$
- Obesity: BMI $\geq$ 30 kg/m$^2$
- Metabolic syndrome (syndrome X):
  - Older age
  - Hypertension
  - Low HDL cholesterol
  - High triglyceride levels
  - High plasma glucose
  - Central obesity (large waist)
  - Insulin resistance

In a multisite study of 12,861 subjects representative of the general noninstitutionalized U.S. population, 22.8% of men and 22.6% of women had metabolic syndrome; 60% of obese men and 50% of obese women had metabolic syndrome (Park et al., 2003).

Weight gain with neuroleptics is related to antihistaminic properties and is most directly the result of increased appetite and decreased activity; interference with insulin signaling and stimulation of 5HT$_7$ receptors may also be factors.

- Meta-analysis of data on weight gain over 10 weeks in 74 antipsychotic trials showed (Allison, Mentore, & Heo, 1999):
  - Patients receiving placebo lost an average of 1.63 pounds.
  - Molindone was associated with slight weight loss.
  - Weight gain on other antipsychotics
    - Clozapine: 4.45 kg (9.89 pounds)
    - Olanzapine: 4.15 kg (9.22 pounds)
    - Risperidone: 2.10 kg (4.67 pounds)
    - Quetiapine: 2.27 kg (5 pounds)
    - Ziprasidone: 0.04 kg (0.09 pounds)
    - Haloperidol: 1.05 kg (2.3 pounds)
- Greatest weight gain occurs with clozapine, olanzapine, and low-potency neuroleptics.
  - More than half of patients taking olanzapine chronically have clinically significant weight gain (defined by convention as gaining > 7% of baseline weight).

- In a prospective follow-up of 82 patients treated with clozapine over 5 years, the average baseline weight was 175.5 pounds (Henderson, Cagliero, Gray, et al., 2000).
  - 52% had at least one elevated fasting blood glucose.
  - 31% of patients developed type 2 diabetes during follow-up.
    - Not correlated with weight gain, concomitant use of valproate, or clozapine dose.
  - Average weight gain was 1.16 pounds/month.
    - Greatest weight gain occurred during first year.
    - Patients continued to gain weight until month 46, when weight gain leveled off.
  - Serum triglycerides increased significantly.
    - Total cholesterol did not change significantly.
- In the Canadian National Outcomes Measurement Study in Schizophrenia, a naturalistic prospective follow-up, supported by the manufacturer of risperidone and consisting of 111 patients taking risperidone, 109 taking olanzapine, and 23 taking quetiapine (McIntyre et al., 2003):
  - Significantly more weight gain with quetiapine
    - Number on quetiapine so small that data may not be reliable.
  - Percentage of patients gaining > 7% of body weight
    - 24% with risperidone, 31% with olanzapine, 56% with quetiapine
  - Percentage gaining > 10% of body weight
    - 13% with risperidone, 19% with olanzapine, 39% with quetiapine
  - Percentage gaining enough weight to move from overweight to obese
    - 11% on olanzapine, 9% on quetiapine, 8% on risperidone
- In 20 adolescent patients with schizophrenia the increase in BMI over 4 weeks was significantly greater with olanzapine (mean dose 14 mg) than haloperidol (mean dose 6.5 mg) (Gothelf, Falk, Singer, et al., 2002).
  - Caloric intake increased by 28% on olanzapine.
  - There was no change in percentage of carbohydrates, fats, or protein ingested.
  - There was no change in resting energy expenditure or level of physical activity.
- Actual weight gain with quetiapine is often somewhat lower than the amount reported in studies.

Management
- It is easier to prevent weight gain than it is to treat it.

- Advise patient to start a diet before starting a medication with a high frequency of weight gain.
  - At least eliminate all low-volume, high-calorie foods.
- Encourage regular exercise.
- Medications:
  - Medicines are generally considered for BMI > 27, with additional risk factors; or BMI > 30 with no risk factors.
  - Topiramate
    - Primarily effective in reducing appetite.
    - Average dose is 100 mg.
    - A review of published studies found that addition of topiramate to ongoing antimanic drugs in bipolar patients resulted in mean weight loss of 0.7–6.2 kg and mean reduction of BMI of 0.6–2.2 (Nemeroff, 2003).
    - Weight loss peaks within 3–12 months.
    - Some patients regain a portion of weight that was lost.
  - Zonisamide
    - Decreases appetite.
    - A 16-week randomized double-blind placebo-controlled trial of zonisamide (mean dose 427 mg) in 51 of 60 patients who completed the trial, all receiving dietary counseling, was followed by a 16-week single-blind extension. Results indicated (Gadde, Franciscy, Wagner, & Krishnan, 2003): (1) In the double-blind phase, the zonisamide group lost 5.9 kg, vs. 0.9 kg for the placebo group ($p < 0.001$). (Considering only the patients who completed this phase, zonisamide patients lost 6.4 kg, and placebo patients lost 1.1 kg [$p < 0.001$].) (2) 10/19 zonisamide patients and none of 17 placebo patients had lost at least 10% of their body weight by week 32 ($p < 0.001$).
    - Adverse effects of zonisamide: fatigue, paresthesias, cognitive impairment, vision problems
  - Orlistat (Xenical)
    - Reduces absorption of fat.
    - 120 mg tid with meals
    - Sustained weight loss of 9.7% at 2 years (Meyer, 2001)
    - Over 3.3 months, 11 of 13 consecutively treated patients lost 35% of weight gained on psychotropic medications; the other 2 discontinued the medication (Schwartz & Beale, 2003).
    - No CNS activity reported.
    - May have GI side effects; add vitamin A and E supplements.

- Sibutramine (Meridia)
  - 5HT and NE reuptake inhibitor
  - Approved for long-term use.
  - Weight loss thought to be related to agonism of beta-3 receptors.
  - Sibutramine 20 mg produced 8.8% weight loss after 24 weeks of treatment (Meyer, 2001).
  - Average dose 20 mg
  - Side effects: increased blood pressure and pulse, dry mouth, insomnia; serotonergic side effects
- Bupropion may reduce weight short term.
  - No long-term data available.
- Fluoxetine 20 mg/day added to 10 mg/day olanzapine was no better than placebo in reducing weight gain over 8 weeks of treatment (mean 7.9 kg with olanzapine + fluoxetine; 6.0 kg with olanzapine + placebo; Poyurovsky, Pashinian, Gil-Ad, et al., 2002).
- A comparison of reboxetine (norepinephrine reuptake inhibitor) 4 mg day or placebo combined with 10 mg/day of olanzapine in patients treated for 6 weeks for first episode schizophrenia with olanzapine found (Poyurovsky, Isaacs, Fuchs, et al., 2003):
  - Weight gain 5.5 kg with olanzapine + placebo (N = 10)
  - Weight gain 2.5 kg with olanzapine + reboxetine
  - Significantly fewer patients with olanzapine + reboxetine (N = 2 of 10) than with olanzapine + placebo (N = 7 of 10) gained at least 7% of initial weight.
- Metformin (Glucophage)
  - Used anecdotally, but risky.
  - Most appropriate for patients with metabolic syndrome.

## Hematologic Side Effects

The most important hematologic effect of antipsychotic drugs involves bone marrow suppression.

### Agranulocytosis

- Defined as granulocyte count $< 500/mm^3$.
- Usually has sudden onset.
- Has been reported at any time during first 18 months of treatment.
- Occurs in $< 0.02\%$ of patients taking neuroleptics.
  - 0.7% of patients taking chlorpromazine
  - Very rare with high-potency neuroleptics and atypical antipsychotics
- Incidence of agranulocytosis is 1–2% with clozapine.

- Common presenting signs and symptoms include:
  - Sore throat
  - High fever
  - Mouth sores
  - Persistent infection
  - Bruising
  - Weakness
  - Lymphadenopathy
  - Skin uleractions
  - Laryngeal, angioneurotic, or peripheral edema
  - Anaphylaxis

Management:
- Routine CBCs only useful with clozapine (see below).
- Discontinue neuroleptic.
- Change to atypical antipsychotic.
- Do not use low-potency neuroleptic if white blood count < 3000.
- Lithium elevates neutrophil count.
- More aggressive interventions rarely necessary.

Clozapine-induced agranulocytosis
- Idiosyncratic medication reaction
- Risk factors include:
  - Women affected twice as frequently as men.
  - Older age
  - Low baseline white blood count
  - Ashkenazi Jewish ethnicity
  - Specific HLA halplotype
  - Coadministration of other medications that can suppress bone marrow.
  - No relationship reported between clozapine dose and agranulocytosis risk.
- Most cases develop within first 6 months of treatment.
  - Similar lower incidence during the second and the third six months of treatment (~0.05%).
  - Risks after 18 months not studied.
- Monitoring:
  - Do not start clozapine if WBC < 3500/m$^3$ or absolute neutrophil count < 1500/m$^3$.
    - Applies to neutropenia of any cause, including cancer chemotherapy and HIV.

- Weekly CBC for 6 months
- CBC every other week for next year
- Subsequent need for routine monitoring not clearly established.
- Obtain CBC for any indication of possible bone marrow suppression.
- Treatment
  - Stop clozapine if WBC < 3000
    - Do not rechallenge.
    - Change to a high-potency neuroleptic or an atypical antipsychotic other than olanzapine. (Prolonged ganulocytopenia reported in some patients.)
  - Lithium may elevate neutrophil count.
  - Granulocyte colony stimulating factor (G-CSF) or granulocyte-macrophage colony stimulating factor (GM-CSF).
  - Bone marrow transplantation necessary if no response.

### LEUKOPENIA

- More common than agranulocytosis
- Usually asymptomatic
- Gradual onset
- Often transient

### EOSINOPHILIA

- Allergic reaction, most commonly in response to clozapine.
- Develops within 3–5 weeks; resolves in 1 month.
- Discontinue clozapine if eosinophil count > 3000/mL.

### VENOUS THROMBOSIS

Venous thrombosis and pulmonary embolism reported with clozapine.

## Renal/Urinary Side Effects

Effects of the medication on renal function must be distinguished from effects of the illness.

### POLYDIPSIA AND HYPONATREMIA

Psychogenic polydipsia is common in schizophrenia.

- With normal renal function, it is necessary to drink > 1 liter/hour to overcome the capacity of the kidneys to excrete water.
- Hyponatremia occurs in 25–50% of chronically psychotic patients with persistent psychogenic polydipsia.
  - Usually attributable to syndrome of inappropriate antidiuretic hormone secretion (SIADH) caused by psychosis.

- Neuroleptics impair renal water excretion and exacerbate hypo-natremia.
- Signs and symptoms of water intoxication include:
  - Confusion
  - Nausea
  - Headache
  - Anorexia
  - Lethargy
  - Myoclonus
  - Cramps
  - Diurnal weight gain
  - Delirium
  - Seizures
  - Increased urinary output
  - Low urine-specific gravity
  - Severe signs more likely with serum sodium < 120 mM
- Treatment of water intoxication:
  - Fluid restriction
    - Difficult to maintain with psychotic patients
  - Furosemide and salt tablets
  - Lithium
  - Demeclocycline

## Urinary Retention

- Anticholinergic effect
- Incidence similar in men and women
- Can increase risk of urinary tract infection.
- Treatment:
  - Switch to a less anticholinergic antipsychotic medication.
  - Reduce use of anticholinergic antiparkinsonian drug.
  - Administer cholinesterase inhibitor (e.g., donepezil 5–10 mg/day).
  - Administer bethanechol 5–75 mg/day.
    - Effective but poorly tolerated.

## Urinary Incontinence

- Can be caused by anticholinergic effects of neuroleptics (overflow incontinence) or alpha-adrenergic blockade (e.g., clozapine).
- Usually improves spontaneously.
- Management:
  - Ephedrine 25–150 mg/day

- Oxybutynin (Ditropan) less reliable
- Bedtime vasopressin (DDAVP) in patients without polydipsia or hyponatremia

### Skin, Allergies, and Temperature Regulation

ABNORMAL BODY TEMPERATURE

- Hypothermia more common than hyperthermia.
- Hypothermia may be risky in patients exposed to cold environment.
- Decreased sweating caused by antiadrenergic and anticholinergic effects.
- Inability to dissipate body heat normally can lead to hyperthermia, especially in patients with polyuria.
  - May predispose to neurotoxicity of concomitant medications, such as lithium.
  - Risk factors for heat stroke:
    - Working in hot weather
    - In seclusion with decreased fluid intake, agitation, and high ambient temperature
    - Excessive use of alcohol
    - CNS disease
- Transient fever occurs in 20–25% of patients with clozapine.
  - Lasts 1–9 days.
  - Does not increase risk of agranulocytosis.

PHOTOSENSITIVITY

- Increased sensitivity to sunburn with neuroleptics
- Management:
  - Wear long sleeves and a hat when out in the sun.
  - Use PABA sunscreen.

SKIN RASH

- Neuroleptic-induced parkinsonism may be associated with seborrheic dermatitis.
- Allergic rashes may occur.

## PREGNANCY AND LACTATION

### Teratogenicity

Women with schizophrenia have an increased baseline level of obstetrical complications, making it difficult to be certain about teratogenicity. Case control studies have not revealed any significant fetal anomalies with antipsychotic drug exposure in utero.

Table 1.10  Drug–Drug Interactions

| DRUGS (X) INTERACT WITH: | ANTI-PSYCHOTICS (A) | COMMENTS |
|---|---|---|
| acetaminophen | X↓ | May overuse acetaminophen. |
| alcohol | X↑ A↑ | CNS depression; haloperidol increases alcohol effect. |
| alpha-methyldopa | X↑ | Increases hypotension and confusion. |
| alprazolam | A↑ | Increases sedation, haloperidol and fluphenazine levels. |
| aluminum hydroxide | A↓ | Give aluminum hydroxide at least one hour before, or 2 h after, antipsychotic agents. (*See also* calcium carbonate.) |
| amphetamines (*see* dextroamphetamine | | |
| anesthetics (general) | X↑ | CNS depression, hypotension. |
| anticholinergics | X↑ A↓ | Added anticholinergic effect. Consider amantadine; may decrease antipsychotic effect. |
| anticonvulsants | X↓? | Carbamazepine level unchanged. Clozapine could interfere with anticonvulsants. |
| antihistamines | X↑ A↑ | CNS depression. Added anticholinergic effect. |
| antihypertensives | X↑ | Increased hypotension, particularly with low-potency neuroleptics. |
| bromocriptine | X↓ A↓ | All neuroleptics except clozapine can reduce effectiveness for reducing prolactin. Increased psychosis. |
| caffeine | A↓ | Increased psychosis in high doses, 600–1000 mg. |
| calcium carbonate | | No effect, unlike aluminum and magnesium hydroxides. |
| citalopram (*see* SSRIs) | | |
| clonidine | X↑ | Hypotension. |
| dextroamphetamine | X↓ A↑ | Chlorpromazine treats dextroamphetamine overdose, but amphetamines should never treat neuroleptic overdose. |
| dichloralphenazone | A↓ | Hastens neuroleptic metabolism. |
| digoxin | X↑ A↑ | Each may increase unbound fraction of the other. |
| diuretics (thiazides) | X↑ | Increased orthostatic hypotension, hypotension, risk of shock. |
| epinephrine | X↓ | Hypotensive phenothiazine-treated patients might do better on levarterenol or phenylephrine. |
| estrogen | A↑ | May increase phenothiazine level. |

*(continues)*

**Table 1.10  Continued**

| DRUGS (X) INTERACT WITH: | ANTI-PSYCHOTICS (A) | COMMENTS |
|---|---|---|
| fluoxetine (*see* SSRIs) | | |
| griseofulvin | A↓ | Speeds neuroleptic metabolism. |
| guanethidine | X↓ | Hypotensive action inhibited by phenothiazines, haloperidol, and possibly thioxanthines. |
| hypnoanxiolytics | X↑ A↑ | CNS depression. |
| isoproterenol | X↓ | Marked hypotension |
| levodopa | X↓ | Antagonizes effects of dopamine agonists; try clozapine or possibly risperidone. |
| lithium | X↑ A? | May cause EPS; extremely rare. Acute neuro-toxicity at normal serum levels, especially with haloperidol or thioridazine. Chronic combina-tion a smaller problem. Lithium and chlorpro-mazine may *lower* levels in both. Increases molindone levels. |
| magnesium hydroxide | A↓ | Give magnesium hydroxide at least one hour before, or 2 h after, antipsychotic agents. (*See also* calcium carbonate.) |
| MAOIs | X↓ A? | Hypotension may result; MAOIs may trigger EPS. |
| methyldopa | X↑ | Hypotension, rarely delirium. |
| methylphenidate (*see* dextroamphetamine) | | |
| nicotine | A↓ | Decreased blood levels. |
| norepinephrine | X↓ | Hypotension. |
| opiates | X↑ A↑ | CNS depression. |
| orphenadrine | X↓ A↓ | Lowers neuroleptic levels; with CPZ may cause hypoglycemia; increases anticholinergic effects. |
| paroxetine (*see* SSRIs) | | |
| phenylbutazone | X↑ A↑ | More drowsiness. |
| phenytoin | X? A↓? | Toxicity may occur. Obtain phenytoin level and adjust; can reduce clozapine and other levels. |
| propranolol | X↑ A↑ | Hypotension, toxicity, and seizures. Monitor serum levels; decrease dose. |
| quinidine | X↑ A↑ | Increased quinidine-like effects with dysrhyth-mias, especially phenothiazines. Increases risperidone levels. |
| rifampin | A↓ | Speeds neuroleptic metabolism. |
| SSRIs (citalopram, fluoxetine, fluvoxamine, paroxetine, sertraline) | A↑ | May increase EPS and plasma levels. Fluvoxam-ine least likely to increase antipsychotic levels. Haloperidol, perphenazine, thioridazine most likely to be increased. |

*(continues)*

## Table 1.10 Continued

| DRUGS (X) INTERACT WITH: | ANTI-PSYCHOTICS (A) | COMMENTS |
|---|---|---|
| stimulants (*see* dextro-amphetamine) | | |
| succinylcholine | X↑ | May have prolonged paralysis. |
| TCAs | X↑ A↑ | Possible toxicity or hypotension; TCAs may diminish EPS. TCA levels increased by pheno-thiazine and haloperidol. |
| trazodone | X↑ A↑ | Additive hypotensive effects. |
| tobacco (*see* nicotine) | | |
| valproic acid | A↑ | Potentially increases levels; reported with risperidone and clozapine. |
| warfarin | X↑ A↑ | Increased bleeding time by increasing warfarin. May increase unbound antipsychotic. |

| DRUGS (X) INTERACT WITH: | ARIPIPRAZOLE (A) | COMMENTS |
|---|---|---|
| carbamazepine | A↓ | Aripiprazole metabolized by CYP3A4, which is induced by carbamazepine |
| fluoxetine, paroxetine | A↑ | Aripiprazole also metabolized by CYP2D6, which is inhibited by fluoxetine and paroxetine |
| hypotensive agents | X↑ A↑ | Additive hypotensive effects |
| ketoconazole | A↑ | Ketoconazole inhibits CYP3A4 |
| quinidine | A↑ | Quinidine inhibits CYP2D6 |

| DRUGS (X) INTERACT WITH: | CHLORPROMAZINE (C) | COMMENTS |
|---|---|---|
| antimalarial agents (amodiaquine, chloroquine, pyrimethamine, sulfadoxine) | C↑ | Chlorpromazine 2–4 times higher levels. |
| anorectic agents | X↓ | Inhibits anorectic effect. |
| antidiabetics | X↓ | Loss of glucose control possible; change neuroleptics. |
| barbiturates | X↑C↓ | CNS depression acute; antipsychotic effects lowered. |
| captopril | X↑ | Hypotension. |
| cimetidine | C↓ | Avoid cimetidine; try ranitidine or nizatidine. |
| enalapril | X↑ | Hypotension. |

(*continues*)

**Table 1.10  Continued**

| DRUGS (X) INTERACT WITH: | CHLORPROMAZINE (C) | COMMENTS |
|---|---|---|
| insulin (*see* antidiabetics) | | |
| meperidine | X↑ C↓ | Hypotension, lethargy, CNS depression; switch one drug. |
| phenmetrazine (*see* anorectic agents) | | |
| sulfonylureas | X↑ | Change neuroleptic. |
| valproic acid | X↑ C↑ | Toxicity; switch to haloperidol. |

| DRUGS (X) INTERACT WITH: | CLOZAPINE (C) | COMMENTS |
|---|---|---|
| carbamazepine | X↑ C↑ | Increases agranulocytosis risk. |
| cimetidine | C↑ | Increases clozapine levels; consider ranitidine as alternative. |
| diltiazem | C↑ | Increases clozapine levels. |
| fluvoxamine | C↑ | Increases clozapine levels. |
| hypnoanxiolytic benzodiazepines | H↑ C↑ | Increased risk of respiratory arrest. |
| phenytoin | C↑ | Increases agranulocytosis risk. |
| risperidone (*see* risperidone below) | | |
| verapamil | C↑ | Increases clozapine levels. |

| DRUGS (X) INTERACT WITH: | HALOPERIDOL (H) | COMMENTS |
|---|---|---|
| carbamazepine | H↓ | Psychosis; 50% lower serum level. |
| indomethacin | H↑ | Drowsiness, tiredness, and confusion; change one agent. |
| buspirone | H↑ | About 26% increase in haloperidol level. |

| DRUGS (X) INTERACT WITH: | LOXAPINE (L) | COMMENTS |
|---|---|---|
| lorazepam | X↑ | Rare respiratory depression, stupor, and hypotension. Switch one drug. No other benzodiazepine apparently interacts with loxapine. |

| DRUGS (X) INTERACT WITH: | THIORIDAZINE (T) | COMMENTS |
|---|---|---|
| phenylpropanolamine | X↑ | One sudden death. Tell patients to avoid common over-the-counter drugs with PPA (e.g., Dexatrim, Allerest, Dimetapp); causal effect not proven. |

(*continues*)

**Table 1.10  Continued**

| DRUGS (X) INTERACT WITH: | RISPERIDONE | COMMENTS |
|---|---|---|
| carbamazepine | R↓ | Decreased level with chronic carbamazepine. |
| clozapine | R↑ | Increased level with chronic clozapine. |
| SSRIs | R↑? | Probable increase in risperidone levels. |
| P4502D6 metabolized drugs<br>haloperidol<br>thioridazine<br>perphenazine<br>dextromethorphan<br>bufaralol<br>propranolol<br>tricyclic antidepressants<br>timolol | X↑ | Increased levels possible. |

↑ Increases; ↓ Decreases

**Table 1.11  Effects on Laboratory Tests***

| GENERIC NAMES | BLOOD/SERUM TESTS | URINE TESTS |
|---|---|---|
| chlorpromazine | LFT**↑ | VMA↓<br>Urobilinogen ↑ |
| clozapine | WBC↓<br>LFT↑ | |
| fluphenazine | LFT↑<br>Cephaline flocculation ↑ | VMA↓<br>Urobilinogen ↑ |
| loxapine | LFT ↑ | None |
| molindone | LFT ↑<br>Eosinophils ↑<br>Leukocytes ↓<br>Fatty acids ↑ | ? |
| perphenazine | Glucose ↑ | Pregnancy tests false + or − |
| risperidone | | Pregnancy tests false + or − |
| thiothixene | LFT ↑<br>Uric acid ↓ | None |
| trifluoperazine | LFT ↑ | VMA↓<br>Urobilinogen ↑ |

*All except clozapine can elevate prolactin levels; ↑ Increases; ↓ Decreases; ** LFT = liver function tests refer to AST/SGOT, ALT/SGPT, alkaline phosphatase, bilirubin, and LDH.

**Table 1.12  Recommendations for Medical Monitoring of Patients Taking Antipsychotic Medications**

| MEDICATION | EPS | TARDIVE DYSKINESIA | WEIGHT | BLOOD SUGAR CHOLESTEROL/ TRIGLYCERIDES | PROLACTIN | EKG |
|---|---|---|---|---|---|---|
| Neuroleptic | Every visit if a problem; otherwise, q 6 months | Q 6 months | 3 months; 1 year | If > 7% weight gain, yearly | Yearly or if any symptoms (e.g., sexual side effects depression | Yearly for thioridazine or mesoridazine, |
| Risperidone | Every visit only if problem | Yearly | 3 months; 1 year | | | NA |
| Olanzapine | Every visit only if problem | Yearly | Every visit for 6 months, then q 3 months | | | |
| Quetiapine | Every visit only if problem | Yearly | Yearly | | | |
| Ziprasidone | Every visit only if problem | Yearly | Yearly | | | Not mandated by FDA |
| Clozapine | Every visit only if problem | Yearly | Every visit for 6 months, then q 3 months | | | NA |

Adapted from Marder et al. (2002).

- A review of published studies between 1996 and 2001 suggests that there could be an increased risk of congenital malformations with exposure to phenothiazines during weeks 4–10 of gestation (Patton et al., 2002).
- Behavioral teratogenicity of neuroleptics has been demonstrated in animals but not in people.
  - Clinical implications are unknown.
- Insufficient experience with atypical antipsychotics to determine safety in pregnancy.

## Neonatal Effects

- Neonatal jaundice has been reported with older preparations of chlorpromazine but not recently.
- EPS in newborn may persist until medication is metabolized; manifestations include
  - Tremor
  - Hypertonicity

  - Hyperreflexia
  - Excessive crying
  - Irritability
  - Vasomotor instability
- Hypotension reported with low-potency neuroleptics.
- Newborns may be oversedated.

### Lactation

Like most psychotropic medications, antipsychotic medications are excreted in breast milk in concentrations that may equal plasma levels.
- Actual dose to newborn is low.
- Antipsychotic side effects may occur in newborn, especially
  - EPS
  - Sedation

## WITHDRAWAL

Antipsychotic drugs do not cause dependence or addiction. However, they can be associated with discontinuation syndromes when they are reduced or stopped abruptly.
- Withdrawal may produce
  - Influenza-like symptoms
  - Insomnia, nightmares
  - Gastrointestinal distress
  - Headaches
  - Diaphoresis
  - Dizziness
  - Hot or cold sensations
  - Tremor
  - Tachycardia
  - Cholinergic rebound with anticholinergic preparations (e.g., low-potency neuroleptics), such as sweating, diarrhea, abdominal pain, nausea, vomiting
- Clozapine withdrawal can cause delirium, agitation, abnormal movements.
- Withdrawal syndromes begin 2–7 days after discontinuation and last 2 weeks.
- Because the duration of action of neuroleptics is longer than that of antiparkinsonian drugs, withdrawing both at the same time often results in acute EPS.

- Maintain antiparkinsonian medication 1–2 weeks after discontinuing neuroleptic.
    - Longer with depot neuroleptics
- Withdrawal dyskinesia, probably caused by dopaminergic rebound, may occur with rapid neuroleptic discontinuation.
    - Prevented by slower discontinuation.
    - Not improved by antiparkinsonian drugs.
- Withdrawal psychosis
    - After withdrawal or reduction of dose in chronic treatment with neuroleptics, some patients experience a rebound of psychosis that is more marked than the original psychotic symptoms.
    - Quantitatively different from original symptoms, return of which would indicate relapse.
    - This may represent dopamine receptor supersensitivity induced by chronic receptor blockade that rebounds when blockade is removed.
    - Occasionally, psychosis may become chronic in nonschizophrenic patients who were treated long-term with neuroleptics.

## TOXICITY AND OVERDOSE

Neuroleptics can be fatal in overdose, but the risk is less than with TCAs.
- Lethality is much greater for low-potency than high-potency neuroleptics.
- Atypical antipsychotic drugs *other than clozapine* seem safer in overdose.
    - Overdoses of ziprasidone have not been associated with adverse cardiac events.
- Most fatalities occur when neuroleptic overdoses are combined with other CNS depressants. For example, an overdose of chlorpromazine + a TCA is three times as likely to induce coma as is an overdose of chlorpromazine alone.

Management of overdose:
- Discontinue antipsychotic drug.
- Discontinue antiparkinsonian medications.
- Determine what other medications/substances have been used recently.
- Provide supportive care (airway, fluids, blood pressure support).
- Administer gastric lavage if patient conscious.
    - Most effective if overdose occurred within 4 hours, but may be useful within 24–36 hours of ingestion.
    - Follow with activated charcoal: 40–50 gm for adults; 20–25 gm for children.
- Observe conscious patient for 8–12 hours after ingestion.

- Do not use emetics because of risk that acute dystonia of head and neck could cause aspiration.
- Hemodialysis not helpful because serum drug concentrations are low, whereas tissue concentrations are high.
- Treat acute effects, which are primarily severe side effects.
  - Hypotension
    - May not appear for 2–3 days.
    - Can develop into shock.
    - Administer fluids.
    - Pure alpha-adrenergic agonist (e.g., norepinephrine, mataraminol, phenylephrine); do not use mixed alpha/beta agonist such as epinephrine, because alpha effect will be blocked by neuroleptic, and more vasodilatation will occur.
  - Urinary retention
    - Catheterize if no urine production.
    - Administer bethanechol 5–10 mg IM or sc (subcutaneous).
  - Seizures
    - Seen especially in children.
    - Administer IV diazepam.
    - Avoid barbiturates, which may aggravate respiratory depression.

## PRECAUTIONS

Antipsychotic medications should be used cautiously in the presence of
- Hypotension
- Cardiovascular disease
- Narrow angle glaucoma
- Concomitant use of CNS depressants
- History of breast cancer
  - Atypicals with low risk of prolactinemia are preferable.
- Prolactinemia
- Bone marrow depression
- Hypersensitivity to neuroleptics
- Parkinson's disease
- Hepatic impairment
- Acute illness (in children; e.g., chickenpox, measles, gastroenteritis, dehydration, Reye's syndrome)
  - Increased susceptibility to EPS
  - Elevated risk of hepatotoxicity

- Older age
- Diabetes mellitus
- Seizure disorder (low-potency neuroleptics, loxapine)
- QTc prolongation (pimozide, thioridazine, ziprasidone)

No dosage adjustment necessary for aripiprazole in renal or hepatic impairment or for age.

## ADVICE FOR CARETAKERS

Nonadherence is a common cause of poor response to treatment. It is important to assess patient acceptance of medication regularly.

### Oral Preparations

Elixirs enhance compliance but often have a bitter taste.
- Haloperidol is tasteless and colorless.
- Taking elixir with milk, orange juice, or food may reduce bitter taste.
- Protect elixirs from prolonged exposure to light.
- Slight discoloration does not indicate reduced potency.
  - Substantial discoloration *does* indicate reduced potency.

### Injections

- Do not keep medication in syringe > 15 minutes because plastic can absorb active drug.
- Administer IM injection slowly.
- Do not let liquid drip on patient's skin.
  - May cause contact dermatitis.
- Administer IM injection in deltoid, thigh, or upper-outer quadrant of buttocks.
  - More rapid absorption from deltoid because of better perfusion.
  - Tell patient that injection may sting.
  - Massage injection site slowly to prevent formation of sterile abscess.
  - Administer in alternating injection sites.
  - Be careful about orthostatic hypotension after injection.
- For depot injections:
  - Do not keep medication in syringe > 15 minutes because plastic can absorb active drug.
  - Use needle no larger than 21 gauge.
  - Give deep IM injection into a large muscle using Z-track method.

- Rotate injection site.
  - Note date of each site in chart
- *Do not* massage injection site.
- Depot preparations can be given sc.

## NOTES FOR PATIENT AND FAMILY

Patients should be warned about common side effects and encouraged to call physician or nurse immediately if symptoms are suggestive of severe acute adverse effects (e.g., hypotension, agranulocytosis, NMS). Patients who are hypervigilant or paranoid or who hear voices telling them not to take medications still must be informed about common and severe side effects, or treatment must be considered involuntary. Psychosis does not invalidate capacity for informed consent if patient can understand illness, why medication is recommended, alternative therapies, and potential consequences of consenting to or refusing treatment.

- Inform patient that medications work best for psychosis when taken regularly.
  - However, prn dosing can be useful for acute exacerbations.
- Explain anticholinergic side effects.
- Tolerance to sedation often develops if dose is raised slowly.
- Show patients how to stand up slowly if they experience postural hypotension or dizziness.
  - Consider elastic stocking for orthostatic hypotension.
- Patient should be warned about acute EPS, especially:
  - Dystonia (sudden, sustained contraction of a group of muscles, often of the neck, trunk, or eyes)
  - Akathisia (uncomfortable inner restlessness)
  - Parkinsonism (stiff muscles, tremor, slowed movement)
- To reduce impairment from EPS
  - Advise patient to wear loose, lightweight clothing that has Velcro fasteners rather than buttons.
  - Shoes that slip on are preferable to laced or zipped shoes.
  - Minimize use of high-heeled shoes or other footwear that makes walking more difficult.
  - Show patient how to walk into turns rather than pivoting, which can result in a fall.
  - If stiffness or rigidity makes it difficult to get out of bed, show patient how to
    - First lie, then sit on the side of the bed.

- Slowly drop one leg over the side of bed while pushing down with elbow of opposite arm.
  - Prevent bathing accidents with
    - No-slip rubber mat
    - Grab bar
    - Removal of glass tub or shower door
    - Shower chair
    - Soap attached to a cord
- It is not necessary to discuss TD risk for acute treatment of an acutely psychotic patient, because the risk is very low in the first few months of treatment, and it is often unclear whether the patient will take the medication chronically. However, TD should be discussed
  - Before 3 months of treatment have elapsed
  - Whenever chronic treatment is planned
  - Although the risk of TD is much lower with atypicals, this risk is still important enough to review.
  - Loose-fitting dentures can mimic TD and can ulcerate gums in patients who do have TD.
- Discuss risk of oversedation and diabetes mellitus when chronic treatment is planned with olanzapine, clozapine, or low-potency neuroleptics.
- Warn patient about risk of psychomotor impairment.
  - Have someone else assess patient's driving for slowed reaction time and poor coordination.
  - Additive psychomotor impairment occurs with alcohol.
- Remind patient to wear a hat and use sunscreen when outside.
- Instruct patient that if a dose is missed
  - Can take the missed dose if up to 3–4 hours late.
  - If more than 3–4 hours late, wait for next scheduled dose.
  - Do not take two doses together if one dose is missed, unless this approach has already been found to be effective.
- Tell patient not to stop medication abruptly.
  - Risk of relapse is the same as with slow discontinuation, but risk of rebound psychosis and withdrawal symptoms is greater.
  - If patient insists on withdrawing a chronically administered antipsychotic, try to take 3–6 months to do so unless severe side effects are present.

# CHAPTER TWO

# Neurological and Neuropsychiatric Medications

Neurological side effects induced by antipsychotic medications can be treated with anticholinergic agents (ACAs), including many antihistamines, alpha-adrenergic blockers, benzodiazepines, and dopamine agonists. Some of these medications (e.g., ACAs) are used primarily to treat extrapyramidal side effects (EPS), whereas others (e.g., propranolol) are used for multiple purposes.

Antipsychotic drugs and a number of other medications are frequently used in the management of delirium and dementia, but neurological side effects are more common in these patients. New treatments have emerged that improve cognitive function in dementia and that are also used to treat certain side effects of psychotropic medications and other neuropsychiatric disorders.

This chapter considers

- Treatment of EPS with antiparkinsonian and other medications
- Treatment of delirium
- Treatment of agitation associated with brain damage
- Treatment of dementia

Table 2.1 provides a basic overview of the drugs addressed in this chapter.

## PHARMACOLOGY

A balance between dopaminergic, cholinergic, noradrenergic, and serotonergic input provides for smooth regulation of motor output by the basal ganglia. When dopaminergic transmission is reduced by blockade of postsynaptic $D_2$ receptors due to antipsychotic medications, the ratio of dopaminergic and cholinergic input is reduced, and the ability to generate and regulate normal movement is impaired; parkinsonism may be the result. Reducing cholinergic tone (e.g., with ACAs) or increasing dopaminergic transmission (e.g., with amantadine) can restore

Table 2.1  Names, Dose Forms, Colors

| GENERIC NAMES | BRAND NAMES | DOSE FORMS (MG)* | COLORS |
|---|---|---|---|
| amantadine | Symmetrel | c: 100<br>s: 50 mg/5 ml | c: red |
| benztropine | Cogentin | t: 0.5/1/2<br>p: 1 mg/ml | t: all white |
| biperiden | Akineton | t: 2<br>p: 5 mg/ml | t: white |
| bromocriptine | Parlodel | t: 2.5<br>c: 5 | t: white<br>c: caramel-white |
| diazepam | Valium | t: 2/5/10<br>p: 5 mg/ml | t: white/yellow/<br>blue |
| diphenhydramine[†] | Benadryl | c: 25/50<br>p: 10/50 mg/ml | c: all pink-white |
| lorazepam | Ativan | t: 0.5/1/2 | t: all white |
| procyclidine | Kemadrin | t: 5 | t: white |
| propranolol | Inderal | t: 10/20/40/80<br>p: 1 mg/ml | t: orange/blue/<br>green/pink/<br>yellow |
| trihexyphenidyl | Artane | t: 2/5<br>sr: 5 mg<br>e: 2 mg/5 ml | t: all white<br>sr: blue |

* c = capsules; e = elixir; p = parenteral; s = syrup; sr = sustained-release sequels; t = tablets;
[†] Can be purchased over the counter only in 25 mg.

coordinated striatal neurotransmission and reduce parkinsonism. An excess of noradrenergic over dopaminergic neurotransmission, corrected by blockade of beta receptors, may be involved in akathisia. With chronic blockade, $D_2$ receptors become supersensitive and the dopamine/acetylcholine ratio reverses itself as new abnormal movements are generated (TD). Increasing the $D_2$ blockade by raising the antipsychotic dose temporarily suppresses the increased expression of $D_2$ signaling, but receptor supersensitivity eventually overrides this effect, and abnormal movements reappear.

Striatal dopaminergic neurons have serotonin $5HT_2$ heteroreceptors that reduce dopamine release. Increased serotonin input to these receptors (e.g., as a result of treatment with SSRIs) reduces dopamine release, resulting in parkinsonism or akathisia. Postreceptor interactions between $5HT_2$ and $D_2$ receptors intensify the effects of decreased dopamine release and enhance $D_2$ up-regulation in response to chronic blockade. Conversely, blockade of $5HT_2$ receptors (e.g., with atypical) mitigates acute EPS and reduces both the risk and expression of TD.

## CLINICAL INDICATIONS AND USE

Treatment of acute EPS is not necessary as frequently with atypical antipsychotics as it is with neuroleptics. Among the atypicals, risperidone is probably most likely to require concomitant treatment for EPS. Although treatment for EPS is usually not initiated prophylactically with the atypicals, the decision to institute prophylactic treatment with neuroleptics is more difficult.

- In favor of prophylactic treatment:
  - EPS can lead to discontinuation of the antipsychotic medication and can mimic negative symptoms.
  - EPS common with high-potency neuroleptics.
  - Antiparkinsonian drugs clearly reduce dystonia, akinesia, and parkinsonism.
- Against prophylactic treatment:
  - Many patients do not develop EPS.
    - Especially with low-potency neuroleptics
  - Antiparkinsonian medications can have significant adverse effects.
  - Antiparkinsonian drugs can be added, if necessary.
  - Antiparkinsonian drugs are not predictably effective for akathisia.

Guidelines for use of medications for EPS include the following considerations.

- Consider prophylactic treatment in the presence of
  - Younger male
  - Past history of severe EPS
  - High-potency neuroleptic
    - Dystonia rate 70% in younger patient treated with haloperidol.
- It may be necessary to add an antiparkinsonian medication when blood levels peak 2–14 days after administration of depot neuroleptic.
- Add a medication for EPS if signs or symptoms develop.
- Acute EPS often remit spontaneously within 6–8 weeks.
  - Attempt to withdraw EPS medication gradually within 6 months to determine if it is still necessary.
    - About 15% experience return of neurological side effects.
    - About 30% feel less agitated if ACA continued.
- Because duration of action of neuroleptics is longer than that of medications for EPS, continue the latter for several days after withdrawing neuroleptic.

## CHOOSING A MEDICATION FOR EPS

Table 2.2 presents a summary of medication choices in relation to type of EPS.

Adjusting dose of medications for EPS:
- Start with divided dose.
  - Once daily dosing effective with chronic treatment with long half-life ACAs (e.g., benztropine, biperiden).
- ACA levels vary 100-fold with similar doses.
  - 25% of patients taking 4 mg/day benztropine have low blood levels.
    - These patients respond when dose is increased to 6–12 mg/day.
    - Monitor carefully for anticholinergic side effects.
  - Some patients experience toxicity at low doses.
- Treatment of EPS has a better correlation with ACA blood levels (> 7 pmol atropine equivalent) than with ACA dose.

## SIDE EFFECTS

Side effects of ACAs and amantadine are considered below; side effects of beta-blockers and clonidine are addressed in Chapter 7.

The most important side effects of ACAs and amantadine involve the CNS and gastrointestinal systems. Because amantadine has some anticholinergic properties, adverse effects overlap.

**Table 2.2 Medications for EPS**

| TYPE OF EPS | MEDICATIONS | COMMENTS |
|---|---|---|
| Akathisia | Beta-blocker | Use lipid soluble beta-blocker (propranolol, metropolol, pindolol, nadolol; *not* atenolol). |
| | | Benzodiazepines second-line choice. |
| | | Clonidine and buspirone occasionally helpful. |
| | | ACAs not reliably effective for acute akathisia but sometimes help tardive akathisia. |
| Dystonia | Diphenhydramine ACA | 25–50 mg IV provides rapid reduction of akathisia. |
| | | Benztropine 1–2 mg IV can be rapidly effective. |
| | | Prophylactic ACA can prevent recurrence. |
| Parkinsonism | Reduce neuroleptic dose; ACA amantadine | Amantadine and other dopaminergic medications can reduce parkinsonism but sometimes aggravate psychosis and cause depression. |
| Rabbit syndrome | ACA | Responds rapidly to any ACA. |

## Table 2.3  Choosing Oral Antiparkinsonian Drugs

| SYMPTOM | MEDICATION |
|---|---|
| Akathisia | Propranolol 10–80 mg or other lipophilic β-blocker (e. g., metoprolol, pindolol, or nadolol, but not atenolol) is first choice if akathisia is an isolated symptom.<br>Amantadine or benzodiazepines (lorazepam or diazepam) are second choices.<br>ACAs are third choices. If other EPS also occur, which are better treated with ACA, use ACA first.<br>Clonidine (0.15–2 mg/qd) also reported to help for "tardive" as well as acute akathisia. |
| Dystonia | Diphenhydramine 25–50 mg IV/IM as first choice; often provides complete relief in minutes and reduces patient anxiety. Hydroxyzine alternative.<br>Benztropine 1–2 mg IV/IM is the second choice, and always works quickly.<br>If patient does not respond to the above, question the diagnosis.<br>Prevent future dystonias with any ACA. |
| Parkinsonism | Reduce neuroleptics to lowest effective dose.<br>Try any ACA.<br>Prescribe amantadine if troublesome anticholinergic symptoms already exist.<br>Consider amantadine in geriatrics and to preserve new memory acquisition in any age group. |
| Rabbit syndrome | Responds well to any ACA. |

## Table 2.4  Doses

| GENERIC NAMES | ORAL DOSES (MG) | IM/IV DOSES (MG) | MAJOR CHEMICAL GROUP |
|---|---|---|---|
| amantadine | 100 bid–tid* | — | Dopaminergic agonist |
| benztropine | 1–3 bid | 1–2 | ACA |
| biperiden | 2 tid–qid | 2 | ACA |
| diazepam | 5 tid | 5–10 | Benzodiazepine |
| diphenhydramine | 25–50 tid–qid | 25–50 | Antihistamine and ACA |
| lorazepam | 1–2 tid | — | Benzodiazepine |
| procyclidine | 2.5–5 tid | — | ACA |
| propranolol | 10–20 tid; up to 40 qid | — | β-blocker |
| trihexyphenidyl** | 2–5 tid | — | ACA |

*Amantadine can often be given 200 mg qd instead of 100 mg bid. In geriatrics, 100 mg qd is usually enough.
**Start with trihexyphenidyl tablets or elixir; only later transfer to sustained-released sequels (capsules). Use sequels as a single dose after breakfast or one dose q12 h. For akathisia, give trihexyphenidyl 6–10 mg qd; other EPS, provide 2–6 mg qd.

## Cardiovascular Side Effects

- Tachycardia
- Palpitations
- Dizziness

## Central Nervous System Side Effects

- Impaired memory
- Confusion
- Delirium
- Psychosis
  - Amantadine may exacerbate psychosis.
    - High doses can cause hallucinations or paranoia in nonpsychotic patients.
  - Psychosis with ACAs usually caused by anticholinergic delirium.
- Restlessness
- Tremors
- Ataxia
- Weakness, lethargy
- Incoherence
- Numb fingers, difficulty moving specific muscles
  - Especially in the elderly and at higher doses
- Excitement, insomnia
- Depression
  - Especially amantadine
- Chronic treatment with ACAs may increase the risk of TD with neuroleptics.

## Endocrine and Sexual Side Effects

- Amantadine can reduce galactorrhea caused by the antidopaminergic effect of neuroleptics.

## Eyes, Ears, Nose, and Throat Side Effects

- Blurred vision
- Sensitivity to light, photophobia
  - Caused by mydriasis

- Precipitation of narrow angle glaucoma
  - Measure intraocular pressure in patients with history of glaucoma.
- Nasal congestion
- Dry throat, thirst
- Aggravation of respiratory ailments

### Gastrointestinal Side Effects

- Constipation
  - Paralytic ileus
- Dry mouth (see pp. 34–35)
- Nausea, vomiting

### Renal/Urinary Side Effects

- Urinary hesitancy
- Urinary retention
- Predisposition to urinary tract infection

### Skin, Allergies, and Temperature Regulation

- Skin rash
- Flushing of skin
- Decreased sweating
- Fever

## PREGNANCY AND LACTATION

No teratogenicity has been reported with ACAs or amantadine, but safety in pregnancy is not established.

### Direct Effects on Newborn

Persistent cholinergic effects can cause neonatal paralytic ileus

### Lactation

- Dopaminergic effect of amantadine can inhibit lactation.
- All medications for EPS are excreted in breast milk.

## INTERACTIONS

Additive anticholinergic effects are common when ACAs or amantadine are combined with low-potency neuroleptics (e.g., chlorpromazine, thioridazine), tricyclic antidepressants, or paroxetine. It is generally inadvisable to add ACAs to these medication classes, unless an ACA is clearly indicated. Delirium, fever predisposing to neurotoxicity, and cardiotoxicity may occur.

## WITHDRAWAL

ACAs are frequently abused for the "spaced out" feeling they can induce (see below). In addition, abrupt withdrawal of any anticholinergic medication can lead to cholinergic rebound lasting up to 2 weeks and characterized by

- Influenza-like symptoms without fever
- Nausea, vomiting, diarrhea
- Sialorrhea
- Headache
- Insomnia
- Nightmares
- Rhinorrhea
- Increased appetite
- Dizziness
- Giddiness
- Tremor
- Hot or cold sensation

### Amantadine Withdrawal

Abrupt discontinuation of amantadine can produce
- Cholinergic rebound and/or rebound EPS
- Acute exacerbation of parkinsonism or neuroleptic-induced EPS

### Prevention of Discontinuation Syndromes

- Gradual tapering of medication reduces risk of withdrawal symptoms.
- If neuroleptic is going to be withdrawn, taper that medication first.
- Amantadine and ACA withdrawal are not life threatening.

## TOXICITY AND OVERDOSE

Overdose of ACAs or amantadine produces extreme anticholinergic side effects. Amantadine overdose also can cause hyperactivity, convulsions, arrhythmias, and hypotension. In addition to general measures described on pages 76–77, management of overdose includes the following:

- Emetics can be used for conscious patient who has taken overdose of ACA or amantadine alone.
- Physostimine 1–2 mg IV q 1–2 hours can reduce acute toxicity.
- Acidifying urine accelerates elimination of amantadine.

## PRECAUTIONS

ACA abuse has been reported with all preparations.
- Up to 17.5% of those taking ACAs
- Most common with trihexyphenidyl
- Promoted by psychic effects
  - Feeling energized
  - Euphoria
  - Sedation
  - Psychedelic and psychotic-like experiences

ACAs should not be used in patients with
- Urinary retention
- Significant prostatic hypertrophy
- Bowel obstruction, paralytic ileus
- Hyperthermia, heat stroke
- Congestive heart failure
- Narrow angle glaucoma
- Hypersensitivity to ACAs
- Dry bronchial secretions
- Delirium and dementia
- Severe hypertension

Use ACAs very cautiously in the presence of
- Cardiac arrhythmias
- Hypotension
- Older age
- Peripheral edema
- Liver or kidney disease

## ADVICE FOR CARETAKERS

Patients may reveal information about problems with ACAs in an off-hand manner, especially

- Abuse of ACAs
- Anticholinergic side effects

It is important to assess continued need for ACAs periodically, as well as adverse effects. The patient should be helped to avoid continuing these medications just because they were felt to be useful initially.

## NOTES FOR PATIENT AND FAMILY

Patients benefit from advice about dosing and management of anticholinergic side effects.

- If blurred vision or impaired cognition occur, do not drive until the side effect is resolved.
- Treat dry mouth with sugar-free candy.
    - Drinking fluid constantly only provides relief as long as liquid is in mouth.
    - Beverages and candy with sugar can cause dental caries and weight gain.
- All anticholinergic medications should be kept away from children.
- Use alcohol sparingly.
- Heat stroke is more likely to occur in hot weather.
    - Exercise cautiously.
    - Drink plenty of fluids.
- If a dose is missed
    - It can be taken up to 2 hours later.
    - After that, skip the dose.
- Benztropine, biperiden, and amantadine can be taken in one daily dose.
- Taking medication on a full stomach may reduce nausea.

## DELIRIUM

Delirium is a syndrome in which the clouding of consciousness is usually acute but sometimes prolonged. It is caused by diffuse CNS depression or depression of the reticular activating system.

Common signs and symptom include
- Disorientation
- Impaired memory and concentration
- Confusion
- Change in affect regulation that produces corresponding behavioral changes
  - Anxiety causes agitation.
  - Anger causes assaultiveness.
  - Depression causes withdrawal and passivity.
- Illusions, hallucinations and delusions often reflect misinterpretation of actual events, such as
  - Smelling gas when oxygen is on
  - Interpreting noises in the corridor as voices of persecutors
  - Paranoia that doctors are trying to kill the patient
- In medically ill patients, delirium is a sign of organ failure and either resolves or progresses to death.
- In psychiatric patients, the most common causes of delirium are
  - Medication side effects and interactions (especially anticholinergic medications and CNS depressants such as benzodiazepines and barbiturates)
    - Any medication that enters the brain can cause delirium.
  - Substance use, especially alcohol, tranquilizers, and PCP
  - Withdrawal from CNS depressants
  - Exacerbation of dementia by a minor physiological anomaly (e.g., urinary tract infection)
  - Postictal states, head injury

### Treatment of Delirium

Delirium is usually reversed by treating the underlying cause. In the meantime, general measures are adopted that include the following:
- Stop all unnecessary medications.
- Orient the patient repeatedly.
  - Easily visible clock and calendar
  - Night light
- Provide adequate hydration.
- Treat reversal of the sleep–wake cycle (a cause of "sundowning") with artificial bright light in the morning (see pp. 157–158).

CNS depressant withdrawal can cause delirium as well as generalized CNS excitability. Diagnosis and treatment of this syndrome with the barbiturate tolerance test is discussed on pages 447–449.

Clues to anticholinergic delirium
- Warm, dry skin with tachycardia
- Dilated pupils
- Dry mucous membranes
- Absent bowel sounds

Treatment of anticholinergic delirium
- Stop anticholinergic medications.
- If diagnosis unclear or patient unresponsive, diagnose/treat with 1–2 mg physostigmine IM or IV no faster than 1 mg/minute.
  - Repeat dose once 30 minutes later, if necessary.
  - Maximum dose 4 mg/day
  - Improvement of consciousness lasts 30–60 minutes.
  - Side effects of physostigmine:
    - Vomiting
    - Sweating
    - Bradycardia
    - Abdominal cramps
    - Urge to urinate or defecate
    - Seizures
    - Bronchospasm in asthmatics
  - Ongoing treatment with physostigmine is usually impractical.
  - Consider using a cholinesterase inhibitor for a few days.

Treatment of delirium is often complicated by agitation, with or without psychosis. This problem typically resolves with specific treatment (e.g., cholinergic medication for anticholinergic delirium, or barbiturate for CNS depressant withdrawal).

Nonspecific treatments for agitation in delirious patients, regardless of cause, include the following:
- Intravenous haloperidol
  - Can produce rapid tranquilization without excessive sedation.
  - Considerable experience but no controlled studies of delirium in acutely ill cardiac or cancer patients.
  - Initial dose 1–5 mg IV repeated every 1–4 hours, as needed.
  - In some cases of life-threatening agitation in coronary care patients, single doses as high as 75 mg have occasionally been used.
  - Most patients are calm after a few doses.
    - Treatment for more than 1–2 days is rarely needed.

- In intractable delirium, a haloperidol drip over several days has been used successfully.
- Do not combine with an ACA, which will aggravate delirium.
  - EPS is less frequent with IV haloperidol, possibly because it skips first-pass metabolism.
- Despite apparent safety on the coronary care unit, Torsades de Pointes sometimes occurs with IV haloperidol.
- IV lorazepam
  - Even though CNS depressant action of benzodiazepines can worsen delirium, IV lorazepam has been used successfully as an acute treatment for agitation that is complicating delirium.
  - Usual dose is 1–5 mg repeated every few hours.
  - For severe delirium use 2–5 mg haloperidol and 1–5 mg lorazepam *in same syringe.*
- If it is not possible to establish an IV route, consider:
  - IM haloperidol or lorazepam
  - IM droperidol
    - Rapid tranquilization with less EPS than IM haloperidol
    - QTc prolongation may occur.
- In an open-label study, quetiapine (mean dose 50 mg) reduced delirium over 5 days without causing significant EPS (Sasaki, Matsuyama, Inoue, et al., 2003).
  - Not clear whether delirium would have remitted over this time without an antipsychotic drug.
- IM ziprasidone could be effective, but no studies.
- Electroconvulsive therapy (ECT):
  - Standard treatment for delirium in Europe
  - Multiple reports and case series over many years support clearing of delirium with 1–4 ECTs (Dubovsky, 1986).
  - Effective for confusion and agitation, regardless of cause of delirium
  - Clears delirium, even if underlying cause not yet treated.
  - Consider for intractable or severe delirium with life-threatening agitation.

## DEMENTIA

Dementia is a syndrome of global cognitive decline characterized by loss of memory, judgment, abstract thinking, executive function, impulse control, and language (without prominent clouding of consciousness, unless delirium is superimposed).

- Dementia may be reversible or irreversible.
  - Common reversible causes include
    - Substance use
    - Hypothyroidism
    - Depression
    - Infection
    - Brain tumor
    - Normal pressure hydrocephalus
  - Common irreversible causes include
    - Alzheimer's disease (50% of cases)
    - Vascular dementia
    - Parkinson's disease
    - Frontotemporal dementia
    - Lewy body dementia
    - Pick's disease
- Behavioral disorders are common in demented patients. Typical manifestations include
  - Agitation
  - Unpredictable aggressive outbursts
  - Screaming
  - Wandering
  - Disinhibition
  - Psychosis

### Treatment of Cognitive Dysfunction

Memory deficits in Alzheimer's disease are associated with loss of cholinergic neurons in the Nucleus Basalis of Meinhert caused by accumulation of beta-amyloid in neurofibrillary tangles and plaques, some of which contain elevated activity of acetylcholinesterase (AChE) and butylcholinesterase (BuChE). Since ACh is a neurotransmitter of memory, inhibiting AChE (and possibly BuChE) can improve memory and other aspects of cognition, although it does not address the primary cause of Alzheimer's disease. Progression of the disease is associated in part with release of high levels of excitatory amino acids (excitotoxicity) from neurons injured by amyloid; these amino acids act on NMDA and other receptors to induce excessive calcium ion influx. In turn, this influx activates proteolytic enzymes and reactive oxygen species, causing further neuronal injury. Treatments for this pathophysiology include the following pharmacological interventions.

*Cholinesterase inhibitors*

- All cholinesterase inhibitors produce moderate improvement and slowing of deterioration of cognition and functioning in patients with Alzheimer's disease.
- May reduce agitation independent of improvement in cognition.
- Benefits decline as more cholinergic neurons are lost.
- A meta-analysis of 29 nonoverlapping controlled trials of cholinesterase inhibitors found
    - Improvement in the Alzheimer's Disease Assessment Scale (ADAS) on the noncog score of 1.72 points compared with placebo, which was statistically significant if small, and 0.03 points in the Neuropsychiatric Inventory (NPI), which was not significant,
        - More diminishment in neuropsychiatric dysfunction than in affective, psychotic, and behavioral symptoms (Trinh, Hoblyn, Mohanty, & Yaffe, 2003).
        - Improvement of Alzheimer's Disease Seventy Index (ADSI) was 0.09–0.1 *SDs,* indicating a small but statistically significant improvement.
        - This is at the very lower end of being clinically detectable, equivalent to preventing a 2-month per year decline.
- Cholinesterase inhibitors also may be useful for cognitive dysfunction associated with other disorders, such as
    - Other forms of dementia (e.g., vascular dementia)
    - Traumatic brain injury
    - Attention-deficit disorder
- Cholinesterase inhibitors may reduce cognitive side effects of other medications.
    - Especially anticholinergic medications
        - Also useful for other anticholinergic side effects, such as constipation, dry mouth, blurred vision.
    - May decrease cognitive side effects of medications that are not primarily anticholinergic.
- Tacrine
    - First cholinesterase inhibitor to be released.
    - High incidence of hepatotoxicity (40%) and other adverse effects and high dropout rate reduce overall efficacy, even though tacrine is as effective as other cholinesterase inhibitors.
    - Supplanted by newer, better-tolerated cholinesterase inhibitors.
- Donepezil
    - There are eight published double-blind randomized placebo-controlled trials, involving 2,664 subjects and lasting 12–52 weeks (Birks, Melzer, & Beppu, 2002).

- These studies demonstrate statistically significant improvement for 5 and 10 mg of donepezil compared with placebo, with 2.9 points on the ADAS-Cog scale for 10 mg at 24 weeks.
  - There was improvement in global clinical state compared with placebo, but no change in patient ratings of quality of life.
- A randomized placebo-controlled 24-week study of donepezil 10 mg in 67 patients with mild–moderate Alzheimer's disease found that donepezil-treated patients had significantly smaller decreases in hippocampal volume at the end of the study and increased neuronal N-acetylaspartate concentrations (vs. decreases with placebo) between weeks 6 and 18, along with significantly greater improvement of cognition throughout the study (Krishnan, Charles, Doraiswamy, et al., 2003).
- Superiority to placebo lasts about 18 months
- Once daily dosing
- Less effective when reinstituted after having been discontinued for 3 weeks or more

- Rivastigmine
  - Inhibits BuChE as well as AchE.
    - More selective for hippocampal AChE
  - Average ADAS improvement about 4 points
  - Adverse effects more significant than donepezil
  - Usual dose 4–12 mg/day
  - Requires bid dosing.

- Galantamine
  - Nicotinic cholinergic receptor agonist as well as cholinesterase inhibitor.
  - Induces release of other neurotransmitters, such as dopamine, norepinephrine, serotonin, GABA, and glutamate
  - Usual dose 16–24 mg/day
    - Must be given in divided doses.
  - Seven placebo-controlled trials were reviewed that were 12 weeks–6 months in duration (Olin & Schneider, 2002).
    - In 6-month trials, only doses of 8 mg/day failed to demonstrate significant improvement. ADAS-Cog improvement was 4 points at 32 mg/day. The magnitude of improvement was similar to other cholinesterase inhibitors. There was no statistically significant correlation between dose and response above 8 mg. Doses of 16 mg seemed to be the best initial target.

- Galantamine was found to be equally effective in improving cognition in Alzheimer's disease in patients who had and had not previously taken cholinesterase inhibitors (Mintzer & Kershaw, 2003).
- A 6-month study in patients with Alzheimer's disease or vascular dementia found that galantamine improved cognition, global function, and behavior (Kurz, 2002).
- Using cholinesterase inhibitors
  - Increase dose slowly to reduce limiting side effects.
  - If nausea is severe, treat with
    - Ginger root pills taken with medication
    - Broth made by grating 2 tablespoons of fresh ginger root into a cup of hot water
    - $5HT_3$ antagonist (e.g., ondansetron 2–4 mg once to three times/day, or 1 mg granisetron once to three times/day)
  - Wait at least 3 months at highest tolerated dose to assess benefit.
  - Lack of deterioration may be a positive effect of medication.
  - When patient inevitably deteriorates, reconsider whether medication is still useful.
  - Discuss with patient and family the benefit of slowing deterioration in a patient who is already markedly impaired.
    - Cholinesterase inhibitors may be useful for behavioral disturbances in such patients.

Memantine
- NMDA receptors mediate excitotoxicity and learning.
  - Phasic activation necessary for learning and synaptic plasticity.

**Table 2.5 Pharmacologic Characteristics of Approved Cholinesterase Inhibitors**

| DRUG | CLASS | TYPES OF CHOLINESTERASE INHIBITION | $t^{1/2}$(SERUM) (H)* | DOSAGE (MG/DAY) |
|------|-------|-----------------------------------|----------------------|-----------------|
| donepezil | Piperidine | Reversible; mixed competitive/noncompetitive | 70–80 | 5–10 (qd) |
| galantamine | Phenentrine alkaloid | Reversible; competitive | 5–7 | 20–50 (tid) |
| rivastigmine | Carbamate | Pseudoreversible | 1.5* | 6–12 (bid) |
| tacrine | Acridine | Reversible; noncompetitive | 1.3–2 | 80–160 (qid) |

* Brain t ½ = 8–10 hrs.

- Tonic (nontemporal) activation increases synaptic "noise."
- Competitive antagonism can interfere with learning and cause psychosis (discussed later).
- Uncompetitive antagonism can be neuroprotective and can reverse learning deficits caused by excess tonic activity.
- Memantine, a derivative of amantadine, is a low-affinity uncompetitive NMDA receptor antagonist.
  - Resembles physiologic activity of Mg2+.
  - Binds rapidly to NMDA receptor with open calcium channel.
  - Does not alter affinity for other ligands (e.g., glutamate).
  - Dissociates quickly from receptor.
  - Voltage dependent blockade.
  - Blocks tonically increased glutamate transmission, causing brain damage.
  - Becomes more active with escalating glutamate neurotransmission.
  - Does not interfere as much with normal NMDA signaling necessary for synaptic plasticity.
  - Alzheimer's disease associated with excessive tonic rather than phasic NMDA activation.
    - Mg2+ ions no longer able to reduce NMDA activity.
  - Memantine restores synaptic plasticity impaired by Mg2+ deficiency at receptor or by excess glutamate (GLU) activity.
    - May have the potential to improve rather than interfere with learning in chronic neurodegenerative disease with excitotoxicity.
    - Activates ascending dopaminergic pathways to increase dopamine in cortex, nucleus accumbens, and posterior striatum.
    - Increases brain derived neurotrophic factor (BDNF).
  - May slow deterioration of any progressive forms of dementia by reducing excitotoxicity.
  - Improves mood, well-being, and functioning better than measures of cognition.
- Generally should be combined with a cholinesterase inhibitor for additive effects.
- Usual dose 10 mg bid.
- In a 28-week double-blind trial, 252 patients with moderate–severe Alzheimer's disease were randomly assigned to memantine 20 mg/day or placebo (Reisberg et al., 2003). At the end of the study, analysis of the last observation carried forward demonstrated:
  - CIBIC Plus (Clinician's Interview-Based Impression of Change Plus Caregiver Input) showed mean difference in decrease of scores of 0.3 (4.5 vs. 4.8 points); $p = 0.03$.

- ADCC-ADLsev (activities of daily living scale) scores showed significantly less deterioration in memantine group, with difference in deterioration between groups of 2.1 out of about 21 points.
- Memantine patients had significantly less deterioration of functioning on the Severe Impairment Battery.
  - Memantine patients had a decrease of 4 out of 66 points.
  - Placebo patients had a decline of 10 out of 68 points.
- Memantine patients had significantly less deterioration in functional Alzheimer's disease stage, with decrease of 0.2 of 2.8 points for memantine vs. 0.6 out of 2.8 points for placebo.
- Significantly more memantine patients had clinically meaningful response (29% vs. 10%).
- The difference between groups in average caregiver time spent assisting patients was 46 hours/month.
- A systematic review of published memantine studies can be found in Areosa and Sheriff (2003).
  - Memantine 20 mg/day improved cognition, activities of daily living, CIBIC-Plus scores, and slowed decline over six months in Alzheimer's disease.
    - Best results seen in agitated patients.
  - Statistically significant but not immediately clinically apparent reduction of cognitive deterioration in mild–moderate vascular dementia with 20 mg/day memantine.
- In a double-blind crossover study (Merello, Nouzeilles, Cammarota, & Leiguarda, 1999) and an open study (Rabey, Nissipeanu, & Korczyn, 1992) with patients with Parkinson's disease, memantine
  - Improved Parkinsonian symptoms.
  - Reduced off episodes in on/off phenomena.
  - Had no effect on drug-induced dyskinesias.
- A study of 166 Alzheimer's disease patients randomly assigned to memantine or placebo (Wimo, Winblad, Stoffler, Wirth, & Mobius, 2003) found that memantine was associated with significantly
  - Less caregiver time (51.5 hours/month less)
  - Longer time to institutionalization
  - Lower caregive cost ($824 less/month)
  - Lower direct nonmedical costs ($431 less/month)
  - Higher cost of medication
- Neuramaxine is an experimental NMDA antagonist currently in phase-III trials.
  - Usual dose 50 mg once daily
  - May have different indications than memantine but similar actions

Nimodipine
- Since excitotoxicity is mediated by excessive $Ca^{2+}$ influx, calcium channel-blockers may have the potential to slow deterioration in Alzheimer's disease and other dementias.
- Pooled data from nine double-blind studies (N = 2,492) lasting 12–24 weeks of nimodipine 90 or 180 mg/day revealed improvement of cognitive function and global functioning but not activities of daily living in patients with Alzheimer's disease or vascular dementia (Lopez-Arrieta & Birks, 2002).
- Multi-center industry-sponsored trial found no superiority to placebo.
- Nimodipine is probably more likely to be helpful early in the course of dementia.

Antidepressants (also see Chapter 3)
- Depression can produce a dementia syndrome that is very difficult to distinguish from neurological dementia.
  - Adequate treatment of depression reverses or improves dementia.
  - Dementia returns within 5 years in the majority of cases.
- Depressive symptoms often masked by comorbid dementia.
  - Presence of depression increases cognitive dysfunction of dementia.
- Empirical trial of an antidepressant should be considered in all newly diagnosed dementia patients.
  - Avoid anticholinergic medications (e.g., TCAs).
  - Bupropion and venlafaxine may have positive effects on cognition.
  - SSRIs are usually well tolerated.

Selegiline (see pp. 218–219)
- Antioxidant properties may be neuroprotective and slow deterioration.
- Amphetamine-like action can improve attention and energy.
- Dosing in Alzheimer's disease not clearly established.
- Mixed results in studies of efficacy.
- Patients may have difficulty remembering dietary restrictions with higher doses.

Estrogen
- Estrogen deficiency is associated with cognitive dysfunction.
  - Improves with estrogen replacement.
- Estrogen has some cholinergic agonist properties.
- Addition of estrogen to donepezil in women improves response to the cholinesterase inhibitor.
- A large controlled trial of estrogen in Alzheimer's disease has not shown superiority to placebo.

NSAIDs

- Inflammatory response may contribute to neurofibrillary tangles.
- Possibly inhibited by antiinflammatory drugs.
- Case control epidemiological studies suggest that chronic use of ibuprofen may reduce risk of Alzheimer's disease.

Vagus nerve stimulation (VNS)

- Studied openly in 10 patients with probable Alzheimer's disease (average MMSE score 21) and minimal depressive symptoms (Sjogren et al., 2002).
  - After 3 months of VNS, ADAS-Cog scores improved by a median of 3 points (mean = 1.9).
  - After 6 months, median ADAS-Cog scores improved by 2.5 points (mean = 2.0).
    - 7 of the 10 patients being considered responders at each time.

Transdermal nicotine patch

- Significantly improved attention in patients with Alzheimer's disease as well as schizophrenia and ADHD (Levin & Rezvani, 2002).
  - Infusion of nicotine in rat hippocampus and amygdale interacts with dopaminergic and glutaminergic systems.

## Treatment of Behavioral Disorders in Demented Patients

Acute agitation in demented patients is usually caused by superimposed delirium or a change in the environment that increases confusion (e.g., change of room or roommate). Treatment of severe acute agitation that does not respond to orientation measures (e.g., reminding patient of location and date, keeping lights on at night to reduce sundowning) and treatment of the underlying illness is described on pages 92–93. Controlling chronic or intermittent unpredictable episodes of agitation also involves minimizing changes in the environment, and avoiding power struggles. There are few controlled studies of medications for chronic agitation in brain-damaged patients. The following medications may be useful.

- SSRIs
  - Serotonergic agents reduce impulsive aggression and agitation.
  - Paroxetine would not be an early choice because anticholinergic properties can be troublesome in dementia.
- Buspirone
  - Higher doses are serotonergic.
  - Animal studies and uncontrolled experience suggest reduction of agitation/aggression at doses of 60–100 mg/day.

- Beta-adrenergic blockers
  - Considerable experience with propranolol demonstrates efficacy for unprovoked aggressive outbursts.
  - May be a result of serotonergic rather than antiadrenergic effect ($5HT_{1A}$ antagonist effect increases 5HT release).
  - High doses of propranolol may be necessary.
    - 80–320 mg/day
    - Some reports note higher doses.
  - Using proproanolol for aggression:
    - Start with 10 mg.
    - Increase gradually to 10 mg qid.
    - Increase each dose by 10–20 mg at a time.
    - Onset of action may take a month or more.
  - Other lipid soluble beta-blockers have also been used.
- Anticonvulsants
  - Many have been found to reduce intermittent agitation.
  - Carbamazepine, valproate used most frequently.
- Lithium
  - Benefit most noticeable in patients with affective symptoms.
  - Serotonergic action may be useful for aggression.
  - Diverse actions on the CNS:
    - Reduces apoptosis and is therefore neuroprotective by (1) inducing nitric oxide release, which decreases excitotoxicity; (2) increasing expression of the neuroprotective protein bcl-2; and (3) decreasing expression of beta catenin, a pro-apoptotic protein.
    - Impairs cognition in some patients.
- Trazodone
  - A few reports of improvement of intractable agitation in demented patients.
  - May help to restore normal sleep–wake cycle.
- Benzodiazepines
  - Although short-acting benzodiazepines such as lorazepam can be useful acutely, these medications are often disinhibiting when given chronically.
- Artificial bright light
  - Sundowning and daytime agitation can result from reversal of the sleep–wake cycle.
    - Hallucinations can be caused by intrusion of REM sleep into waking state.

- Morning artificial bright light can reset sleep–wake cycle and reduce agitation.
- Ambient artificial bright ceiling light (at least 2500 lux) during first part of the day in common rooms can normalize sleep and behavior in nursing room residents.
    - Not effective in patients with cataracts and reduced entry of light into the eye.

- Neuroleptics
    - Frequently used to treat chronic agitation in demented patients, but controlled trials have repeatedly shown that they are no better than placebo when used to treat chronic nonpsychotic agitation.
        - Low-potency neuroleptics should especially be avoided, because anticholinergic and sedative properties aggravate cognitive dysfunction, and hypotensive effects are troublesome for older patients.
        - Haloperidol 0.25–1 mg once to three times/day may be helpful for refractory agitation.

- Atypical antipsychotics
    - Risperidone (0.5–2 mg/day) and olanzapine (1.25–5 mg/day) are effective for nonpsychotic agitation in demented patients.
    - A randomized double-blind placebo-controlled 12-week trial of risperidone in flexible doses up to 2 mg (mean dose 0.95 mg) for aggression in 337 elderly patients with Alzheimer's disease, vascular dementia, or both (Brodaty, Ames, Snowdon, et al., 2003) found that risperidone was significantly better than placebo in reducing
        - Aggression
        - Agitation
        - Psychosis
        - Lower doses were better tolerated but less effective.
    - Olanzapine 5 mg/day was effective in reducing agitation in demented patients and reduced emergence of psychosis (Buckley, 2001).
        - The soluble tablet is preferable for elderly patients with difficulty swallowing.
    - Quetiapine has produced similar benefit at doses of 50–300 mg/day (Buckley, 2001).
    - In a 10-week multicenter study of 208 outpatients with Alzheimer's disease and psychosis (De Deyn, 2003) using placebo vs. aripiprazole (mean dose 10 mg/day) found that
        - Aripiprazole produced significantly more improvement of psychosis.
        - No falls, injuries, or changes in EKG or weight occurred.

## Treatment of Behavioral Disorders in Other Neurological Illnesses

Parkinson's disease
- Psychosis a common side effect of L-dopa.
- Treatment with atypicals is preferable because of lower risk of exacerbation of parkinsonism.
  - Clozapine best studied.
    - Average dose 25 mg/day, starting with 6.25 mg.
  - Olanzapine may be better tolerated than risperidone, but both can worsen motor dysfunction.
  - Quetiapine has low risk of exacerbating motor dysfunction.
    - Usual dose 12.5–150 mg/day.

Huntington's disease
- Clozapine, risperidone, and olanzapine have been found to decrease depression, anxiety, and obsessive symptoms without worsening chorea.

## SIDE EFFECTS

Side effects of cholinesterase inhibitors are discussed here; anticholinergic side effects are discussed earlier in this chapter (pp. 84–87). Antidepressants, beta-blockers, antipsychotic drugs, and bright light are discussed in Chapters 1, 3, and 6.

Side effects of cholinesterase inhibitors are mostly attributable to increased cholinergic activity.

### Gastrointestinal Side Effects

GI consequences of vagal stimulation include
- Nausea
  - Can be treated with ginger root capsules taken with medication or ginger root broth made by grating 2 tablespoons fresh ginger root into cup of hot water.
  - Coca-Cola syrup or Emetrol is sometimes helpful.
  - Ondansetron or granisetron can be helpful for intractable nausea in patient who is otherwise doing well.
- Vomiting
- Diarrhea
- Abdominal cramps
- Decreased appetite and weight

## Cardiovascular Side Effects

Increased vagal tone results in

- Cardiac slowing
  - Do not prescribe if resting heart rate < 55.
- Syncope
- Worsening of congestive heart failure

## Central Nervous System Side Effects

- Dizziness
- Fatigue
- Headache
- Insomnia
- Tremor

# DRUG INTERACTIONS

Table 2.6 Drug–Drug Interactions Cholinesterase Inhibitor (CI)

| DRUG (X) | EFFECT | COMMENTS |
|---|---|---|
| Anticholinergic drugs, including<br>  Anticholinergics<br>  Amantadine<br>  Cyclobenzaprine<br>  Sedating $H_1$ blockers | X ↓, CI ↓ | Cholinesterase inhibitors and anticholinergics have opposing actions; anticholinergic drugs interfere with the therapeutic effect of cholinesterase inhibitors. |
| Other cholinesterase inhibitors | X ↑ | Additive cholinergic actions |
| Digoxin | X ↑ CI ↑ | Additive cardiac slowing |
| Succinylcholine | X ↑ | CI inhibits pseudocholinesterase, which metabolizes succinylcholine. More likely with rivastigmine, which inhibits butylcholinesterase (closer in structure to pseudocholinesterase). |
| NSAIDs | X ↑ | Additive pharmacodynamic GI side effects |
| CYP2D6 inhibitors, for example:<br>  Fluoxetine<br>  Paroxetine<br>  Quinidine<br>  Amioradone<br>  Ethanol | CI ↑ | Cholinesterase inhibitors are metabolized by CYP2D6; inhibition of this enzyme increases CI bio-availability by 40%, leading to increased adverse effects. |

(*continues*)

## Table 2.6 Continued

| DRUG (X) | EFFECT | COMMENTS |
|---|---|---|
| CYP 3A4 inhibitors, for example:<br>Nefazodone<br>Fluvoxamine<br>Erythromycin<br>Ketoconazole<br>Protease inhibitors<br>Cimetidine<br>Verapamil<br>Quinine | CI ↑ | Cholinesterase inhibitors are also metabolized by CYP3A4; bioavailability increased by 12–30% when combined with 3A4 inhibitors, with increased adverse effects. |

## Table 2.7 Drug–Drug Interactions*

| COMMONLY PRESCRIBED MEDICATIONS | NONPSYCHIATRIC ANTICHOLINERGIC AGENTS | ANTIHISTAMINES |
|---|---|---|
| codeine<br>coumadin<br>digoxin<br>dipyridamole<br>disopyramide<br>isosorbide<br>meperidine<br>nifedipine<br>prednisone<br>procainamide<br>quinidine<br>ranitidine | anisotropine (Valpine)<br>atropine<br>belladonna alkaloids<br>clidinium (Quarzan)<br>dicyclomine (Bentyl)<br>ethopropazine (Parsidol)<br>glycopyrrolate (Robinul)<br>hexocyclium (Tral)<br>homatropine<br>hyoscyamine<br>ipratropium<br>isopropamide (Darbid)<br>mepenzolate (Cantil)<br>methantheline (Banthine)<br>methscopolamine (Pamine)<br>orphenadrine (Disipal)<br>oxyphencyclimine (Daricon)<br>propantheline (Pro-Banthine)<br>scopolamine<br>tridihexethyl (Pathilon) | brompheniramine (Dimetane)<br>chlorpheniramine (Chlor-Trimeton)<br>clemastine (Tavist)<br>cyproheptadine (Periactin)<br>dexchlorpheniramine (Polaramine)<br>diphenhydramine (Benadryl)<br>hydroxyzine (Atarax, Vistraril)<br>methdilazine (Tacaryl)<br>promethazine (Phenergan)<br>trimeprazine (Temaril)<br>triprolidine (Actidil) |

| DRUGS (X) | ANTICHOLINERGICS (A) | COMMENTS |
|---|---|---|
| acetaminophen | X↓ | May increase acetaminophen use. |
| amantadine | X↑ A↑ | Increased amantadine and ACA effects. |
| antihistamines | X↑ A↓ | Increased anticholinergic effects. |
| antipsychotics | X↑ A↑ | ACAs may slow antipsychotic actions. ACAs enhance anticholinergic effects of antipsychotics, particularly low-potency phenothiazines. |

(continues)

**Table 2.7 Continued**

| DRUGS (x) | ANTICHOLINERGICS (A) | COMMENTS |
|---|---|---|
| atenolol | X↑ | May increase atenolol's concentration. |
| cocaine | A↓ | Decreased anticholinergic effects. |
| digoxin | X↑ | Increases level, more slowly dissolved digoxin tablet. |
| levodopa (L-dopa) | X↓ | May reduce L-dopa's availability; when ACAs stopped, L-dopa's toxicity may erupt. |
| methotrimeparazine | A↓ | Combination may increase EPS. |
| MAOIs | A↑ | May increase anticholinergic effects. |
| nitrofurantoin | X↑ | ACA may increase nitrofurantoin effects. |
| primidone | X↑ | Excessive sedation. |
| procainamide | X↑ | Increased procainamide effect. |
| propranolol | X↓ | ACAs can block β-blocker's bradycardia. |
| TCAs | A↑ X↑ | May diminish EPS; increased risk of anticholinergic toxicity. |
| tacrine | X↓ A↓ | Interfere with each other's effects. |

| DRUGS (x) | AMANTADINE (A) | COMMENTS |
|---|---|---|
| alcohol | X↑ | Increased alcohol effect; possible fainting. |
| anticholinergics | X↑ A↑ | Increased amantadine and ACA effects. |
| anti-emetics | X↓ | Possible decreased efficacy. |
| antipsychotics | X↓ | May interfere with antipsychotic effect. |
| cocaine | X↑ | Major overstimulation. |
| sympathomimetics | X↑ | Increased stimulation and agitation. |
| trimethoprim, sulfa-methoxazole (Bactrim, Septa) | X↑ A↑ | May increase each other's levels; CNS toxicity possible. |
| quinidine[†] | A↑ | Modest increase in amantadine levels. |
| quinine[†] | A↑ | Modest increase in amantadine levels. |
| triamterene (in Dyazide)[†] | A↑ | Modest increase in amantadine levels. |

Moderately important reaction; ↑ Increases; ↓ Decreases; [†] Decreases renal clearance of amantadine. Additive anticholinergic effects can occur with many medications used in psychiatry and in general medicine, as well as with over the counter cold medicines and sleep aids. Examples are listed below.

**Table 2.8  Effects on Laboratory Tests**

| GENERIC NAMES | BLOOD/SERUM TESTS* | URINE TESTS |
|---|---|---|
| amantadine | WBC↓<br>Leukocytes ↓ | |
| benztropine | None | None |
| diphenhydramine | WBC ↓, RBC ↓,<br>Platelets ↓ | |
| trihexyphenidyl | None | None |

No effect on urine tests found for benztropine and trihexyphenidyl; others not known
*↑ Increases; ↓ Decreases

## TOXICITY AND OVERDOSE

Acute toxicity of the cholinesterase inhibitors is an extension of their pharmacological effects, including

- Excessive cholinergic muscarinic stimulation causes
  - Miosis
  - Salivation
  - Sweating
  - Broncoconstriction
  - Vomiting
  - Diarrhea
  - Bradycardia
- Nicotinic effects cause
  - Neuromuscular blockade
  - Fasciculations
  - Respiratory depression

Management of poisoning with cholinesterase inhibitors includes the following:

- Maintain or assist respiration.
- Remove secretions.
- Administer oxygen.
- Atropine antagonizes muscarinic but not nicotinic effects.
  - 2–4 mg initially
  - Then 2 mg every 5–10 minutes
- Administer pralidoxime (Protopam) for nicotinic effects.
  - Reactivates acetylcholinesterase.

- 500 mg/minute infused over 15–30 minutes for total dose 1–2 grams
- maximum dose 12 gm within 24 hours

## PRECAUTIONS

Use cholinesterase inhibitors cautiously in the presence of
- Anticholinergic medications
- Asthma
- AV block
- Bradycardia
- Cardiac arrhythmia
- Cardiac disease
- Chronic obstructive pulmonary disease (COPD)
- GI disease, especially GI bleeding
- Hepatic disease
- Hypotension
- Jaundice
- Parkinson's disease
- Peptic ulcer disease
- Renal dysfunction
- Sick sinus syndrome

## ADVICE FOR CARETAKERS

Behavioral interventions are essential for managing agitation in brain-damaged patients.
- Patients are not likely to remember long, complicated discussions.
  - Keep interactions brief and focused, using short sentences.
- Remind patient who you are and where patient is located.
- Medications patient is already taking frequently contribute to confusion and agitation.
  - Review medications.
  - Address demands of patient and family for more or different medicines.
- Help patient to keep regular hours, but avoid excessive insistence that patient stay on schedule (e.g., time of taking medication) unless it is absolutely necessary.
  - Power struggles related to patient's routine often precipitate episodes of aggression.

- Explain that premature grieving for loss of the person the patient once was can make it difficult to maintain emotional connection to patient.
- A single clinician should coordinate the patient's care and maintain record of all treatments.

## NOTES FOR PATIENT AND FAMILY

Cholinesterase inhibitors slow deterioration and improve functioning to some extent, but they are not cures.

- New treatments for Alzheimer's disease are the subject of intense research.
- Current treatments hopefully will slow deterioration sufficiently for more definitive therapies to be developed.
- Do not take any medications from other physicians or any over-the-counter preparations without consulting with case manager or primary physician.
- Minimize use of alcohol.

# CHAPTER THREE

# Antidepressants

The classification of antidepressants can be confusing. Some antidepressants are classified according to structure (e.g., tricyclic antidepressants or TCAs) and others according to a known action (e.g., serotonin reuptake inhibitors) or when they were released (e.g., atypical or second-generation antidepressants). A common scheme categorizes antidepressants as

- Heterocyclic antidepressants (HCAs):
  - Contain three or four benzene rings with at least one noncarbon atom.
  - All but maprotiline have a three-ring structure.
    - Maprotiline has four rings (i.e., it is a tetracyclic).
  - For simplicity, all heterocyclics are referred to as TCAs because they have similar actions and side effects.
- Selective serotonin reuptake inhibitors (SSRIs)
- Second- and third-generation antidepressants
- Monoamine oxidase inhibitors (MAOIs)

This chapter addresses the first 3 groups; MAOIs are discussed in Chapter 4.

Conditions and therapies covered in this chapter include:

- Major depression and dysthymia (see pp. 122–124)
- Electroconvulsive therapy (ECT) (pp. 149–154)
- Repetitive transcranial magnetic stimulation (rTMS) (pp. 154–156)
- Vagal nerve stimulation (VNS) (pp. 158–159)
- Artificial bright light (pp. 157–158)
- Seasonal affective disorder (p. 157)
- Refractory depression (pp. 165–177)
- Chronic pain (pp. 133–134)
- Premenstrual dysphoric disorder (pp. 135–136)

- Eating disorders (pp. 131–132)
- Bereavement (p. 128)
- Dementia syndrome of depression ("pseudodementia"; p. 129)
- Somatization (p. 164)
- Medical illnesses in adults (pp. 129–130)
    - Allergies
    - Cardiac conduction abnormalities
    - Cataplexy
    - Congestive heart failure
    - Constipation
    - Diabetes
    - Diarrhea
    - Epilepsy
    - Irritable bowel syndrome
    - Migraine headache
    - Narrow angle glaucoma
    - Neurogenic bladder
    - Parkinson's disease
    - Peptic ulcer disease
    - Sleep apnea
    - Tardive dyskinesia
- Childhood stage-4 sleep disorders (pp. 136–137)
    - Enuresis
    - Night terrors
    - Sleepwalking

Conditions treated with antidepressants discussed elsewhere include:
- Agoraphobia (Antianxiety, Chapter 7)
- Attention-deficit disorder (Stimulants, Chapter 9)
- Atypical depression (MAOIs, Chapter 4)
- Borderline personality disorder (Lithium, p. 136; Chapter 5)
- Narcolepsy (Stimulants, Chapter 8)
- Obsessive–compulsive disorder (pp. 384–390)
- Panic disorder (Antianxiety, Chapter 7)
- Schizoaffective disorder (Lithium, Chapter 5)
- Social phobia (Antianxiety, Chapter 7)

Table 3.1 provides a basic overview of the drugs addressed in this chapter.

Table 3.1  Names, Classes, Dose Forms, Colors

| GENERIC NAMES | BRAND NAMES | DOSE FORMS (mg) | COLORS |
|---|---|---|---|
| | | HETEROCYCLICS | |
| *Tertiary amine* | | | |
| amitriptyline | Elavil | t: 10/25/50/75/ 100/150 p: 10 mg/ml | t: blue/yellow/ beige/orange mauve/blue |
| | Endepryl | t: 10/25/50/75 100/150 | t: orange/orange/ orange/yellow peach/salmon |
| clomipramine | Anafranil | c: 25/50/75 | c: ivory-melon-yellow/ ivory-aqua-blue/ ivory-yellow |
| doxepine | Sinequan | c: 10/25/50 75/100/150 o: 10 mg/ml | c: red-pink/blue-pink/ peach-off-white/ pale pink-light pink blue-white/blue |
| imipramine | Tofranil | t: 10/25/50 p: 25 mg/2 ml | t: triangular coral/ round biconvex coral/round biconvex coral |
| | Janimine | t: 10/25/50 | t: orange/yellow/ peach |
| imipramine pamoate | Tofranil-PM (sustained-release) | c: 75/100/125/150 | c: coral/dark yellow-coral/light yellow-coral/coral |
| trimipramine | Surmontil | c: 25/50/100 | c: blue-yellow/blue-orange/blue-white |
| *Secondary amine* | | | |
| desipramine | norpramin | t: 10/25/50/75 100/150 | t: blue/yellow/green/ orange/peach/white |
| nortriptyline | Pamelor | c: 10/25/50/75 o: 10 mg/5 ml | c: orange-white/ orange-white/ white/orange |
| | Aventyl | c: 10/25 | c: cream/gold |
| protriptyline | Vivactil | t: 5/10 | t: orange/yellow |
| | | TETRACYCLICS | |
| amoxapine | Asendin | t: 25/50/100/150 | t: white/orange blue/peach |
| maprotiline | Ludiomil | t: 25/50/75 | t: oval orange/ round orange/ oval white |

*(continues)*

**Table 3.1  Continued**

| GENERIC NAMES | BRAND NAMES | DOSE FORMS (mg) | COLORS |
|---|---|---|---|
| citalopram | Celexa | t: 20/40 | t: pink/white |
| fluoxetine | Prozac | c: 10/20<br>o: 5 mg/ml | c: green-gray/<br>off-white |
| fluvoxamine | Luvox | t: 50/100 | t: yellow/beige |
| paroxetine | Paxil | t: 20/30 | t: pink/blue |
| sertraline | Zoloft | t: 50/100 | t: light/blue<br>light yellow |
| SECOND AND THIRD GENERATION | | | |
| bupropion | Wellbutrin SR | t: 100/150 | t: blue/purple |
| mirtazapine | Remeron | t: 15/30/45 | t: yellow/red-<br>brown/white |
| nefazodone | Serzone | t: 100/150/200/250 | t: white/peach/<br>light yellow/white |
| trazodone | Desyrel | t: 50/100/150/300 | t: orange/white/<br>orange/yellow |
| venlafaxine | Effexor | t: 25/37.5/50/<br>75/100 | t: all peach |
| | Effexor XR | c: 37.5/75/150 | gray/pink pink/red |

## PHARMACOLOGY

Antidepressant effects are generally thought to be attributable to enhancement of neurotransmission with norepinephrine, serotonin, or dopamine by inhibition of neurotransmitter reuptake into the presynaptic neuron. However, neurotransmitter reuptake inhibition is immediate, whereas onset of antidepressant action may take a month or more. In addition, some antidepressants (e.g., mianserin, available in Europe) and ECT have no direct effect on neurotransmitters, whereas tianeptine, an effective tricyclic antidepressant available in Europe, is a serotonin reuptake enhancer. The time course of $5HT_2$ down-regulation and $\beta$-receptors by antidepressants is more consistent with the onset of clinical effect, but these actions are inconsistent and at times contradictory. Research is investigating the effects of antidepressants on expression of neuroprotective and other genes (e.g., BDNF [brain-derived neurotropic factor]) as a possible mechanism of action. For example, chronic treatment with antidepressants increases neurogenesis in the rat hippocampus (Santarelli, Saxe, Gross, et al., 2003) and alters expression of eight genes involved in neuronal plasticity in this region (Chen, Wang, Sun, & Young, 2003), including:

- Increased expression of neuromodulin (growth-associated protein 43)
  - Regulates growth of axons and formation of new neuronal connections.
  - Key element in making and reorganizing synapses.
- Decreased expression of somatostatin
- Up-regulation of cAMP signaling
- Increased expression of BDNF
- Increased expression of transcription factors that regulate expression of other genes, such as
  - cAMP responsive element binding protein (CREB)
  - c-Fos
    - Involved in learning and oncogenesis

### Placebo Response Rates

Most antidepressant trials compare new agents with placebo; more recent trials often include an established antidepressant as an active comparator. It is therefore necessary to understand placebo response rates to evaluate antidepressant efficacy.

- An evaluation of 75 placebo-controlled trials in adult depression conducted between 1981 and 2000 found that the mean percentage of patients responding to the active antidepressant was 50% (range 32–70%), and the placebo response rate was 30% (range 13–52%; Walsh, Seidman, Sysko, & Gould, 2002).
- In another review of 29 multicenter studies, remission rates at different sites ranged from 0 to 71% with active antidepressant and 0 to 75% with placebo (Schneider & Small, 2002).
  - Response rates to both medication and placebo were higher in private research sites than in academic sites, probably reflecting lower severity of illness in the former.
- Response rates to both antidepressants and placebo have increased significantly over the past 20 years, but the placebo response rate has increased significantly more than the antidepressant response rate (Walsh et al., 2002).
  - Increased rate of placebo response is probably related to the changing characteristics of patients recruited into clinical trials.

More severely depressed patients who have less of a placebo response are in treatment and are less likely to enter clinical trials.

- More subjects who are mildly depressed and have a high rate of spontaneous improvements are recruited from advertisements.

- A meta-analysis of 38 phase III placebo-controlled studies between 1987 and 1999 of six antidepressants (widely reported in the media) argued that because antidepressants produced an average 10-point reduction in Hamilton Rating Scale for Depression (HRSD) scores and placebo produced an 8-point decrease, the antidepressant only accounted for a 2-point increment over placebo (Kirsch, Moore, Scoboria, & Nicholls, 2002).
  - However, placebo response is higher in milder depression, which accounts for a greater percentage of subjects in recent antidepressant trials.
  - Placebo response rate is very low in severe, chronic, bipolar, and psychotic forms of depression.
  - Placebo response usually wears off within 3 months.
  - Placebo does not prevent relapse, whereas antidepressants do prevent relapse.
- Other problems interpreting antidepressant research:
  - Statistical significance is emphasized more than clinical significance.
  - Industry-sponsored trials not always adequately powered to detect small effect size.
  - Endpoint is often response (50% symptom reduction) rather than remission (patient has minimal symptoms and no longer meets illness criteria).
  - Subsyndromal symptoms and functional improvement are usually not assessed.

## Features of Antidepressant Classes

### Heterocyclics

- TCAs are characterized as tertiary (i.e., three methyl groups) or secondary (i.e., two methyl groups) amines.
  - Secondary amines (e.g., desipramine, nortriptyline) tend to be
    - More noradrenergic
    - Less anticholinergic
    - Less hypotensive
    - Less sedating
  - Tertiary amines tend to be
    - Noradrenergic and serotonergic
    - More sedating
    - More anticholinergic
    - More likely to cause weight gain

- Because they are not as well tolerated and more likely to be lethal in overdose, TCAs are usually not first-line treatments for outpatient depression.
- TCAs have elimination half-lives in excess of 24 hours.
  - All can be given in one daily dose.
  - Protriptyline half-life is around 80 hours.
- All TCAs are type Ia antiarrhythmics (see pp. 35–37, 195–196).

## SSRIs

- SSRIs account for 80–90% of antidepressant prescriptions.
- The drug class has considerable variation in structure.
- Differences in selectivity and potency for the 5HT transporter do not predict differences in selectivity of antidepressant potency.
  - Paroxetine is more potent than fluoxetine in inhibiting serotonin re-uptake, but it is not more potent as an antidepressant (i.e., it does not have the same clinical effect at a lower dose, and it is not more effecive).
  - Sertraline is more selective for inhibition of serotonin over norepinephrine reuptake but it is not more selective as an antidepressant.
- Some SSRIs also affect reuptake of other neurotransmitters
  - Paroxetine blocks norepinephrine reuptake at approximately 50 mg.
  - Sertraline has modest dopamine reuptake inhibition at higher doses.
  - These effects to not seem to translate into different clinical applications or tolerability.
- All SSRIs have similar side-effect profiles related to enhancement of serotonergic activity centrally and systemically (see pp. 182–193).
- Different preparations have different patterns of inhibition of CYP450 isoenzymes (see pp. 198–204).
  - Not much is known about actions on other enzyme systems or on P-glycoprotein, an important drug extrusion protein that affects absorption and penetration into the CNS of some drugs.
- Most SSRIs have elimination half-lives around a day and can be given in a single daily dose.
  - Fluoxetine has a half-life of 3 days and has an active metabolite with a half-life of 6 days.
  - Fluvoxamine has a half-life around 15 hours and usually requires bid dosing.
- SSRIs are relatively selective for serotonin reuptake inhibition, but they are not selective clinically.
  - SSRIs are not more effective than other antidepressants in the treatment of depression.

- SSRIs are useful for many other conditions, especially anxiety disorders.
- SSRIs seem to be selective clinically in the treatment of OCD.
  - The only medication that is not an SSRI that is effective for OCD is clomipramine, which is a potent serotonin reuptake inhibitor as well as a norepinephrine reuptake inhibitor.
  - However, OCD is associated with increased rather than decreased central 5HT turnover, and SSRIs reduce rather than increase serotonin turnover in the CNS in patients with OCD; this finding suggests that SSRIs enhance a natural compensatory mechanism that reduces intrusive thought in response to a primary dysfunction that is probably neuroanatomical.

### SECOND- AND THIRD-GENERATION ANTIDEPRESSANTS

This is a diverse group of antidepressants with different actions, interactions, and adverse effects.

- Some medications (e.g., venlafaxine) inhibit reuptake of serotonin (at lower doses), norepinephrine (at doses above 75–150 mg), and dopamine (at higher doses).
  - Bupropion increases norepinephrine and dopamine availability.
- Nefazodone combines serotonin reuptake inhibition with $5HT_2$ antagonism.
  - It also has some $5HT_{1A}$ partial agonism.

Some antidepressants have no direct effect on neurotransmitter reuptake.

- Trazodone is primarily a $5HT_2$ antagonist without any effect on neurotransmitter reuptake.
  - Can be combined safely with MAOIs.
- Mirtazapine antagonizes $5HT_2$, $5HT_3$, and alpha-2 receptors.
  - Effect on adrenergic autoreceptors increases norepinephrine release.
    - This probably explains side effects (e.g., anxiety/agitation) rather than the mechanism of clinical action.
    - Increased serotonin release secondary to increased norepinephrine release may not be a mechanism of action but warrants caution with MAOIs.

Many antidepressants (other than nefazodone, mirtazepine, trimipramine, doxepin) disrupt slow-wave sleep and suppress REM sleep.

## CLINICAL INDICATIONS

The superiority of antidepressants to placebo is more marked in moderate–severe than in mild depression. Antidepressants are as effective as manualized psychotherapies (cognitive–behavioral therapy and interpersonal therapy) for less severe forms of depression. In more severe depression, antidepressants and psychotherapy have additive effects (e.g., antidepressants work faster against vegetative symptoms, and psychotherapy works faster against suicidal thinking).

A full response takes 10–30 days with most antidepressants.

- Some patients may require 2–3 months at therapeutic doses to recover.
  - Sleep and energy often improve before other symptoms.
  - Patients who have no response to an SSRI in 6 weeks may begin to demonstrate recovery at 8 weeks.
  - Inadequate treatment trials (i.e., insufficient time, insufficient dose) are common causes of treatment failure.

The presence or absence of a precipitant does not predict antidepressant response. Predictors of a good response to an antidepressant include

- Melancholic features
- Shorter duration of depression
- Family history of depression
- Past history of response to an antidepressant

Predictors of a poorer response to an antidepressant include

- Psychotic features
  - Responds to antipsychotic drug + antidepressant.
- Bipolar depression
- Active substance abuse
- Comorbid ongoing illness
  - Especially medical illness
- Severe Axis II pathology
- Atypical depression
  - Responds better to SSRIs and MAOIs.

Laboratory testing

- No laboratory test predicts response to specific antidepressants.
- Thyroid function tests can be useful in assessing treatment refractoriness (see pp. 165–174).
- Dexamethasone suppression test (DST):
  - About 40% of depressed patients do not normally suppress cortisol after administration of cortisol.
    - 1 mg of dexamethasone administered at 11 P.M.; serum cortisol measured the next day at 4 P.M.
    - Post-dexamethasone cortisol $\geq$ 5 $\mu$g/dL indicates nonsuppression.

Table 3.2  Doses

| GENERIC NAMES | EQUIVALENT DOSES (MG) | USUAL THERAPEUTIC DOSES (MG/DAY) | LOW AND HIGH DOSES (MG/DAY) | GERIATRIC DOSES (MG/DAY) |
|---|---|---|---|---|
| amitriptyline | 100 | 100–300 | 25–450 | 25–100 |
| amoxapine | 100 | 200–400 | 50–600 | 100–150 |
| bupropion | 150 | 225–450 | 100–450 | 75–150 |
| citalopram | 20 | 20–40 | 10–80 | 10–20 |
| clomipramine | 100 | 125–300 | 25–500 | 50–150 |
| desipramine | 150 | 150–300 | 25–400 | 20–100 |
| doxepin | 150 | 150–300 | 25–350 | 30–150 |
| escitalopram | 20 | 10–20 | 5–40 | 5–20 |
| fluoxetine | 20 | 20–40 | 20–80 | 5–40 |
| fluvoxamine | 100 | 100–300 | 50–400 | 50–200 |
| imipramine | 150 | 150–300 | 25–450 | 30–100 |
| maprotiline | 75 | 150–225 | 25–225 | 50–75 |
| mirtazapine | 30 | 15–45 | 10–90 | 7.5–30 |
| nefazodone | 150 | 300–600 | 100–600 | 200–600 |
| nortriptyline | 50 | 75–150 | 20–200 | 10–75 |
| paroxetine | 20 | 20–40 | 10–50 | 10–40 |
| protriptyline | 20 | 30–60 | 10–80 | 10–30 |
| sertraline | 50 | 50–150 | 25–200 | 25–150 |
| trazodone | 150 | 200–600 | 50–600 | 50–200 |
| trimipramine | 100 | 150–300 | 25–350 | 25–150 |
| venlafaxine | 100 | 75–225 | 25–350 | 25–225 |

- Higher rates of nonsuppression in melancholic, severe, psychotic, and bipolar depressions.
- False positives with hospitalization or smoking.
- Nonsuppressed DST usually a state variable.
- Failure of DST to normalize predicts increased risk of relapse within weeks if antidepressant withdrawn.

### Severe Depression

Contradictory data emerge from comparisons of SSRIs to TCAs in the treatment of severe depression.

Table 3.3  Specific Antidepressant Doses

| GENERIC NAMES | STARTING DOSE (MG/DAY) | DAYS TO REACH STEADY-STATE | ACTIVE METABOLITE |
|---|---|---|---|
| amitriptyline | 25–75 | 4–10 | Nortriptyline |
| amoxapine | 50–150 | 2–7 | 8-hydroxyamoxapine |
| bupropion | 200–225 | 4–15 | — |
| citalopram | 20 | 4–10 | Desmethylcitalopram |
| clomipramine | 75–225 | 7–14 | Desmethylclomipramine |
| desipramine[†] | 25–75 | 2–11 | — |
| doxepin | 25–75 | 2–8 | Desmethyldoxepin |
| escitalopram | 5–10 | 4 | — |
| fluoxetine | 20 | 21–35 | Norfluoxetine |
| fluvoxamine | 100 | 3–8 | — |
| imipramine | 25–75 | 2–5 | Desipramine |
| maprotiline | 25–75 | 6–10 | Desmethylmaprotiline |
| mirtazapine | 15–30 | 3–9 | 8-hydroxymirtazapine N-desmethylmirtazapine N-oxidemirtazapine |
| nefazodone | 100 | 4 | Hydroxynefazodone |
| nortriptyline[†] | 20–40 | 4–19 | — |
| paroxetine | 20 | 5–10 | — |
| protriptyline | 10–20 | 10 | — |
| sertraline | 50 | 4–21 | Desmethylsertaline |
| trazodone | 50–100 | 7–14 | Oxotriazolo-pyridin-propionic acid |

- In a prospective study of 536 patients in a primary care practice, fluoxetine, imipramine, and desipramine produced similar results, but fluoxetine had fewer adverse effects, and patients were more likely to reach adequate doses (Club, 1997).
- A review of 18 clinical trials comparing SSRIs with TCAs and 5 comparing SSRIs with placebo found that SSRIs were as effective as TCAs for severe depression (Hirschfeld, 1999).
- Fluvoxamine was studied in a double-blind multicenter study in 86 severely depressed patients (HRSD score ≥ 25) randomized to fluvoxamine or clomipramine (100–250 mg/day; Zohar, Keegstra, & Barrelet, 2003).
  - After 8 weeks, 71% of fluvoxamine patients and 69% of clomipramine patients responded, but fluvoxamine was better tolerated.

- In 136 parallel group randomized controlled trials comparing TCAs and SSRIs in depression, there were fewer patients dropping out of SSRI treatment (odds ratio [OR] of remaining in trial 1.21), an advantage that was statistically significant but modest clinically (Barbui, Hotopf, Freemantle, et al., 2003).
- Another review of 315 randomized controlled trials comparing newer antidepressants with older antidepressants, placebo, or psychosocial interventions in depression found that SSRIs and TCAs had similar response rates and similar dropout rates, although specific side effects differed (Club, 2000).
- Recent data justify using an SSRI first for more severe depression. Venlafaxine, nefazodone, mirtazepine, or a TCA should be tried in this setting if a single SSRI is not effective.

### Psychotic Depression

There is virtually no placebo response rate and a very low rate of spontaneous improvement in psychotic depression. Furthermore, there is a low probability of response to antidepressant alone (25%).

- An 8-week open label trial of sertraline up to 200 mg/day in 25 patients with psychotic and 25 with nonpsychotic depression reported (Simpson, Sheshai, Rady, Kingsbury, & Fayek, 2003):
  - Nonpsychotic depression had significantly better response and remission rates.
    - By week 8, 4 psychotically depressed and 16 nonpsychotically depressed patients had remitted.
    - In total, 8 psychotically depressed and 17 nonpsychotically depressed patients responded.
  - Psychosis predicted lack of sertraline response independent of severity of depression or general psychopathology.

However, a few small studies find response to antidepressant monotherapy.

- Double-blind study of sertaline and paroxetine monotherapy in 46 patients with psychotic depression (32 unipolar, 14 bipolar) found (Zanardi, Franchini, Gasperini, Perez, & Smeraldi, 1996):
  - 75% responded to sertaline.
  - All patients completed trial.
  - 46% responded to paroxetine.
  - 41% dropped out because of side effects.
- One study suggested that combination therapy is not always necessary for older patients with psychotic depression (Mulsant, Sweet, Rosen, et al., 2001).

- 30 patients aged $\geq$ 50 with delusional depression were openly treated with nortriptyline for at least 4 weeks with a target level of 100 ng/mL.
- After nortriptyline was started, patients were randomly assigned in a double-blind protocol to perphenazine or placebo for at least 2 weeks.
    - Perphenazine dose gradually raised to response, EPS, or maximum dose of 24 mg/day.
- Overall response rates were similar with perphenazine (50%) vs. placebo (44%) addition.
- Dose of neuroleptic may have been too low.
    - Response with antidepressant alone was similar to other studies of antidepressant monotherapy.
- In an older population, this kind of depression may be a prodrome of dementia and a lower response rate to any treatment.

A low rate of response to neuroleptic alone (40%) has been found.

Very good response reported to combination of antidepressant and antipsychotic drug ($\sim$70%).
- Loxapine and amoxapine have been found to be effective as monotherapies for psychotic depression, but response rate lower than with TCA + neuroleptic.
    - Loxapine (a neuroleptic) is metabolized to the antidepressant amoxapine, which has about 1 mg of haloperidol potency/25 mg.
- High neuroleptic doses (32–80 mg perphenazine) may be necessary.
- Neuroleptics raise TCA levels.
    - May increase levels of nortriptyline and desipramine outside therapeutic window.
- TCAs raise neuroleptic levels.
    - Not clinically important
- Neuroleptics and antidepressants can have additive quinidine-like effects.
- Atypical antipsychotics are better tolerated and have more antidepressant effects than neuroleptics.
    - Chart reviews and case series suggest that atypical antipsychotics can be effective in combination with antidepressants and as monotherapy in psychotic depression:
        - No controlled studies available (Wheeler, Jason, Mortimer, & Tyson, 2000).
    - Nevertheless, atypicals are first choice for this indication.
- Most studies have included TCAs.

- Small studies suggest efficacy of SSRI + antipsychotic medication.
    - An open trial of fluoxetine + perphenazine for 5 weeks in 30 patients with psychotic depression reported a response rate of 73% (Rothschild, Samson, Bessette, & Carter-Campbell, 1993b).
    - In a 6-week open trial of 27 patients with psychotic unipolar depression treated with olanzapine (mean dose 10 mg/day) plus fluoxetine (mean dose 53–57 mg/day), response rate was 56% and remission rate 41% (Matthews, Bottonari, Polania, et al., 2002).
- Best response to ECT (80%).

### Mild Depression

- Psychotherapy equivalent to antidepressant.
- Initial treatment depends on patient preference and clinician expertise.
- Combining treatment modalities does not increase response rate, because of high rate of response to either one alone.

### Dysthymic Disorder

- Differences between dysthymia and fluctuating levels of major depression can be a matter of interpretation.
- Dysthymic disorder responds as well to antidepressants as major depressive episode.
- Double depression (dysthymia with superimposed episodes of acute major depression) has good prognosis for response of acute depression to antidepressants but poor prognosis for improvement of chronic depression.

### Depression and Anxiety

- Most antidepressants other than bupropion are predictably effective for anxiety.
    - Bupropion can be effective for anxiety secondary to depression.
        - A retrospective analysis of pooled data from two 8-week placebo-controlled parallel group studies of bupropion SR (N = 234), sertraline (N = 225), and placebo (N = 233) found that both medications were similarly superior to placebo in reducing ratings of both anxiety and depression (Trivedi, Rush, Carmody, et al., 2001).
- Many antidepressants (including SSRIs) acutely increase anxiety because of an early noradrenergic action.

## Bipolar Depression

- Risk of induction of hypomania/mania and rapid cycling traditionally thought to be greatest with TCAs, less with SSRIs, and least with bupropion.
  - These figures are probably a function of better recognition and exclusion of bipolar patients from studies involving newer drugs rather than a true difference in the destabilizing effects of the various antidepressants.
  - Bupropion found to induce mania in 50% of bipolar depressed patients within 1 year of starting medication.
  - In several published trials, all antidepressants have been found to have the same risk of inducing mania.
- Bipolar depression is treated with mood stabilizers with or without an antidepressant.

## Geriatric Depression

- First onset of major depression in late life often associated with cerebrovascular disease.
- Geriatric major depression responds to same treatments as depression earlier in life.
- Some older patients need lower doses than younger adults, but some need the same or higher doses.
- Similar TCA levels are necessary for older and younger patients.
  - Older patients treated with TCAs should have EKG.
  - Tertiary amine TCAs should be avoided in older patients because of poorly tolerated hypotensive and anticholinergic effects.
- Bupropion and venlafaxine may be useful for older depressed patients with cognitive impairment.
- SSRIs are well tolerated but can be associated with increased postural sway and falls.
  - Elderly patients taking antidepressants have twofold increase in risk of falls.
    - Especially if demented
  - Risk of falls with antidepressants similar to benzodiazepines (Mendelson, 1996). Falls per dose: nortriptyline, 0.0021; sertraline, 0.0012; diazepam, 0.00052.
- Some older depressed men have low testosterone levels.
  - Supplemental testosterone improves antidepressant response.

### Pediatric Depression

TCAs

- TCAs have consistently been equivalent to placebo in childhood depression and inferior to placebo in adolescent depression. Possible explanations include:
  - Once daily dosing may be inadequate for younger patients because of more rapid elimination.
  - Serum levels may have to be higher than those generally used in this population.
  - Younger patients may be more sensitive to adverse effects, leading to withdrawal from treatment before a response occurs.
  - Higher rate of bipolarity in early-onset depression may result in lower treatment response and more dropouts because of induction of dysphoric hypomania.
  - Environmental factors play a greater role in childhood depression.
- TCAs are effective for childhood anxiety disorders and enuresis.
- Children receiving TCAs should have EKG before and after starting medication.
  - QRS duration should be < 0.12 seconds.
  - QTc should be < 450 msec.
  - Heart rate should be < 120.
- A small number of children has had sudden death with desipramine.
- Maximum TCA dose usually 4–5 mg/kg/day of impipramine
  - Adult blood level may be necessary.
- Children and younger adolescents need more frequent dosing of all antidepressants because of rapid elimination.

SSRIs

- Fluoxetine and sertraline have been found effective for pediatric major depression.
  - In two multicenter randomized controlled trials supported by the manufacturer, sertraline (mean dose 131 mg/day) was significantly more effective than placebo in 376 patients ages 6–17 years (Wagner, Ambrosini, Rynn, et al., 2003).
    - Mean reduction of depression rating scale scores (Child Depression Rating Scale-Revised [CDRS-R]) was −22.84 on sertraline and −20.19 on placebo at 10 weeks.
    - Patients who completed the entire 10-week trial had greater reductions in CDRS scores (−30.24 vs. −25.83).
    - 69% of sertraline patients vs. 59% of placebo patients had 40% reduction in CDRS scores.

- Concerns have recently been raised about increased suicidal ideation in depressed children taking SSRIs and venlafaxine.
  - May reflect inadequate exclusion of patients with bipolar depression from these populations.
  - Suicide rates in adolescents have decreased in association with increased antidepressant use in that population.
  - No increase in suicides.

## Postpartum Depression

- A spectrum of postpartum mood changes may occur (see Table 3.4).
  - No treatment necessary for indifference or blues.
- Postpartum depression has increased risk of bipolar outcome.
  - Careful evaluation for bipolarity is necessary.
- Risk of recurrence of postpartum depression following another pregnancy is 50%.
- Antidepressants are effective for postpartum unipolar depression.
  - Dopaminergic agents (e.g., bupropion) may inhibit lactation.
  - SSRIs may increase lactation.
  - Most antidepressants, except for MAOIs, can be started during pregnancy to prevent postpartum recurrence and continued during breast feeding (see pp. 206–207).
- Estrogen supplementation prevented postpartum unipolar and bipolar recurrences in one small study
- Calcium supplementation may reduce recurrences of depression during pregnancy

## Postpartum Psychosis

- Rare but serious affective episode.
- Likelihood of bipolar outcome increased 3,000 times.
- Rarely indicative of schizophrenia.
- Risk factors:
  - Primiparous

**Table 3.4 Spectrum of Postpartum Mood Disorders**

| DISORDER | INCIDENCE | ONSET | DURATION |
|---|---|---|---|
| Maternal indifference | 40% of primips | 1 day | 3 days |
| Blues | 25–85% | 3–7 days | < 10 days |
| Major depression | 7–17% | 6 weeks–1 year | 3–6 months or longer |
| Psychosis | 0.1–0.4% | 3 days–1 month | months |

- Previous postpartum psychosis
- Bipolar disorder
- Significant risk of suicide/infanticide
  - Infanticide less likely if mother and baby hospitalized together.
- 90% recover completely from acute episode.
- Risk of psychosis during a subsequent pregnancy: 21–75%.
- Average number of episodes: 2.5
- Problems in baby:
  - Attention-deficit disorder
  - Behavioral problems
  - Depression
- Treatment is with mood stabilizer.
  - Initially often with antipsychotic medication

### Recurrent Brief Depression

- Depressive episodes meeting symptom but not duration criteria for major depressive disorder:
  - Episodes last about 1 week and recur at least 12 times/year.
    - Not in association with menstrual cycle
  - Antidepressants are not useful.
    - Fluoxetine was not effective in preventing recurrences of recurrent brief depression or in decreasing or increasing the number of suicide attempts, compared with placebo (Montgomery et al., 1994).
  - Lithium has been shown to reduce recurrences (Angst & Hochstrasser, 1994).

### Bereavement

Antidepressants are not useful for uncomplicated grief.
- Prescribing an antidepressant immediately after bereavement may promote the idea that experiencing sadness after a loss should be suppressed.
- Brief treatment with a hypnotic may be helpful for persistent insomnia.
- Indications for antidepressants following bereavement include:
  - Symptoms do not improve with support and encouragement of expression of grief.
  - Past history of depression in response to loss
  - Multiple depressive recurrences
  - Emergence of persistent vegetative symptoms of depression
- Usual antidepressant doses are utilized in these settings.

**Table 3.5 Treatment of Depression with Comorbid Conditions**

| DISORDER | PREFERRED | AVOID |
|---|---|---|
| Allergies | doxepine<br>mirtazapine<br>trimipramine | |
| Cardiac conduction problem | bupropion<br>citalopram<br>fluoxetine<br>fluvoxamine<br>paroxetine<br>sertraline | TCAs |
| Cataplexy | desipramine<br>fluoxetine<br>imipramine<br>protriptyline<br>tranylcypromine | |
| Congestive heart failure | bupropion<br>SSRIs | trazodone<br>nefazodone<br>TCAs or venlafaxine? |
| Constipation (chronic) | fluoxetine<br>fluvoxamine<br>sertraline<br>trazodone<br>venlafaxine | amitriptyline<br>doxepin<br>protriptyline<br>trimipramine |
| Dementria, delirium,<br>cognitive disorder | bupropion<br>fluoxetine<br>fluvoxamine<br>nefazodone<br>paroxetine<br>sertraline<br>trazodone<br>venlafaxine | amitriptyline<br>clomipramine<br>doxepin<br>imipramine<br>protriptyline<br>trimipramine |
| Diabetes, type II | fluoxetine | amitriptyline<br>doxepin |
| Diarrhea (chronic) | amitriptyline<br>doxepin<br>protriptyline<br>trimipramine | bupropion<br>SSRIs (except paroxetine)<br>venlafaxine |
| Epilepsy | desipramine<br>doxepin<br>phenelzine<br>SSRIs | amoxapine<br>bupropion<br>maprotiline<br>trimipramine |
| Impotence | bupropion (MH)<br>nefazodone (MH)<br>trazadone | fluoxetine<br>fluvoxamine<br>paroxetine<br>sertraline<br>phenelzine |

*(continues)*

**Table 3.5  Continued**

| DISORDER | PREFERRED | AVOID |
|---|---|---|
| Irritable bowel syndrome | amitriptyline<br>desipramine<br>doxepin<br>nortriptyline<br>phenelzine<br>trazodone | |
| Migraine headache | amitriptyline<br>doxepin<br>fluoxetine<br>imipramine<br>mirtazapine<br>paroxetine<br>phenelzine<br>sertraline<br>tranylcypromine<br>trazodone<br>trimipramine | |
| Narrow-angle glaucoma | bupropion<br>fluoxetine<br>fluvoxamine<br>nefazodone<br>sertraline<br>trazodone<br>venlafaxine | amitriptyline<br>clomipramine<br>doxepin<br>imipramine<br>paroxetine<br>trimipramine |
| Neurogenic bladder | bupropion<br>fluoxetine<br>sertraline<br>venlafaxine | |
| Parkinson's disease | amitriptyline<br>bupropion<br>doxepin<br>imipramine<br>protriptyline<br>selegiline<br>trimipramine | amoxapine<br>SSRIs? |
| Peptic ulcers | doxepin<br>trimipramine | |
| Sleep apnea | protriptyline<br>tranylcypromine | |
| Tardive dyskinesia | desipramine<br>imipramine<br>nefazodone<br>trazodone<br>trimipramine<br>venlafaxine | amoxapine |

### Anorexia Nervosa

There is no proven pharmacological treatment for anorexia nervosa. However, certain medications may be targeted at dimensions of this condition.

- SSRIs are safest and may reduce obsessive preoccupation with eating and weight.
  - Body image also may improve.
  - SSRIs with reputation for weight loss (e.g., fluoxetine) are sometimes abused by anorexia patients in attempt to lose weight.
- Atypical antipsychotic medication can be useful for overvalued ideas about body image and eating.
- Medications that promote weight gain (e.g., TCAs, paroxetine, mirtazepine) may be focus of power struggle with patient and should only be used after careful evaluation of the meaning of the medication to the patient.
  - Patients also may resent sedating medications.
- TCA cardiovascular side effects can be dangerous in patient with starvation.

### Bulimia Nervosa

Psychotherapy is a cornerstone of treatment for bulimia. Antidepressants can be useful as adjuncts for the eating disorder and as primary treatments for the frequently comorbid depression, but by themselves they are often less effective than psychotherapy.

- SSRIs in higher doses (e.g., fluoxetine 60–80 mg/day) can reduce binge eating and purging.
  - Increase the dose slowly to minimize risk of nausea.
- If one SSRI does not help, another may be effective.
- A comprehensive literature review found 19 antidepressant trials in bulimia nervosa (Bacaltchuk & Hay, 2002):
  - TCAs, MAOIs, mianserin, trazodone, bupropion.
  - Pooled relative risk for remission of bingeing was 0.87.
  - Similar benefit from all antidepressants.
  - Patients treated with antidepressants were more likely to discontinue treatment because of side effects.
  - Based on side effects, fluoxetine seemed preferable to TCAs.

Other medications that are sometimes helpful

- Lithium
  - Problematic for patients with self-induced vomiting.

- Naltrexone
  - May reduce craving.
- Anticonvulsants
  - Topiramate (median dose 212 mg) produced significantly greater re-duction in binge frequency than placebo (94% vs. 46%) in a 14–week double-blind study in 61 obese (BMI $\geq$ 30 kg/m$^2$) outpatients with binge eating disorder (McElroy et al., 2003).
  - 64 outpatients with Diagnostic and Statistical Manual-IV bulimia nervosa were randomly assigned to placebo or topiramate starting at 25 mg and gradually increased to 400 mg/day for 10 weeks (Hoopes et al., 2003).
    - Mean weekly binge and/or purge days decreased 45% with topi-ramate vs. 11% with placebo ($p = 0.004$).
- A review of 16 placebo-controlled trials, including 6 with TCAs, 3 with fluoxetine, 4 with MAOIs, and 3 with mianserin, trazodone, or bupropion, found that all were equally effective (Bacaltchuk & Hay, 2002).
  - RR for at least 50% reduction in binge episodes was 0.63.
    - Number needed to treat (NNT) for duration of 9 weeks was 4.
  - RR for remission of binge episodes was 0.88.
    - NNT for duration of 8 weeks was 9.
  - Fluoxetine had lowest dropout rates, TCA highest.

Minimize use of antidepressants that stimulate appetite.

Bupropion does not have an increased seizure risk at doses < 450 mg, but since seizures are more likely in bulimics, and electrolyte imbalance can lower the seizure threshold, it is not an initial choice at any dose.

Cyproheptadine is ineffective in bulimia and may stimulate appetite.

### Chronic Fatigue System

CFS may be a manifestation of a mood disorder, or it may be comor-bid with a mood disorder. Patients with profound fatigue and hyper-somnia associated with CFS may have a prodrome of a bipolar mood disorder. When CFS is associated with major depression

- More stimulating antidepressants (e.g., bupropion) are more likely to increase energy.
- Venlafaxine and SSRIs also can be useful.
- Consider MAO inhibitor for refractory CFS.
- Be alert for treatment-emergent hypomania.

### Chronic Pain

Antidepressants can reduce (but not eliminate) chronic pain but have no effect on acute pain.

TCAs
- Have been found most clearly to alleviate chronic pain.
  - Equal efficacy in depressed and nondepressed patients.
  - Average 50–60% improvement seen in about 50% of patients.
  - Most TCAs seem equally effective.
    - Most frequently studied are desipramine, amitriptyline, and doxepin.
    - Prescribe usual doses if patient is depressed.
    - In the absence of comorbid depression, lower TCA doses (e.g., 25–75 mg desipramine) are effective.
    - Addition of a low dose of a neuroleptic (e.g., 1 mg fluphenazine) can augment antidepressant, possibly by slowing transmission through polysynaptic pain pathways.
    - No data on atypical antipsychotics.
    - Augmentation with gabapentin or carbamazepine is safer and often more effective.
  - TCAs can augment opiate analgesia.

SSRIs
- Not as effective as TCAs for chronic pain.
  - SSRIs that inhibit CYP2D6 (e.g., fluoxetine, paroxetine) block conversion of codeine to morphine, rendering it ineffective.

Nefazodone
- Can be effective for fibromyalgia.
  - Correction of sleep disorder.
  - Mirtazepine also could be useful.

Venlafaxine
- Reduced pain in a laboratory model.

Anticonvulsants
- Carbamazepine
  - Especially useful for neuropathic pain
- Gabapentin
  - Antidepressant/anxiolytic as well as antinociceptive effects

Narcotics

- Long-term treatment with narcotics is usually not recommended for chronic benign (noncancer) pain because of frequent tolerance.
- Long-term opioid use can cause hypersensitivity to pain (sensitization).
  - May be mediated by NMDA receptor.
- Chronic opioid use alters hormonal function.
  - Testosterone depletion
    - Replacement may be helpful.
  - Infertility
- Some patients are able to avoid dosage escalation and other adverse outcomes with chronic opioid therapy. Recommended protocol (Ballantyne & Mao, 2003):
  - Evaluate risk of substance misuse.
  - Confirm inadequacy of nonopioid therapies.
  - Explain risks and benefits thoroughly.
  - Start treatment at low dose and increase gradually over 8 weeks.
    - Discontinue if unsatisfactory benefit or side effects.
  - Maintain stable, moderate dose.
  - Regularly evaluate pain relief, dosage, functioning, and adverse effects.
  - Methadone may be preferable as initial medication.
    - Inexpensive
    - Low street value
    - NMDA antagonist may reduce tolerance and help neuropathic pain.
    - However, accumulation may cause respiratory depression.
  - Switch between opioids if one does not work well.
    - Diversity of μ-opioid receptors may result in lack of complete cross-tolerance.
    - Start new medication at half the equivalent dose of the previous one, because tolerance to the new medication will be lower than to the original one.
    - Opioid rotation may help when tolerance develops repeatedly.
  - If illness escalates, it may be necessary to increase dose cautiously.
  - Usual doses are listed in Table 3.6.
  - Doses > 1 gm/day of morphine equivalent (five times dose validated in literature) are no more effective than lower doses and are not considered safe.
  - Buprenorphine 2–8 mg has analgesic and antidepressant properties.

**Table 3.6  Doses of Commonly Used Opioids**

| GENERIC NAME | TRADE NAME | USUAL INITIAL DOSE | USUAL ANALGESIC DOSE |
|---|---|---|---|
| Codeine | | 30 mg q 3–4 h | Same |
| Fentanyl patch | Duragesic | 25 μg/hour patch q 72 h | Same |
| Hydrocodone | Vicodin | 10 mg q 3–4 h | Same |
| Hydromorphone | Dilaudid | 2–4 mg q 3–4 h | 7.5 mg q 3–4 h |
| Meperidine | Demerol | 50–100 mg q 3 h | 100–300 mg q 3 h |
| Methadone | Dolophine | 5 mg q 8–12 h | 20 mg q 6–8 h |
| Morphine | | 15 mg q 3–4 h | 30 mg q 3–4 h |
| Morphine SR | MSContin | 15 mg q 8–12 h | Same |
| Oxycodone | Percocet Percodan | 5 mg q 3–4 h | Same |
| Oxycodone CR | OxyContin | 10 mg q 8–12 h | Same |

Data from Ballantyne and Mao (2003).

### Fibromyalgia

Fibromyalgia and major depression have similar sleep disorders and family histories of depression; fibromyalgia may combine the physiology of depression with the physiology of arthritis.

- Antidepressants can improve fibromyalgia symptoms.
- First choice is a medication that can increase (or at least not decrease) slow-wave sleep.
  - Nefazodone
  - Mirtazepine

### Premenstrual Dysphoric Disorder (PMDD)

- Most mood disorders are worse premenstrually.
- Serotonin reuptake inhibitors.
- Fluoxetine, sertraline, clomipramine, paroxetine, fluvoxamine effective in blinded or open trials.
- SSRIs superior to other antidepressant classes.
- Effective chronically or during luteal phase.
  - Using just premenstrually reduces side effects.
  - Not as effective when taken prn.
- Prescribe usual doses of SSRIs.
  - Lower doses of clomipramine

- Nefazodone
  - Open-label trial
  - Average dose 245 mg/day
- Alprazolam
  - Small N studied
  - 0.25–0.5 mg qid
  - Effective when taken premenstrually
- Subcutaneous or intranasal gonadotropin-releasing hormone (GnRH) agonists
  - Teuprolide acetate, nafarelin acetate, goserelin acetate
  - Result in anovulation, decreased estrogen, and progesterone
  - Adverse effects limit use to otherwise refractory cases.
- Oral micronized progesterone
  - Widely utilized but studies all show no better than placebo.
  - Synthetic progestins also ineffective.

### Hot Flashes

- A six-week multicenter randomized double-blind placebo-controlled trial of controlled-release paroxetine 12.5 or 25 mg/day in 165 menopausal women found median reduction in hot flashes of 62% with 12.5 mg, 65% with 25 mg, and 38% with placebo (Stearns, Beebe, Iyengar, & Dube, 2003).
  - Benefit may be due to effects on $5HT_{2A}$ receptors, which mediate hyperthermia, and $5HT_{1A}$ receptors, which mediate hypothermia.

### Borderline Personality Disorder (BPD)

- A double-blind study of fluvoxamine in 38 patients with BPD included 6 weeks of random assignment to fluvoxamine (150–250 mg/day) or placebo, then single-blind crossover of placebo patients to fluvoxamine for 6 weeks, followed by 12 weeks of open fluvoxamine treatment (Rinne, Van den Brink, Wouters, & van Dyck, 2002).
  - Fluvoxamine had significantly greater reduction in rapid mood changes, with most improvement occurring during the first 6 weeks.
  - Results were independent of comorbid affective disorder or PTSD.

### Childhood Stage-4 Sleep Disorders

Common stage-4 sleep disorders in children include
- Enuresis
- Night terrors
- Sleepwalking

Effective treatments for enuresis include

- Imipramine
- Desipramine
- Amitriptyline
- Nortriptyline
- Lower doses are often necessary.
  - For example, imipramine 10–25 mg hs
    - Maximum dose 50–75 mg
- 80% of children have 50% reduction in enuresis within 1 week.
- Enuresis returns when antidepressant discontinued.

Night terrors and sleepwalking may be reduced by TCAs.

- Benzodiazepines may be more effective than antidepressants.
  - For example, 3.75–15 mg oxazepam

### Smoking Cessation

Nicotine substitution by itself is only occasionally effective for smoking cessation. Antidepressants may promote smoking cessation when combined with behavior therapy.

- Bupropion SR plus a nicotine patch produces more abstinence from smoking than either one alone or placebo.
- Out of 144 smokers, significantly more stopped smoking after 6 weeks treatment with 75 mg/day nortriptyline than with placebo (56% vs. 23%).
  - Each was combined with cognitive–behavioral therapy (Da Costa, Younes, & Lourenco, 2000).
  - At a 6-month follow-up, many patients had relapsed, but significantly more patients treated with nortriptyline than placebo were still abstinent from smoking (21% vs. 5%).
- Nicotine gum and patch useful for withdrawal symptoms once patient has stopped smoking.
  - Swallowing saliva after chewing nicotine gum leads to gastric discomfort and reduced efficacy.
- Clonidine may reduce preoccupation with smoking, but does not increase smoking cessation > placebo.
- $5HT_3$ antagonists (e.g., ondansetron, granisetron) may reduce craving for nicotine as well as other substances.
  - Ondansetron 4–8 mg tid

### Premature Ejaculation

- SSRIs have treated premature ejaculation in double-blind controlled studies (Segraves, 2003).

- Clomipramine taken 6 hours prior to sexual activity also is effective for premature ejaculation (Segraves, Saran, Segraves, & Maguire, 1993).

## CHOOSING AN ANTIDEPRESSANT

All antidepressants are equally effective. Choosing a particular agent depends on factors that are intrinsic (e.g., past and family history of response, comorbid conditions) and extrinsic (e.g., cost, insurance coverage) to the patient.

### History and Nature of Depression

- Initial choice is usually a medication to which the patient or a family member has responded in the past.
- Side-effect profile of antidepressant may inform treatment in specific settings
  - Elderly and medically ill patients do better with antidepressants that are less anticholinergic, hypotensive, and sedating (e.g., the SSRIs, bupropion, venlafaxine).
  - TCAs are poorly tolerated by older patients.
    - If a TCA is used in this population, start with desipramine or nortriptyline.
  - Because stimulation of $5HT_2$ heteroreceptors on striatal dopaminergic neurons reduces dopamine release and enhances the response of $D_2$ receptors to blockade, SSRIs can aggravate parkinsonism.
    - Dopaminergic antidepressants such as bupropion should improve parkinsonism, although research has not confirmed this.
    - Selegiline can be effective for depression and Parkinson's disease (see Chapter 4).
  - Antidepressants with anticholinergic properties (e.g., most TCAs, paroxetine) can aggravate cognitive dysfunction in demented patients.
    - Initial choices are stimulants, bupropion, venlafaxine.
  - Nonspecific reduction of intrusive thoughts and unpredictable, impulsive aggression make SSRIs useful for depression associated with rumination, and for depression in brain-damaged patients with explosive outbursts.
  - TCAs, trazodone, and mirtazepine can be effective for migraine prophylaxis.
    - SSRIs sometimes reduce migraines because of decreased platelet serotonin uptake, but increased circulating serotonin may aggravate migraines in some cases.

- TCAs are riskier for patients with coronary heart disease than are the newer antidepressants.
- Depressed diabetic patients should receive antidepressants with a lower risk of weight gain.
  - SSRIs *other than* paroxetine, bupropion, venlafaxine, nefazodone
- SSRIs may aggravate both bleeding disorders and clotting disorders.
- $5HT_3$ antagonist properties similar to ondansetron make mirtazepine a good choice for patients with severe nausea caused by cancer chemotherapy or other medications.
- Venlafaxine and mirtazepine are not first choices for hypertensive patients.
- Risk of successful suicide is much higher with TCAs ($LD_{50}$ = 1 week supply) than with newer antidepressants.
  - If the suicide risk is so high that the physician wants to prescribe small amounts of medication, the patient should probably be hospitalized or receive ECT.
- Patients who are likely to be noncompliant or have trouble remembering medication should receive antidepressants that are effective in a single daily dose.
- Expense and insurance coverage can be limiting factors.
  - Many formularies do not include all SSRIs or extended release forms of bupropion and venlafaxine.
    - SSRIs are equally effective in large studies, but some patients have a preferential response to one preparation.
  - TCAs are available as generics, but increased cost of laboratory studies and more frequent doctor visits to monitor side effects offset the cost savings.
  - The only generic SSRIs currently available are fluoxetine, paroxetine, and fluvoxamine.
    - Cost varies, but may not be substantially cheaper than brand name.
  - The cost of 100 mg sertraline tablets is the same as for 50 mg tablets.
    - Patients prescribed 50 mg should take half of a 100 mg tablet.
  - Many manufacturers have free medication programs for low-income patients.
- Strategies for dealing with insurance denials of an antidepressant that is effective for a patient:
  - Always appeal initial denial.
  - Document need for the specific antidepressant.
  - Provide references on efficacy of desired antidepressant.

- Have patient and family call insurance reviewer.
- For managed care companies, file complaint with National Committee on Quality Assurance (NCQA).

### Antidepressant Comparisons

TCAs

- Nortriptyline and probably desipramine have therapeutic windows.
  - Reported range for nortriptyline (50–150 ng/mL) may be too broad; optimal level around 100 ng/mL.
  - Despiramine therapeutic level around 125–200 ng/mL.
- Desipramine is lowest in anticholinergic effects and weight gain.
- Trimipramine and doxepin have antihistaminic properties equivalent to ranitidine.
- Amoxapine is effective as monotherapy for psychotic depression, but it is impossible to adjust neuroleptic and antidepressant doses independently, and TD may occur.
- Clomipramine is the only TCA effective for OCD.

SSRIs

- Similarities are more important than differences, especially with respect to adverse effects.
- Fluoxetine
  - Longer half-life
  - More activating
  - Potent CYP450 2D6 inhibitor
  - Generally weight neutral, but can cause slight weight loss or substantial weight gain.
- Sertraline
  - Half-life about 1 day
  - Active metabolite and 2D6 inhibition usually not clinically important.
  - Reuptake inhibition of dopamine in addition to 5HT at high doses probably not noticeable clinically.
  - Low risk of weight gain
- Paroxetine
  - About as anticholinergic as nortriptyline
  - More weight gain than other SSRIs
  - Potent 2D6 inhibitor
  - Associated with more severe discontinuation syndromes.

- Data from 36 outpatients with major depression treated with 60 mg/day paroxetine or 30 mg desipramine (Gilmor, Owens, & Nemeroff, 2002) demonstrated that
  - Paroxetine decreased norepinephrine uptake by 27% at 100 ng/mL and by 43% at 200 ng/mL, whereas serotonin uptake was decreased by 85% of control.
  - Low dose of desipramine reduced norepinephrine uptake by 85% and decreased serotonin uptake by 18–51%.
  - Clinical implications of modest norepinephrine reuptake inhibition by higher paroxetine doses are not apparent.
- Sustained release form (paroxetine CR) administered in somewhat higher doses.
  - May have slightly less severe adverse effects associated with peak levels (e.g., nausea) than immediate release form, but both forms are given in one daily dose.
  - Available in 12.5, 25, and 37.5 mg tablets
  - Initial dose 25 mg, maximum dose 62.5 mg
  - Food does not affect absorption.
  - Dropout rates in clinical trials of paroxetine CR are 10% vs. 16% with immediate-release paroxetine and 10% with placebo.
- Fluvoxamine
  - Shorter half-life requires bid dosing.
  - Effective as antidepressant, even though primarily studied for OCD.
  - Potent CYP450 3A4 inhibitor
- Citalopram
  - No reported P450 effects
  - No active metabolites
  - Useful for older and medically ill patients
  - Same side effect profile as other SSRIs
- Escitalopram
  - S-enantomer of citalopram
  - Better binding to 5HT transporter than citalopram
    - Does not necessarily predict better antidepressant effect.
  - Low in potential for weight gain and CYP450 interactions
  - An 8-week fixed-dose comparison of escitalopram 10 mg, escitalopram 20 mg, citalopram 40 mg, and placebo found both doses of escitalopram to be significantly more effective than placebo and equivalent to 40 mg citalopram at endpoint, with similar discontinuation rates for adverse effects in all groups (Burke, Gergel, & Bose, 2002).

- Report of faster onset of action than citalopram is based on earlier statistically significant separation of HRSD scores from placebo, but the difference was not clinically meaningful.

## TRAZODONE

- Effective for depression at doses of 300–600 mg/day, given on bid and hs basis because of short half-life.
  - Many patients cannot tolerate daytime sedation at these doses.
- Short half-life and high sedation make this a useful hypnotic.
- Risk of priapism 1:6000
  - Not dose related
  - All men should be informed of this risk.

## NEFAZODONE

- Requires at least two doses/day at 400–600 mg.
  - Daytime sedation can be substantial.
- Potent inhibitor of 3A4
- Anxiogenic metabolite (mCPP) accumulates in about 10% of people, leading to agitation and increased anxiety.
- Does not disrupt sleep architecture, as do most other antidepressants.
  - Useful for severe insomnia
- Can reduce symptoms of fibromyalgia and other forms of chronic pain.
- Risk of severe hepatotoxicity appears to be 18/10,000,000.
  - Routine liver function tests are not likely to identify problem.
  - Brand name preparation (Serzoue) withdrawn from market; generic is available.

## BUPROPION

- Low in potential for sedation and sexual side effects
- No cardiotoxicity
- Dopaminergic effect is activating and useful for parkinsonism.
- Initial choice for some demented patients
- May also be helpful for smoking cessation.
- Bupropion SR often requires bid dosing at higher doses to minimize peak blood levels.
- Seizure risk about 5% at doses > 450 mg
  - Primarily in patients with bulimia, head injury, epilepsy
  - Lower doses have same seizure risk as other antidepressants.
- Not particularly effective for anxiety
  - Sometimes makes anxious patients more jittery.

- Higher serum levels may not work as well.
  - But therapeutic level not established.
- Traditionally thought to have lower risk of mania induction, but some studies show same risk as other antidepressants at equivalent doses.

VENLAFAXINE

- Effective for depression refractory to other antidepressants.
- May be more effective for severe depression.
- May produce higher remission rate than SSRIs.
  - A review sponsored by the manufacturer of multicenter double-blind randomized comparisons of venlafaxine or venlafaxine XR with SSRIs using HRSD scores $\leq 7$ or $\leq 10$ as criterion for remission found
    - Remission was statistically more likely with venlafaxine than with SSRIs or placebo (Rudolph, 2002).
  - A meta-analysis of 32 randomized controlled trials involving 5,562 patients, with follow-up ranging from 4 to 48 weeks (mean 10 weeks) found that response and remission rates in depression with venlafaxine were higher than SSRIs and equivalent to TCAs (Smith, Dempster, Glanville, Freemantle, & Anderson, 2002).
    - There was no difference in dropout rates between venlafaxine and SSRIs.
    - Studies may have been biased by recruiting more patients who failed to respond to SSRIs, which are used more frequently as first-line treatments.
    - The main outcome measure was the HRSD rather than functional or global outcome.
  - Findings from examination of pooled data from 8 double-blind randomized trials in major depression, lasting 8 weeks or less, in which patients were assigned to venlafaxine (75–375 mg/day) or venlafaxine XR (75–225 mg/day) vs. fluoxetine (20–80 mg/day), paroxetine (20–40 mg/day), or fluvoxamine (100–200 mg/day), four of the trials also including placebo arms, and all supported by the manufacturer of venlafaxine (Stahl, Entusah, & Rudolph, 2002):
    - Significantly greater reduction in depression scores found with venlafaxine: (1) 14.5-point decrease on HRSD, (2) 12.6-point decrease with SSRIs, and (3) 11.3-point decrease with placebo.
    - Significantly higher response rate found with venlafaxine (64%) than with SSRIs (59%) and placebo (41%).
    - Dropouts because of adverse effects: venlafaxine = SSRIs > placebo.
    - Clinical significance of difference not clear.
- No effect on P450 enzymes.

- Geriatric dose similar to younger patients.
- Extended release form (venlafaxine XR) can be given once daily at doses < 150 mg.
  - Higher doses should be divided.
- Withdrawal symptoms can persist for weeks after abrupt discontinuation.
  - Influenza-like symptoms
  - Rebound depression
  - Interdose withdrawal may occur, even with XR form.
- Side effects related to NE, 5HT, and DA (at higher doses):
  - Jitteriness, sweating, tremor
  - Sedation, nausea, headaches sexual dysfunction
  - Occasional hypertension as dose approaches 375 mg

## Mirtazepine

- $5HT_2$, $5HT_3$, NE alpha-2 receptor antagonist
  - $5HT_3$ antagonism provides antiemetic effect.
  - Alpha-2 effect increases NE release.
- Most common side effects are sedation and weight gain.
  - Occasionally causes activation/jitteriness (noradrenergic effect) combined with sedation (antihistaminic effect).
- Useful for patients with insomnia, weight loss, and nausea (e.g., those undergoing cancer chemotherapy).
  - Especially effective for depression, nausea, and insomnia caused by carcinoid (serotonin-secreting tumor).
- Not a good choice for patients who cannot afford to gain weight.

## Duloxetine

- 5HT and NE uptake inhibitor, both beginning at low doses
- Half-life 10–15 hours
- CYP450 2D6 substrate and inhibitor
- Lower risk of hypertension at high doses than venlafaxine, because no dopamine reuptake inhibition.
- Effective in a double blind multicenter study of major depression (Karpa, Cavanaugh, & Lakoski, 2002):
  - Greater efficacy in more severe depression
- A multicenter double-blind parallel group study of placebo (N = 122) or 60 mg duloxetine (N = 123) found that
  - Duloxetine was significantly superior in reducing HDRS scores, starting at week 2.

- Remission rates were 44% for duloxetine and 16% for placebo (Detke, Lu, Goldstein, Hayes, & Demitrack, 2002).
- Remission rates were reported to be
  - 45% for duloxetine 120 mg/day vs. 30% for fluoxetine 20 mg/day and 27% for placebo (Tran, Bymaster, McNamara, & Potter, 2003).
- Open-label year-long follow-up (performed by the manufacturer) of 520 patients taking 80–120 mg/day duloxetine (given bid) estimated probability of remission 82% at 52 weeks (Raskin, Goldstein, Mallinckrodt, & Ferguson, 2003).

REBOXETINE

- NE reuptake inhibitor
- In an 8-week multicenter clinical trial of reboxetine in major depression (Andreoli, Caillard, Deo, Rybakowski, & Versiani, 2002):
  - 381 patients were assigned to reboxetine 8–10 mg/day, fluoxetine 20–40 mg/day, or placebo.
  - Both active treatments were significantly more effective than placebo in reducing mean HRSD scores and in producing response.
    - Response rates: 56% for reboxetine, 56% for fluoxetine, and 34% for placebo
    - Remission rates: 48%, 45%, and 27%, respectively
  - Reboxetine was effective in more as well as less severely depressed patients.
- Adverse effects included:
  - Agitation
  - Nausea
  - Constipation
  - Dry mouth
  - Headache
  - Sweating
  - Hypotension
  - Paresthesias
  - Sexual dysfunction

## Dosage

TCAs

- TCAs are metabolized by CYP450 2D6.
  - Interindividual variability in 2D6 activity results in 20-fold interindividual variation in serum level at the same dose.

- Serum levels are only useful for adjusting dose of a few TCAs.
    - Measure when patient is in steady state.
        - 90% steady state is reached in four half-lives.
        - Obtain levels about a week after dosage change.
        - Blood should be drawn 10–14 hours after last dose.
- Nortriptyline has therapeutic window (50–150 ng/mL).
    - Optimal serum level is probably around 100 ng/mL.
        - Achieved with average dose around 75 mg.
- Desipramine probably has therapeutic window around 125–200 ng/mL.
    - Average dose 150–300 mg/day
- Imipramine has onset of action at level around 225 ng/mL of imipramine + desipramine.
    - Desipramine is major active metabolite of imipramine
- Serum levels of other antidepressants are usually only useful to assess adverse effects at low doses or lack of benefit at usual therapeutic doses.
- Doses in children usually are 3.5–5 mg/kg.
- Most TCAs can be administered in one bedtime dose.
    - Protriptyline is more activating and should be taken in the morning.
- Average starting dose generally 25 mg, with dosage increased according to response and side effects.
    - Anxious patients often become overly activated by noradrenergic effect of TCAs and do better with lower starting doses (e.g., 10 mg).
- All antidepressants can induce seizures at high levels.
    - With most TCAs, therapeutic doses are lower than doses that cause seizures.
    - TCAs for which therapeutic and epileptogenic doses overlap:
        - Maprotiline: > 225 mg/day
        - Clomipramine: > 250 mg/day
- TCAs induce their own metabolism.
    - Initial improvement followed by loss of efficacy often caused by decrease of serum level.

## SSRIs

- Some patients can start with average therapeutic dose, but others do better with gradual dosage increase.
    - Anxious patients are hypervigilant for anything that can go wrong and have lower threshold for noticing adverse effects.
    - Slow dosage escalation promotes tolerance to side effects.

- Start with
  - 10 mg fluoxetine or paroxetine
  - 25–50 mg sertraline
  - 10 mg citalopram or escitalopram
  - 50 mg fluvoxamine
- Dose may be increased once/week or less frequently to
  - 40 mg fluoxetine
  - 50 mg paroxetine
  - 200 mg sertraline
  - 40 mg citalopram
  - 20–40 mg escitalopram
  - 150–300 mg fluvoxamine
- Fluoxetine sometimes develops a therapeutic window months to a year or more after a good response.
  - Raising dose only helps briefly.
  - Reducing dose or stopping medication and restarting at lower dose a few weeks later can restore response.
  - May be caused by gradual accumulation of a long-acting metabolite that interferes with therapeutic effect of parent drug.

## BUPROPION

- Start with 25–37.5 mg in outpatients.
- Target dose 300–450 mg/day
- Bupropion and bupropion SR administered two or three times per day.
  - Single doses > 150–200 mg may cause activation or seizures.
- Bupropion XL administered once daily.

## VENLAFAXINE

- Starting dose 37.5–75 mg
- Broad dosage range: 75–375 mg/day
- Doses > 150 mg should be divided, even with XR form.
- Higher doses should be divided to bid or tid, even with XR form.

## TRAZODONE

- Start with 50 mg hs.
- If used as a hypnotic, increase dose to 100–300 mg, as tolerated.
- If used as an antidepressant, add two daytime doses.
- Target dose 300–600 mg/day in three doses/day.

NEFAZODONE

- Start with low dose (e.g., 50 mg) and increase slowly to facilitate tolerance to sedation.
- For antidepressant efficacy
  - Must be administered two or three times/day at total doses of 400–600 mg.

MIRTAZEPINE

- Some patients experience improvement of sedation with increasing doses.
  - May be manifestation of adrenergic effect.
- For other patients, slow dosage escalation permits tolerance to sedation.

## Duration of a Therapeutic Trial

Most antidepressants require at least 4 weeks at a therapeutic dose.
If no improvement in any symptoms (e.g., sleep) after 2 weeks, increase dose.

Data from a multicenter placebo-controlled discontinuation study (N = 840) were reanalyzed to determine how long to continue an SSRI (Quitkin et al., 2003).
- Patients treated openly with 20 mg/day of fluoxetine for 12 weeks (607 completers).
- Patients with remission (N = 424) were randomized to active medication or placebo for another 14 weeks.
- 51% of patients who were unchanged after week 4 attained remission by week 12.
- 41% of patients who were unimproved after 6 weeks had remission by week 12.
- 48% of patients with partial improvement at 6 weeks had remission at week 12.
- 77% of responders at week 6 had remission by week 12.
- 23% of patients with no improvement at 8 weeks were in remission at week 12.
- 42% of patients with partial improvement had remission at week 12.
- 72% of patients with response had remission at week 12.
- During the discontinuation phase:
  - 44% of patients assigned to placebo relapsed.
  - 18–27% of patients on fluoxetine relapsed.
    - Level of improvement at week 6 did not predict relapse risk.

- The results suggested that a minimum of an 8-week trial of fluoxetine is indicated because
  - Patients with no improvement at week 6 had 31–41% chance of remission by week 12.
  - Patients with partial improvement at week 8 had 38% chance of remission 4 weeks later, suggesting 10-week trial for partially improved patients at 8 weeks.
  - Whereas most antidepressants show some response by 8 weeks, fluoxetine may require a 12-week trial.

## NonPharmacological Somatic Therapies

### Electroconvulsive Therapy (ECT)

- Requires electrical but not motor seizure.

  Most important indication for ECT is major depression.
- Also effective for
  - Mania
  - Bipolar depression
  - Rapid cycling
  - Catatonia
  - A review of published studies of ECT for schizophrenia found that "there is some limited evidence" to support the use of ECT combined with antipsychotic medications for patients who have unsatisfactory response to antipsychotics alone (Tharyan & Adams, 2002).
  - Delirium
- Most effective for patients who cannot tolerate antidepressants.
  - Response rate 90% in patients who have not had adequate antidepressant trials, but 50% in patients who have had two or more adequate antidepressant trials.
- Medications that were not effective prior to ECT are no more effective following ECT.
  - However, medications that were poorly tolerated before ECT may be better tolerated subsequently.
- ECT is administered acutely two or three times per week until patient has a complete response.
  - Minimum effective seizure duration may be around 20–30 seconds.
  - EEG seizure > 180 seconds associated with excessive confusion, without added benefit, and should be terminated.
  - There is no relationship between seizure duration or seizure threshold and response to ECT (Abrams, 2002).

- The conventional wisdom that the minimum effective seizure duration is 25–30 seconds is not supported by empirical data.
- Do not continue acute ECT after depression has remitted.
- Twice-weekly ECT decreases cognitive side effects without reducing efficacy (Lerer et al., 1995).
- Nondominant (right-sided) unilateral (RUL) ECT is better tolerated than bilateral (BL) ECT.
  - RUL has a dose–response relationship, with greater likelihood of response at stimulus intensity three times seizure threshold.
    - RUL ECT was as effective as BL ECT if the stimulus intensity was six times the seizure threshold (Sackeim, Prudic, & Devanand, 2000).
    - In another study by the same group comparing fixed RUL high-dose ECT and RUL ECT with dose titrated above seizure threshold, the degree to which the stimulus intensity exceeded the seizure threshold predicted treatment response from 6–13 times the seizure threshold (McCall, Reboussin, & Weiner, 2000).
  - A review of published RUL ECT dosage studies found that higher stimulus doses (> 195–378 mC) are consistently more effective (Abrams, 2002).
    - No study found > 65% efficacy with doses < 195 mC.
    - No study found < 65% efficacy with doses > 378 mC.
    - Fewer ECTs are needed at higher doses (6.8 for high dose vs. 8.9 for low dose).
    - High dose studies used fixed rather than titrated doses.
    - More adverse effects at higher stimulus intensity.
    - Based on stimulus–dosage findings, Abrams recommends starting RUL at maximum device capacity, with a 0.25–0.5 msec pulse width, adjusting the frequency to produce the maximum number of pulses. If the patient does not improve, switch to BL ECT (Abrams, 2002).
  - In 24 patients who failed to respond to 5–8 RUL ECTs at 150% above seizure threshold, those randomly assigned to RUL at 450% above seizure threshold had as much as those randomly assigned to BL, but cognitive side effects were greater with BL (Tew et al., 2002).
  - BL has not demonstrated the same dose–response relationship.
  - If correctly applied, bifrontal ECT has fewer cognitive side effects (Abrams, 2002).
    - Focuses stimulus on prefrontal region with less spread to temporal cortex, which produces cognitive side effects.

- A review of 52 case reports and case series of acute ECT in 213 patients with movement disorders found (Kennedy, Mittal, & O'Jile, 2003):
  - Most reports suggest a positive response in Parkinson's disease.
    - Results are probably not a function of improvement of psychomotor retardation.
    - Not dependent on co-administration of L-dopa.
    - ECT may increase dopaminergic transmission, mainly through receptor actions.
  - ECT also may improve drug-induced parkinsonism and possibly TD.
  - ECT is effective in refractory Parkinson's disease (Andrade & Kurinji, 2002).
  - Maintenance ECT may be an alternative to surgery in refractory Parkinson's patients who have responded acutely to ECT.
  - Risk of cognitive side effects may be increased.
- Most common adverse effects are confusion and memory loss.
  - Confusion often clears within a few hours of each treatment.
    - May become cumulative with frequent treatment.
  - Anterograde and retrograde amnesia may occur.
  - Loss of a single autobiographical memory sometimes occurs.
  - No evidence from imaging, biochemical (e.g., markers of neuronal damage), or pathological studies in humans and animals that ECT, as it is currently administered, causes brain damage.
    - Animal studies suggest that 3 hours of continuous ECT without anesthesia and muscle relaxant, or 6 hours with anesthesia and muscle relaxant, are necessary to cause neurological damage.
  - Cognitive impairment caused by depression improves following successful ECT.
- Methohexital most frequently used barbiturate anesthetic.
  - Usual dose 0.67 mg/kg
    - Higher dose for patients who are tolerant to CNS depressants.
  - In a randomized double-blind crossover trial in seven patients (mean age 42), methohexital (0.625 mg/kg) + remifentanil (1 μg/kg) produced longer seizure durations than methohexital alone (1.25 mg/kg; Smith, Angst, Brock-Utne, & DeBattista, 2003).
    - Consider substituting remifentanil for a portion of methohexital in patients needing longer seizure duration.

Muscle relaxants used to prevent convulsion:
- Succinylcholine
  - 0.4–0.7 mg/kg

- Higher dose for patients with higher ratio of muscle/adipose tissue.
- Stimulus administered 1–2 minutes after injection.
  - As soon as fasciculations stop
- EEG monitoring more accurate than inflating blood pressure cuff > systolic pressure on one extremity to observe localized movement.
- Succinylcholine precautions:
  - Hyperkalemia in patients with damaged muscle (e.g., after stroke, burn, or other muscle injury)
  - Prolonged paralysis in patients with increased or decreased serum $K^+$
  - Prolonged respiratory depression in patients taking cholinesterase inhibitors (block pseudocholinesterase, which metabolizes succinylcholine); may be more likely with rivastigmine, because pseudocholinesterase is similar to BuChE.
  - Use mivacurium (short-acting nondepolarizing agent) for these patients.
- Suxamethonium
  - 1 mg/kg IV

Adjunctive agents
- Beta-blockers
  - Used to prevent hypertension and tachycardia.
  - Most commonly used: labetolol (4-min. half-life), esmolol (9–min. half-life)
  - Risks
    - Aggravation of vagal stimulation by stimulus causes severe bradycardia or hypotension.
- IV nitroglycerine
  - More effective acutely than beta-blocker for hypertension caused by stimulus.
  - May increase heart rate.
- Anticholinergics
  - Central effect of stimulus increases vagal activity.
    - Can cause bradycardia, asystole, escape rhythms, hypersalivation in 30–70% of treatments.
  - IV preparations
    - Atropine 0.4–1.0 mg
    - Glycopyrrolate 0.2–0.4 mg (preferable for excess secretions)
  - Consider using in presence of
    - High-seizure threshold (vagal hyperactivity a function of stimulus intensity).

- Failed seizure (absence of catecholamine release caused by seizure results in reduced offset of increased vagal activity).
- Use of beta-blockers can aggravate cardiac slowing
- Past cardiac slowing during ECT
- Adverse effects: tachycardia, relaxation of lower esophageal sphincter (can cause gastroesophageal reflux/aspiration), confusion (atropine but not glycopyrrolate crosses the blood–brain barrier).

- Seizure augmentation
  - Used for excessively short or failed seizures.
  - Hyperventilation: (1) hyperventilate patient for 2–3 minutes before stimulus; (2) apply moderate decrease in seizure threshold and increase in seizure duration.
  - Caffeine 500–1000 mg IV reduces seizure threshold but does not increase seizure duration.
  - Sustained-release theophylline 200 mg the night prior to ECT prolongs seizure time.

- Medications that raise seizure threshold and reduce ECT efficacy:
  - Anticonvulsants
  - Benzodiazepines
  - Barbiturates
    - Methohexital
    - Thiopental
  - Propofol
  - Lidocaine
  - High doses of beta-blockers (e.g., > 20 mg labetolol)

- Medications that can prolong seizures:
  - Ketamine
  - Etomidate
  - Theophylline
  - Caffeine
  - Clozapine
  - Some antidepressants
    - Bupropion
    - Maprotiline
    - Amoxapine
    - Clomipramine

- Use of psychotropic agents during ECT:
  - Neuroleptics may potentiate ECT.
    - Low-potency phenothiazines sometimes decrease seizure threshold.

- Antipsychotic drugs are well tolerated with ECT.
- Lithium prolongs action of succinylcholine and results in increased confusion and other signs of neurotoxicity.
  - Due to increased entry of lithium into brain during seizure.
- Antidepressants do not potentiate ECT and occasionally increase neurotoxicity and poor treatment response.
- Anticonvulsants and benzodiazepines can decrease ECT efficacy.
  - Carbamazepine prolongs action of succinylcholine.
- CNS stimulants may prolong seizures and increase the risk of dysrhythmias.

*Relapse after ECT:* Common without some form of continuation/maintenance treatment.

*Continuation ECT:* Treatments once/week–once/month following acute course of ECT to prevent relapse.

*Maintenance ECT:* Extension of continuation ECT beyond 6 months.

## Repetitive Transcranial Magnetic Stimulation (rTMS)

In rTMS, a magnetic field penetrates the scalp and skull unattenuated because these tissues are nonconducting, and depolarization of the neural tissue just under the coil is induced perpendicular to the magnetic field. Local action potentials propagate to other parts of the brain along existing neural networks.

Because magnetic field declines with square of distance from coil, rTMS stimulates superficial levels of cortex. However, rTMS applied to the cortex stimulates cortical–limbic connections. It is not clear whether this is actually the therapeutic mechanism of the treatment.

- Prefrontal rTMS
  - Modulates frontal–limbic circuits that are abnormal in major depression.
  - Promotes subcortical dopamine release.
  - Acts on the HPA (hypothalamic–pituitary–adrenal) axis.
- Slow rTMS (1 Hz) decreases cortical excitability and regional blood flow, and the inhibition spreads to other areas, whereas fast rTMS ($\geq$ 10 Hz) increases amplitude of motor-evoked potentials (Gershon, Dannon, & Grunhaus, 2003).
  - Depressed patients who respond well to one frequency do poorly with the other.
  - If depression is associated with relative hypofunction of the left frontal lobe, left excitatory stimuli or right inhibitory stimuli would be expected to reduce depression.

- Other patients might have the reverse pattern of lateralization and respond to inhibitory stimulus to left prefrontal cortex or excitatory stimulus to the right.
- Slow rTMS is approved by the FDA but is less reliable than fast rTMS (10–20 Hz), which is not yet approved by the FDA and therefore is an experimental treatment.
- Dosing approach uses motor threshold (MT).
  - MT is the minimum amount of current necessary to produce movement of the contralateral thumb when coil is placed over the primary motor cortex.
    - Assessed with an electromyography or visual observation.
- The best results in treatment of depression with fast rTMS appear to be correlated with daily left prefrontal stimulation (Gershon et al., 2003).
  - However, it is often difficult to place the coil precisely over the left dorsolateral prefrontal cortex without using MRI.
- A group of patients who requested ECT was randomly assigned to ECT or rTMS (Grunhaus, Dolberg, Polak, & Dannon, 2002). ECT was superior to rTMS for psychotically depressed patients, and the two treatments were similarly effective for nonpsychotic patients. The absence of a control group limited interpretation of the results.
  - It is not clear whether rTMS is less effective for psychotic depression or whether different parameters are necessary for response of psychotic depression (e.g., higher frequency, longer treatment; Gershon et al., 2003).
- A meta-analysis of 10 published double-blind studies using left prefrontal rTMS found an effect size of 0.53 in major depression (Kozel & George, 2002).
  - Taken together, published meta-analyses suggest an overall effect size of 0.65.
    - Represents a moderate effect similar to the results of antidepressant trials.
- Four studies compared ECT and fast rTMS to the left prefrontal cortex (Gershon et al., 2003). Response rates in the four studies were
  - 45–69% with rTMS
  - 56–80% with ECT
- Parameters associated with a better response in pooled data from available studies (Gershon et al., 2003):
  - Treatment administered for > 10 days.
  - More intense magnetic pulse administered: 100–110% of motor threshold.
  - More pulses per day administered: 1200–1600 pulses/day.

- Six months following an acute course of ECT or rTMS, patients maintained on similar medication regimens had equivalent low relapse rates (about 20%; Dannon, Dolberg, & Schreiber, 2002).
- There is limited information about the use of rTMS in bipolar disorder, but preliminary experience suggests that it may be helpful.
  - Mania has been treated with fast rTMS to right prefrontal cortex.
    - On the other hand, rTMS may induce mania in some patients.
  - A randomized trial in 23 patients with bipolar I or II depression found no antidepressant effect over 2 weeks of left prefrontal rTMS or sham treatment (Nahas, Kozel, Li, Anderson, & George, 2003).
  - In 25 hospitalized manic patients, there was no benefit either of right prefrontal rTMS or sham treatment (Kapstan, Yaroslavsky, Applebaum, Belmaker, & Grisaru, 2003).
- 1 Hz rTMS for 15 minutes reduces activity in the brain area that is directly stimulated and in functionally connected areas.
  - During auditory hallucinations, the left temporoparietal region is activated.
  - 24 patients with schizophrenia or schizoaffective disorder and medication-resistant auditory hallucinations were randomly assigned to 9 days of sham rTMS or 1 Hz rTMS for 8–16 minutes to the left temporoparietal cortex at 90% of motor threshold (Hoffman et al., 2003).
  - Reductions in frequency and severity of hallucinations were significantly better with real than with sham rTMS, and improvement was maintained for 15 weeks in 52% of patients.
- Adverse effects
  - Headache
  - Seizures reported in 12 patients.
    - Seizure risk may be higher in patients with a history of epilepsy, although attempts to induce seizures in epileptic patients have not been successful.
  - Peak magnetic field strength is equivalent to an MRI (2 tesla).
    - No evidence of neuronal damage
    - No cognitive impairment
  - As with MRI, patients with metallic or electronic implants should not receive rTMS because the magnetic field may exert torque on the implant and cause bleeding.

## MAGNETIC SEIZURE THERAPY

- rTMS is used to induce a seizure.
- Because magnetic fields pass through tissue unimpeded, the stimulus can be focused on relevant brain areas, thereby reducing spread to medial–temporal structures involved in the cognitive side effects of ECT.

- Uses general anesthesia and muscle relaxant.
- No controlled efficacy studies, but a feasibility study showed less robust seizures than ECT, with less cognitive impairment (Lisanby, 2002).

ARTIFICIAL BRIGHT LIGHT

- Bright-light therapy is as effective as antidepressants for seasonal affective disorder (SAD).
- Helpful for seasonal exacerbation of chronic depression.
- Sometimes effective for bipolar depression.
- Minimum effective intensity is 2500 lux.
  - Intensity of 10,000 lux requires shorter duration of exposure to light.
    - 30 minutes vs. 2 hours for 2500 lux
- Begin with administration of light in the morning, especially for patients who tend to sleep late.
- Response usually occurs within 3–5 days of starting light.
- Relapse develops 1–3 days after discontinuing light.
- Starting light when days get shorter (e.g., September) and continuing until days get longer (e.g., April) prevents recurrence of winter depression.
- Use of artificial bright light to treat sleep-phase changes.
  - The best cue to the sleep–wake cycle is exposure to bright light in the morning.
  - Hypnotics may induce sleep but do not change the time the patient's brain wakes up.
  - Sleep-phase delay is treated with morning bright light or exposure to bright light as sleep is delayed around the clock to a normal hour (see pp. 433–435).
  - Sleep-phase advance is treated with morning bright light moved gradually later each day.
  - Some people who work at night and sleep during the day never entrain their sleep to the new schedule.
    - Exposure to bright light upon awakening to go to work can improve alertness and productivity.
  - To treat jet lag:
    - Traveling west to east over multiple time zones (overnight flight): (1) Go to sleep at the time corresponding to bedtime at the new time zone; (2) wake up at the time of waking at the new time zone; (3) use artificial bright light or go out in the sun as soon as is practical upon arrival in the morning; and (4) do not take a nap the first day in the new time zone.

- Traveling east to west over multiple time zones (overnight): (1) Go to sleep at the time corresponding to the new time zone (usually soon after take-off); (2) wake up at the time corresponding to the time of waking in the new time zone; (3) stay awake until the new bedtime; and (4) use artificial bright light or go out in the sun the next morning.
- Use of artificial bright light to treat demented patients:
  - Increased confusion/agitation at night and somnolence during day indicates reversal of sleep–wake cycle.
  - Exposure to bright light in the morning improves sleep at night and reduces daytime confusion.

## Vagus Nerve Stimulation (VNS)

- VNS is approved for the treatment of refractory epilepsy and has been used in over 13,000 patients.
  - Hyperpolarizes neurons.
  - Mechanism of action in epilepsy unknown.
  - Median reduction in seizure frequency with high-stimulation VNS at 3 and 12 months is 34% and 45%, respectively (Schacter, 2002).
  - Improves mood in patients treated for epilepsy.
  - The vagus nerve has afferent connections to limbic and cortical regions.
  - Approved in the European Union for major depressive episode in adults.
- VNS was studied openly in 30 outpatients with unipolar or bipolar depression refractory to at least two robust medication trials or ECT (Rush et al., 2000).
  - Single-blind run-in with no stimulation followed by 10 weeks of VNS
  - 40% responded by HRSD and CGI and 50% by Montgomery Asberg Depression Rating Scale (MADRS) scores.
- In an open study of VNS in 59 patients with major depressive episodes refractory to an average of 4.8 treatments, patients on stable medication regimens received 2 weeks with no stimulation after implantation of the device, followed by 10 weeks of VNS (Sackeim et al., 2001).
  - Response rate was 31% for HRSD, 34% for MADRS, and 37% for CGI.
  - Patients who had never received ECT were four times as likely to respond.
  - No patients who had failed to respond to seven adequate antidepressant trials responded to VNS, vs. 39% of the remaining patients.
  - VNS therefore was not beneficial for patients with severe treatment resistance.

- In 30 outpatients with treatment-resistant nonpsychotic major depressive episodes who received open treatment with 3 months of acute VNS followed by 9 months of maintenance VNS (Marangell et al., 2002):
  - Response rate remained about the same (40% and 46%, $p$ = NS) over the extended treatment.
  - Remission rate (HRSD score ≤ 10) increased from 17% to 29% ($p$ = 0.045).
  - Functioning improved over the year of total treatment.
- A 10-week industry-sponsored double-blind study found VNS to be no better than sham treatment for the primary outcome measure in major depression (Carpenter, Friehs, & Price, 2003).
  - Stimulus intensity may have been too low.
- Difference between negative findings in a controlled study and positive findings in longer open studies suggests that VNS may be effective for selected patients, but the benefit may not be evident for a year.
- Use of VNS for dementia is discussed on page 101.
- Adverse effects
  - Transient asystole during implantation
    - No arrhythmias reported with long-term treatment.
  - Hoarseness common
  - No cognitive side effects

## SLEEP DEPRIVATION

- Sleep deprivation produces improvement in depression the next day.
- Similar benefit with sleep deprivation for entire night or second half of night.
- Depression returns with recovery sleep.

### Summary of Antidepressant Treatment Choices

## UNCOMPLICATED OUTPATIENT DEPRESSION

- SSRI
- Bupropion SR
- Venlafaxine XR

## SEVERE DEPRESSION

- Venlafaxine
- Nefazodone
- Mirtazepine
- TCA
- ECT

PSYCHOTIC DEPRESSION: ECT OR ANTIPSYCHOTIC DRUG PLUS

- TCA
- Venlafaxine
- Nefazodone
- Mirtazepine

BIPOLAR DEPRESSION (also see Chapters 5 & 6)

- Artificial bright light
- Lamotrigine
- Stimulant
- Bupropion
- Short-acting SSRI
- MAOI

SEASONAL AFFECTIVE DISORDER (SAD)

- Artificial bright light (also see pp. 157–158)
- Bupropion
- SSRI

DEPRESSION WITH ANXIETY

- SSRI
- Nefazodone
- Mirtazepine
- Venlafaxine
- MAOI
- Increase antidepressant dose very slowly (e.g., 1–5 mg of fluoxetine).
- Start benzodiazepine or buspirone first; add antidepressant after anxiety decreases.
    - Findings of a review of all published randomized controlled trials of antidepressant–benzodiazepine combinations vs. antidepressants alone for adults with major depression, including data from nine studies involving 679 patients (no trial lasted longer than 8 weeks; Furukawa, Streiner, & Young, 2002):
        - Combination therapy resulted in decreased likelihood of dropping out of treatment (RR 0.63) because patients had fewer side effects to antidepressants.
        - A response was more likely with combination therapy (RR 1.63 at 1 week and 1.38 at 4 weeks), in part, because those who dropped out had the worst outcome.

- Differences between combination treatment and antidepressant alone were no longer significant after 6–8 weeks.
- Adding a benzodiazepine can keep depressed patients in treatment until they respond, and until tolerance develops to activation caused by antidepressant.
- A double-blind study of augmentation of 20 mg fluoxetine with placebo or 0.5–1 mg clonazepam for 18 weeks found earlier reduction of depression, better reduction of insomnia, and reduced side effects associated with increasing the fluoxetine dose, but no extended effect on anxiety or core depressive symptoms (Smith, Londborg, Glaudin, & Painter, 2002b).

## Depression with Rumination

- SSRI

## Major Depression with Schizophrenia

- Depressive symptoms occur in ⅓–½ of patients with schizophrenia.
- A review of 11 controlled studies, each with < 30 patients/group, suggested that antidepressants were statistically significantly better than placebo in some of these trials in reducing depressive symptoms in schizophrenia, mostly right after an acute psychotic episode (Whitehead, Moss, Cardno, & Lewis, 2002).
  - There was no evidence that antidepressants worsened psychotic symptoms.

## Depression and Chronic Medical Illness

- Cytokine immunotherapy for cancer and hepatitis C frequently induces depression, possibly because of effects of cytokines on mood.
  - Antidepressants can reverse this depression, reduce production of pro-inflammatory cytokines, and decrease production of anti-inflammatory cytokines (Capuron, Hauser, Hinze-Selch, Miller, & Neveu, 2002).
- SSRIs improve glycemic control in depressed diabetic patients, probably because of better compliance.
- Findings of a meta-analysis of 18 randomized trials of patients with cancer, diabetes, head injury, heart disease, HIV disease, MS (multiple sclerosis), renal disease, and stroke found (Gill & Hatcher 2002)
  - Antidepressants significantly > placebo.
  - Medications studied:
    - SSRIs: 6 studies
    - TCAs: 9 studies
    - Other new antidepressants: 3 studies

- Four patients would have to be treated to produce one recovery from depression that would not occur with placebo.
- Ten patients would have to be treated to produce one dropout that would not occur with placebo.
- TCAs slightly more effective than SSRIs, but slightly less well tolerated.
- Depression remits on discharge in 50% of medical inpatients.
- Do not defer treatment of depression if patient remains ill.
- Stimulants rapidly effective and well tolerated.
  - Tolerance to antidepressant effect develops after a few months, but patient may remain well if illness improves.
- SSRIs good initial choices.
  - Monitor interactions with drugs for the medical illness.
- Bupropion and venlafaxine do not have clinically significant P450 effects.

## Depression in Demented Patients

- Bupropion
- Venlafaxine
- Stimulant
- SSRI other than paroxetine
- Selegiline (if patient can remember diet)
- ECT not contraindicated

## Depression in Patients with Cancer

- Mirtazepine
- SSRI
- Bupropion

## Depression and Fatigue in HIV Patients

- Bupropion
- Stimulant (if no history of substance abuse)
- Mirtazepine
- Nefazodone
- MAO inhibitor

## Depression with Parkinson's Disease

- Selegiline (see pp. 218–219)
  - Higher doses may interact with L-dopa.
- SSRI may aggravate parkinsonism.

- Bupropion theoretically helpful for parkinsonism but sometimes exacerbates symptoms.
- Nefazodone
- Trazodone
- ECT treats both depression and on–off phenomenon in Parkinson's disease.
- rTMS has seemed helpful for parkinsonism in a few reports.

### DEPRESSION AND MIGRAINE

- $5HT_2$ antagonists reduce vasoconstriction and platelet aggregation.
  - Trazodone
  - Nefazodone
  - Mirtazepine
  - TCAs
- Variable effect of SSRIs
  - Blockade of platelet serotonin uptake may reduce migraines.
  - Serotonergic effect may stimulate platelets and increase migraines.

### DEPRESSION IN PATIENTS WITH HYPERTENSION

- Captopril
  - Only antihypertensive with reports of antidepressant effect
- Pindolol
  - Early experience suggesting augmentation of antidepressants not clearly confirmed.
- Propranolol may not increase depression, but it does cause lethargy, sexual dysfunction.
- Avoid methyldopa, reserpine.
- SSRI
- Nefazodone, trazodone
- MAOI lowers blood pressure if diet is followed.
- Blood pressure may be increased by TCAs, bupropion, venlafaxine, mirtazepine.

### DEPRESSION AND STROKE

- Left-sided stroke more frequently associated with depression.
- SSRIs
  - Positive studies of citalopram, sertraline, fluoxetine
  - Mixed effect on platelet aggregation
    - Bleeding or thrombosis
- Bupropion
  - May improve cognitive function.

- Check blood pressure.
- TCAs
  - Nortriptyline repeatedly demonstrated effective.
  - Not as well tolerated.
- MAO inhibitors
  - Selegiline may be neuroprotective.
  - Stimulant effect may improve cognition.
  - Hypertension can be a problem.

### DEPRESSION AND EPILEPSY

- MAOI
- SSRI
  - May alter anticonvulsant level.
- Gabapentin
- Lamotrizine
- ECT
  - Raises seizure threshold.
  - Anticonvulsants may interfere with antidepressant action.
- Avoid amoxapine, maprotiline, bupropion, tertiary amine TCAs.

### DEPRESSION AND TRAUMATIC BRAIN INJURY (TBI)

- SSRIs may reduce impulsivity and irritability as well as depression.
- Venlafaxine may improve cognition.
- Moclobemide (reversible MAO inhibitor not available in United States) found effective for depression in TBI.
- Bupropion well tolerated if no seizure risk.
- Increased risk of serious adverse events with TCAs.
  - Seizures in as many as 20%
  - Anticholinergic effects further impair cognition.

### DEPRESSION AND CHRONIC PAIN (SEE PP. 133–134)

- TCAs most effective for chronic pain.
  - Additive effect with analgesics.
- Venlafoxine, nefazodone & duloxetine may be useful

### DEPRESSION WITH SOMATIZATION

- SSRIs may reduce rumination and preoccupation with minor physical symptoms.

### POSTPARTUM DEPRESSION

- Exclude bipolar disorder.
- Dopaminergic agents (e.g., bupropion) may inhibit lactation.

- SSRIs may increase lactation due to antidopaminergic effect.
- Breast milk concentrations of antidepressants are 50–100% of serum levels.
  - Actual dose to nursing infant usually very low, with serum levels < threshold for detection.
  - Lower milk:serum ratio with drugs that are
    - Less lipid soluble
    - More protein bound (protein concentration is higher in serum than milk)
  - Milk: plasma ratio low for sertraline and paroxetine.
    - Higher with fluoxetine
  - Study of nursing mothers taking 50–200 mg of sertraline and their infants (Epperson et al., 2001) found:
    - 70–90% reduction of maternal platelet serotonin levels
    - No change in infant platelet serotonin
    - Maternal levels of sertraline and desmethyl-sertraline 31 and 45 ng/mL
    - Infant levels undetectable
  - Prospective study of infant, maternal, and breast milk fluoxetine levels in 11 women taking 20–40 mg fluoxetine (Heikkinen, Ekblad, Kero, Ekblad, & Laine, 2003):
    - Mean estimated daily maternal-weight-adjusted daily dose of fluoxetine to nursing infants was 2.4% at 2 weeks and 3.8% at 2 months.
    - Infant fluoxetine and norfluoxetine levels decreased from 65–72% at birth to below the limit of detection over several months.
    - No adverse effects or developmental abnormalities were noted over 1 year of follow-up.
  - Occasional oversedation and respiratory depression seen when mother takes doxepin.
  - Occasional colic seen with SSRI exposure.
- Use a single medication at the lowest effective dose.
- Use short half-life antidepressant.
- Nurse baby before taking antidepressant.

### Treatment Refractoriness

About 60% of depressed patients respond to a given antidepressant. The rate of remission is lower (around 30–50%), partly because patients are often undertreated. Treatment to remission is important because residual symptoms increase the risk of relapse and recurrence; social dysfunction is a common residual symptom. Most antidepressant studies emphasize symptomatic but not psychosocial remission.

Questions to ask when a depressed patient has had an inadequate response to an antidepressant include the following:

- Is the dose sufficient?
    - Even though SSRIs have simpler dosing schedules, the range of effective doses can be significant.
    - Divided dosing necessary for trazodone, nefazodone, bupropion, venlafaxine, fluvoxamine.
- Is the patient taking the medication?
    - Rates of nonadherence in depressed patients average 50%.
    - Common causes of nonadherence include:
        - Medication cost
        - Problems authorizing refills through managed care company
        - Complicated regiments
        - Side effects
        - Belief that medications only have to be taken if patient feels depressed that day.
        - Reluctance to depend on medications or the person who prescribes them.
- Is the diagnosis accurate?
    - Depressed mood may occur in
        - Personality disorders
        - PTSD
        - Anxiety disorders
        - Schizophrenia
- Is the patient using a substance that interferes with the antidepressant?
    - Alcohol is the most common self-treatment for depression.
        - Directly induces depression and accelerates antidepressant metabolism.
    - Stimulants cause withdrawal and rebound depression.
- Are psychotic features present?
    - Patient may not report, or may even conceal, psychosis.
    - Antipsychotic drug usually must be added to antidepressant.
    - Clues to covert psychosis in a depressed patient:
        - Severity
        - Confusion
        - Gross pseudodementia
        - Idiosyncratic thought

- Marked agitation or psychomotor retardation
- Dissociation without abuse
- Post-dexamethasone cortisol $> 10$
- REM latency $< 20$ minutes
- Is the depression bipolar?
  - An antidepressant produces initial improvement followed by increased depression, often mixed with dysphoric hypomania (see pp. 263–270).
  - Clues to bipolarity:
    - Early onset
    - High rate of recurrence
    - Sluggish, hypersomnic depression in adult
    - Increased recurrences on antidepressants
    - Abrupt onset
    - Intense irritability
    - Extreme interpersonal sensitivity
    - Overstimulation in interactions
    - Psychosis before age 50
    - Mood-incongruent psychotic symptoms
    - Hallucinations without delusions
    - Appearance and behavior not as bad as subjective depression
    - Family history of mood disorder in three consecutive generations
- Are psychological issues being ignored?
  - Antidepressant alone effective for milder forms of depression.
    - More severe and complex depression usually requires psychotherapy and antidepressant.
  - Patients who feel that clinician only wants to hear about target symptoms for medication may emphasize these symptoms to communicate lack of response of psychosocial dimensions of depression.
- Is the patient's family involved?
  - Family members may either facilitate or interfere with treatment.
  - Relatives and spouses of depressed people are more likely to be depressed themselves.

## TREATING INADEQUATE RESPONSE

- Treat substance abuse before, or concomitant with, treating depression.
- Augmentation of antidepressant vs. changing antidepressant:
  - No proven rationale for one over the other.
  - Augmentation may work better when there has been a partial response.

- Changing antidepressant may be indicated when no response at all has occurred.

## AUGMENTATION STRATEGIES

### Lithium

- Best studied augmenting agent.
- More effective in bipolar than unipolar depression.
- Improves antidepressant response in ⅓–⅔ of patients.
- Some patients respond to low doses (300–600 mg); some require usual therapeutic levels.
- Response occurs in 2–4 weeks.

### Buspirone

- Has antidepressant properties at doses of 45–90 mg/day.
- Most useful for anxious depression.

### Stimulant

- Most useful in geriatric depression and depression in brain-damaged patients.
- Can also be used to treat sedative side effects and elevate serum level of medications patient has difficulty tolerating at therapeutic doses.
    - Eliminates some side effects associated with first-pass metabolism.
    - May increase nortriptyline or desipramine level outside therapeutic range.
- Usual doses for augmentation:
    - Methylphenidate 10–30 mg/day
    - Dextroamphetamine 5–20 mg/day

### Thyroid supplementation

- Adding thyroxine is most useful for hypothyroid patients.
    - Some patients with low-normal T4 and non-suppressed TSH have subclinical hypothyroidism demonstrated on TRH stimulation test.
    - Some euthyroid patients become more depressed with addition of thyroxine.
- $T_3$ 25–50 μg/day has been found to augment partial antidepressant response in 50% of patients.
    - Most studies and reports did not control for subclinical hypothyroidism.
    - Many studies did not allow sufficient time on antidepressant alone to be certain that longer duration without augmentation would not have been effective.
- Chronic treatment with $T_3$ results in suppressed serum TSH and $T_4$ and increased serum $T_3$.

Anticonvulsant

- Carbamazepine reported to augment antidepressants in some cases of unipolar depression.
- Gabapentin has antianxiety and antidepressant properties useful for augmenting antidepressant in anxious depression.
  - Usual dose 900–3600 mg/day given tid.
- Lamotrigine 100–200 mg/day sometimes augments antidepressant.
  - Retrospective chart review of 37 patients with chronic or recurrent major depression, who had not responded to an average of 13 previous antidepressant trials (Barbee & Jamhour, 2002), revealed that
    - Adding lamotrigine (mean dose 113 mg) to antidepressants produced much or very much improvement in 41% and mild improvement in 22%, using intent-to-treat analysis.
  - 40 patients with major depressive episode taking paroxetine had lamotrigine 200 mg/day or placebo added for 9 weeks (Normann et al., 2002).
    - Adjunctive lamotrigine with paroxetine did not decrease HRSD scores significantly, compared with paroxetine plus placebo.
    - However, lamotrigine did produce significantly greater reduction of depressed mood, guilt, and work and interest, and of the CGI severity of illness scale.
    - Superiority to placebo might not have been demonstrated because all patients had decreased depression, and patients were not truly refractory.
  - Another prospective study randomly assigned 23 inpatients with a major depressive episode (8 bipolar, 15 unipolar) refractory to at least one prior antidepressant trial and taking 20 mg/day fluoxetine to 6 weeks addition of placebo or lamotrigine 100 mg/day (Barbee & Jamhour, 2002):
    - The lamotrigine group had significantly greater improvement, measured by CGI-I.
    - However, there were no differences between groups in final depression rating scale scores.
- Valproate is usually not effective.

Testosterone

- 19 men (mean age 47) with at least 4 weeks persistence of major depression, despite adequate antidepressant dose who had low or borderline serum testosterone and normal prostate specific antigen (PSA) received addition of either 8 weeks of testosterone gel or placebo gel (Pope, Cohane, Kanayama, Siegel, & Hudson, 2003).
  - Starting testosterone dose 10 gm/day for 1 week, then reduced to 7.5 gm/day if testosterone levels increased too much.

- Testosterone augmentation was associated with significantly greater reductions of HRSD and CGI severity scores. There was similar reduction in psychological symptoms such as depressed mood and guilt and vegetative symptoms such as sleep, appetite, and libido.
- Risks of testosterone treatment include benign prostatic hypertrophy (BPH), oligospermia, cancer, hyperlipidemia, aggression, psychosis, paranoia.

Antipsychotic
- Usually necessary for psychotic depression.
  - The antipsychotic dose may need to be higher in psychotic depression than in schizophrenia.
    - For example, 30–80 mg perphenazine equivalent (Dubovsky & Thomas, 1992).
  - No controlled studies of atypical antipsychotics, but accumulating experience (Wheeler et al., 2000) indicates that these are still first choices in psychotic depression because of
    - Antidepressant as well as antipsychotic effect
    - Better tolerability
    - Low doses of atypicals may be more effective than low doses of neuroleptics in psychotic depression.

Some patients with refractory nonpsychotic depression respond to augmentation with an atypical antipsychotic medication.
- An open-label 76-week multicenter study conducted by the manufacturer followed 560 patients with major depressive disorder, 145 or 26% of whom had failed to respond to at least two adequate antidepressant trials (Corya et al., 2003).
  - Patients received a combination of olanzapine and fluoxetine.
    - Starting doses 6 mg olanzapine + 25 mg fluoxetine
    - Dose then adjusted according to clinician preference to 6, 12, or 18 mg/day olanzapine + 25, 50, or 75 mg fluoxetine.
  - Response defined as ≥ 50% decrease in MADRS score.
  - Remission defined as MADRS score ≤ 8.
  - Relapse defined as MADRS ≥ 16 after first meeting remission criterion.
  - In the treatment-resistant group
    - 53% response rate
    - 44% remission rate
    - 25% relapse rate
  - Mean weight gain was 5.6 kg.
    - 31% gained ≥ 10% of their baseline body weight.

- Methodological limitations:
  - Aggressiveness of previous antidepressant trials not assessed.
  - Responders not characterized precisely.

No clearly demonstrated predictors of benefit from antipsychotic drug, but features associated with psychosis may be indicators.
- Failure to respond to multiple antidepressant trials
- Severe symptoms
- Dissociation without significant history of abuse
- Gross psychomotor changes
- Marked pseudodementia
- Pervasive rumination
- Post-dexamethasone cortisol $> 10$ μg/dL

### Pindolol
- Improved speed of antidepressant response and augmented antidepressants in some case series.
- Usual dose 2.5–5 mg bid–tid.
- Potentially useful for patients with hypertension or migraine.
- Recent studies have been negative.

### Testosterone
- Discussed on pages 522–524.

### Dopamine receptor agonist: pramipexole, bromocriptine, pergolide
- Useful for anergic, withdrawn depression and possibly for bipolar depression.
- Of 37 inpatients with refractory major depression (16 unipolar, 21 bipolar) who received addition of pramipexole (mean dose 0.95 mg/day) to a TCA or an SSRI, 31 had at least some treatment and 19 completed a 16-week trial (Lattanzi et al., 2002).
  - Mean MADRS scores decreased from 33 to 14, and 68–74% responded.
- A randomized double-blind trial in 174 patients with nonpsychotic major depression compared pramipexole 0.375, 1, or 5 mg and fluoxetine 20 mg (Corrigan, Denahan, Wright, Ragual, & Evans, 2000):
  - By week 8, 1 mg pramipexole produced significant improvement compared with placebo and similar to fluoxetine.
  - Pramipexole 5 mg was more effective but had such a high dropout rate that statistical comparison could not be done.
- No controlled studies
- May cause agitation of psychosis.

Mifepristone (RU-486)

- Progesterone antagonist at low doses and glucocorticoid receptor antagonist at higher doses.
- 30 psychotically depressed patients at six sites had open addition to antidepressant treatment for 1 week of mifepristone in doses of 50 mg (at which dose it antagonizes progesterone but not glucocorticoids), 600 mg, or 1200 mg (Belanoff et al., 2002).
  - Serum cortisol levels increased significantly more in the higher-dose groups, indicating successful blockade of cortisol receptors and decreased feedback inhibition.
  - 68% of patients who received the two higher doses had at least a 30% reduction in BPRS scores, and 63% had a decrease of at least 50% on positive symptoms on the BPRS.
    - Only 36% of low-dose patients had a 30% BPRS reduction, and only 27% had a 50% decrease in positive symptoms.
  - A response ($\geq$ 50% decrease in HRSD scores) of depression occurred in 42% of high-dose patients vs. 18% of low-dose patients.
- Probably not a practical long-term treatment.

ANTIDEPRESSANT COMBINATIONS

TCA + SSRI

- Low dose of one can improve response to therapeutic dose of the other.
  - For example, 10–25 mg nortriptyline + 200 mg sertraline, or 25–50 mg sertraline + 75 mg nortriptyline.
- Fluoxetine and paroxetine are likely to raise TCA levels significantly.

Mirtazepine + other antidepressant

- 26 patients with major depression unresponsive to an antidepressant at maximum tolerated dose of SSRIs, bupropion, or effexor for at least 4 weeks had random double-blind addition of 15 or 30 mg of mirtazepine or placebo for 4 weeks (Carpenter, Yasmin, & Price, 2002).
  - Significantly more patients responded to mirtazepine than placebo (64% vs. 20%).
  - Mirtazepine augmentation also resulted in significantly better improvement of functioning and quality of life.

TCA + MAOI

- Combination not found superior to TCA or MAOI alone.
  - However, these findings come from studies of patients who did not have refractory depression and were randomly assigned to either medication alone or to both.
    - Response rate was too high to detect additional contribution from the combination.

- TCA + MAOI combination produces more complete response in some refractory cases.
- Any TCA, except imipramine and clomipramine, can be combined with MAOIs.
- Serotonergic interactions contraindicate adding new antidepressants with MAOIs.
  - Possible risk of hypertensive interactions is a likely contraindication to combining bupropion and any MAOI.
- Start both medications together or add the MAOI to the TCA.
  - Severe interactions have occurred when a TCA is added to an MAOI.
- Increase doses of both medications gradually.
- TCA–MAOI combination can be augmented with stimulant, lithium, or anticonvulsant but not with buspirone.

A review of 27 studies of antidepressant combinations in refractory depression, including 5 randomized, controlled trials and 22 open-label trials (Lam, Wan, Cohen, & Kennedy, 2002), found evidence in favor of

- *MAOI + TCA:* 48–70% response rate, but a long-term study found only 50% continued to respond after 3 years.
- *SSRI + TCA:* response rate 35–65%
- *Two SSRIs:* Two small studies (six and seven patients) showed response of 85–100%, but a second SSRI was added about 3 weeks after starting the first one.
  - Improvement could be attributed to the initial antidepressant alone.
- *Bupropion + SSRI or venlafaxine:* Case series suggest superiority to monotherapy, with response rate 74–83%.
- *Venlafaxine + TCA:* Addition of venlafaxine 75–300 mg to TCA administered for 2 months resulted in 82% response rate and 64% rate of remission.
  - It is possible that improvement would have been similar with venlafaxine alone.

CHANGING ANTIDEPRESSANTS

- How to change antidepressants:
  - No rationale for NE–5HT switch.
  - Switching between SSRIs may work.
  - Try something with a different structure.
  - Consider venlafaxine if one or two other antidepressants have been ineffective.
- Duloxetine
  - No direct comparisons or controlled studies in refractory depression.

- Unless a serotonergic antidepressant is being changed to an MAOI, the new antidepressant can usually be overlapped with the old one.
  - Reduces rebound depression when ineffective antidepressant is withdrawn.
  - Permits determining whether new antidepressant will be tolerated before old antidepressant is discontinued.
  - Mild serotonin syndrome may occur when two serotonergic medications are combined.
  - Gradually increase the dose of the new medication and slowly discontinue the old one.

## ECT in Refractory Depression

- Response rate is only 50%.
- Use stimulus intensity at least three times seizure threshold for unipolar depression.
- Possibly need for lower stimulus intensity for bipolar depression.
- Bilateral ECT especially useful for bipolar depression.
- Use longer trial with less frequent treatments.
- Confusion can aggravate or mimic depression.
- Stop antidepressants.
- Try again 6 months later.
  - A second trial is sometimes effective after an initial course of ECT does not work.

## MAINTENANCE THERAPY

Antidepressants facilitate remission but do not alter its time course. In unipolar depression, the antidepressant therefore should be continued until the depression would have been expected to remit anyway—usually about 6–9 months. Maintenance antidepressants clearly reduce the risk of a recurrence, but some patients wish to discontinue treatment once they feel well. The decision about maintenance antidepressant therapy depends on several factors:

- The need for ongoing treatment may not be compelling following a single episode of nonpsychotic depression that has not been accompanied by significant suicidality or self-defeating behavior.
- After a third major depressive episode, further recurrences are virtually inevitable if an effective antidepressant is withdrawn.
  - The potential benefit outweighs the risk of the medication.
- If a single major depressive episode was psychotic, caused a dangerous suicide attempt, was very difficult to treat, or had catastrophic psycho-

social consequences (e.g., impulsively quitting a job or getting a divorce), the potential benefit of preventing a recurrence is greater than the trouble of continuing an antidepressant.

- Any residual symptoms, including subtle symptoms such as poor role adjustment, anhedonia, and insomnia, increase the risk of major relapse if the antidepressant is withdrawn.
  - These residual symptoms are indications for more aggressive acute treatment and for maintenance therapy.
    - "Blips" in mood that represent normal reactions to stress do not increase the risk of relapse, but distinct depressive symptoms in response to stress or hormonal changes (e.g., premenstrual depression) are indications that the physiology of depression is not fully remitted.
- Persistent DST nonsuppression increases the risk of relapse if an antidepressant is withdrawn.
- Significant adverse reactions may be an indication to withdraw or at least change the antidepressant.

Maintenance antidepressant treatment should be considered for

- Recurrent unipolar depression
- Chronic depression
- A single severe or psychotic major depressive episode
- Residual symptoms

### Principles of Maintenance for Antidepressant Treatment

- The therapeutic dose is usually the antidepressant dose.
  - Reducing the antidepressant dose after remission increases the risk of recurrence
- Eliminate all symptoms as completely as possible.
  - Major depression is more likely to recur even with a therapeutic maintenance regimen if mild symptoms or role dysfunction remain.
- Discuss adherence in advance.
  - Many patients stop antidepressants or take them irregularly once they feel better.
  - If adverse effects will limit compliance, gradually change to an antidepressant the patient can tolerate.
- When an antipsychotic drug is necessary acutely:
  - Discontinuing or reducing dose of neuroleptic within a year of remission was associated with relapse of psychotic depression in a retrospective review (Aronson et al., 1988).
    - Depression may relapse without psychosis.
    - Restarting neuroleptic not always effective.

- Another study suggested that the antipsychotic drug may be withdrawn sooner in some patients (Rothschild & Duval 2003).
  - 40 patients with unipolar psychotic depression who had not previously been unresponsive to SSRIs were treated openly with 20 mg of fluoxetine (increased to 40 mg if no response within 3 weeks) and up to 32 mg of perphenazine.
  - After 5 weeks of a mean of 32 mg fluoxetine and 31 mg perphenazine, 30 patients (75%) had 50% decrease in HRSD and BPRS scores, a final HRSD < 12, and no psychotic symptoms.
  - In patients who continued to meet response criteria for a total of 4 months of combination therapy, the perphenazine dose was decreased by 25%/week over the next month.
  - After taper of perphenazine, 73% of the responders had no signs of relapse over the next 11 months.
  - The 27% who relapsed responded to readdition of perphenazine.
- Risk of neurological side effects is increased in depression compared with schizophrenia, especially with the higher neuroleptic doses that may be necessary for psychotic depression.
- Attempt to reduce antipsychotic dose very slowly (e.g., 1–2 mg/perhpenazine equivalent every 2–4 weeks) 1 year after remission.
- Continue antidepressant indefinitely for psychotic unipolar depression.

Maintenance augmentation
- There are few controlled discontinuation studies to guide duration of augmentation.
- Lithium (mean dose 348 mg/day, serum level 0.3–0.7) added to antidepressant reduced relapse rates > placebo in depressed elderly patients following a major depressive episode (Wilkinson, Holmes, Woolford, & Stammers, 2002).
- Stimulants and lithium can sometimes be withdrawn 3 months after remission.
- If it is well tolerated, the augmenting agent generally should be continued indefinitely with the antidepressant.
- *Maintenance antipsychotic medication in psychotic depression:*
  - In an open trial of fluoxetine + perphenazine for 5 weeks in 30 patients with psychotic depression (Rothschild et al., 1993b):
    - 22 patients (73%) did not relapse and were continued on fluoxetine monotherapy for another 8 months (Rothschild, Samson, Bessette, & Carter-Campbell, 1993a).
    - 8 patients relapsed and were restarted on perphenazine.
    - 5 remained relapse-free when perphenazine was withdrawn after 8 months.

- *Maintenance antipsychotic medication in nonpsychotic depression:* A chart review identified 55 nonpsychotically unipolar depressed patients who were taking low doses of maintenance neuroleptics (Mortimer, Martin, Wheeler, & Tyson, 2003).
  - 40 patients were contacted by the authors 12–18 months after the chart audit.
  - 25 had discontinued the neuroleptic.
  - Patients who continued the neuroleptic had been ill for more than twice as long as those who discontinued it.
  - Patients who discontinued the neuroleptic were significantly less symptomatic and had fewer side effects than those who continued it.
    - This could reflect a more severe illness in patients who still needed a neuroleptic.
    - However, after the neuroleptic was discontinued in 13 of the 15 patients who were still taking that medication, there were significant improvements in symptoms, side effects, and self-care.
- *Maintenance treatment following ECT:*
  - Medications that were ineffective prior to ECT are no more effective following a successful course of ECT.
  - Successful ECT may improve the patient's ability to tolerate antidepressants that could not be taken in a therapeutic dose previously.
  - Consider antidepressant maintenance for patients who have not had multiple failed medication trials prior to ECT.
    - Gradually add antidepressant toward latter portion of course of ECT.
  - Institute maintenance ECT when medication trials before ECT have been problematic.
    - Gradually increase time between ECTs to duration that prevents recurrence; reassess patient after each treatment.
    - Relapses during maintenance ECT may respond to administration of the next treatment earlier than scheduled, or to 3–4 acute ECTs (Andrade & Kurinji, 2002).
    - Some experts suggest that bilateral ECT may be preferable in maintenance treatment because it is more reliable and cognitive impairment is not as problematic with less frequent treatments (Andrade & Kurinji, 2002).

### Treatment Discontinuation

Patients who have recovered from an episode of depression often consider withdrawing the antidepressant, because they are not certain that the medication is still necessary or they do not like "depending" on it. The risk of recurrence or relapse is lower if all symptoms (including psychosocial dysfunction) have remitted completely. An antidepressant that was effective previously and withdrawn may work just as well when it is restarted later, but sometimes the antidepressant is no longer as well tolerated or effective when it is reinstituted for a recurrence.

The risk of both rebound depression with withdrawal of the antidepressant and discontinuation-induced refractoriness can be reduced by very slow withdrawal of the antidepressant.

- Decrease the dose by the smallest amount possible once a month or less frequently.
  - For example, 25 mg of a TCA, 5–10 mg of fluoxetine
- If symptoms begin to return, reduce rate of withdrawal.
- If symptoms continue to relapse, reinstitute the previous dose.

## SIDE EFFECTS

### Anticholinergic Side Effects

The TCAs all have anticholinergic properties, with tertiary amines being more anticholinergic than secondary amines. However, paroxetine (SSRI) is about as anticholinergic as nortriptyline.

- TCAs are generally more anticholinergic than neuroleptics, although low-potency neuroleptics such as thioridazine have more anticholinergic side effects than secondary amine TCAs such as desipramine.
- Anticholinergic side effects are discussed in detail in Chapter 2.
- Anticholinergic properties warrant caution using TCAs with
  - Older and demented patients
  - Urinary retention
  - Narrow angle glaucoma
  - Constipation
- Management of anticholinergic side effects:
  - Tolerance may develop in a few weeks.
  - Consider changing to a less anticholinergic antidepressant class.
    - Desipramine and nortriptyline are the least anticholinergic TCAs.
  - Cholinesterase inhibitors (e.g., donepezil 5–10 mg/day) often can reverse anticholinergic side effects, including cognitive effects (see Chapter 2).
    - No effect on mood
  - Bethanechol, which is sometimes used to treat urinary retention caused by anticholinergic side effects, is not as well tolerated as the cholinesterase inhibitors.

### Hematologic Effects

SSRIs can have variable effects on coagulation.

- Increased circulating serotonin may stimulate platelets and cause coagulopathy.
- More frequently, inhibition of platelet 5HT uptake impairs platelet function and causes bleeding.
- Five children ages 8–15 developed bruising or epistaxis 1 week–3 months after starting SSRIs (Lake, Birmaher, Wassick, Mathos, & Yelovich, 2000).
- There were no abnormalities of measures of platelet aggregation, hematopoiesis, or coagulation profile repeated 2 and 4 weeks after starting treatment in seven adults treated with fluoxetine and one with paroxetine (Alderman, Seshadri, & Ben-Tovim, 1996).
- The risk of GI bleeding is increased three times or more in patients on SSRIs.
  - A database study of all people taking antidepressants in Denmark during a 5-year period found risk of hospitalization for GI bleeding was 3.6 times greater than expected in patients taking SSRIs vs. no antidepressants and 12.2 times higher in patients taking SSRIs + NSAIDs or low-dose aspirin (Dalton et al., 2003).
    - Risk of GI bleeding requiring hospitalization increased 2.3 times in patients taking non-SSRI serotonergic antidepressants (e.g., clomipramine).
    - No increased risk was found with other antidepressants.
  - Risk factors include
    - History of GI bleeding
    - Concomitant use of aspirin, NSAIDs, anticoagulants
- 2D6 inhibition can increase coumadin levels and promote bleeding.
- Increased bleeding may be problematic following hemorrhagic stroke or surgery.

### Cardiovascular Side Effects

Hypertension

- Venlafaxine
  - Slight diastolic hypertension common but not significant.
  - Sustained diastolic blood pressure > 90
    - 300 mg/day: 13%
    - 200–300 mg/day: 7%
    - 100–200 mg/day: 5%
    - placebo: 2%

- Occasional hypertension seen with bupropion.
- Alpha-2 receptor antagonism conveys risk of hypertension with mirtazepine
- Noradrenergic effect of TCAs occasionally elevates blood pressure

### HYPOTENSION

- Most common form of hypotension is orthostatic hypotension.
- Most marked with TCAs and MAOIs
    - Tertiary amines > secondary amines
    - Hypotension with MAOIs discussed in Chapter 4.
- Risk of hypotension very low with SSRIs, bupropion.
- Hypotension more common in
    - Cardiovascular disease (14–24%)
    - Elderly patients
        - Risk of injury 4%
- Management of hypotension
    - Tell patient to stand up slowly if dizzy or lightheaded.
        - Sit up.
        - Put feet on floor.
        - Wait at least 60 seconds, then stand up.
    - Wear support hose.
    - If patient taking antihypertensive, reduce dose.
    - Should have high fluid intake with adequate sodium intake if not medically contraindicated.
    - Add stimulant.
    - Change antidepressant.
    - The mineralocorticoid fludrocortisone (0.1 mg daily bid) can be considered if the only acceptable antidepressant causes intractable hypotension.

### CARDIAC CONDUCTION

- EKG changes with TCAs:
    - Dose related
    - Nonspecific ST- and T-wave changes
    - PR interval prolongation
    - Widened QRS
        - Prolongation of QTc interval is attributable to QRS widening and reflects slowing of depolarization, not repolarization.
        - QTc prolongation with antipsychotic drugs is attributable to slowed repolarization.

- Risk of TCAs in the presence of heart block:
  - Minimal risk with first-degree AV block
  - Some risk with bundle-branch block
  - Risk of cardiac arrest with second- and third-degree AV block
- Death from TCA overdose is better correlated with QTc prolongation than with serum level.
- Patients taking TCAs who should have a baseline and follow-up EKG:
  - Children
  - Elderly patients
  - Patients with a history of heart disease
- Antidepressants with a low risk of altering cardiac conduction include
  - SSRIs
  - Bupropion
  - Venlafaxine
  - Mirtazepine
  - Nefazodone

## ARRHYTHMIAS

- Anticholinergic and adrenergic effects of TCAs cause sinus tachycardia.
- Tachycardia also can occur with venlafaxine and mirtazepine.
- Bradycardia occurs in 1.5% of patients taking nefazodone.
- Occasional bradycardia seen with fluoxetine and other SSRIs.
- All TCAs are type Ia antiarrhythmics.
  - Imipramine equivalent to quinidine as an antiarrhythmic agent.
  - Useful for ventricular arrhythmias.
  - Can aggravate heart block and cause new arrhythmias at toxic doses.
  - CAST (Cardiac Arrhythmia Suppression Trial) I and II found increased risk of sudden cardiac death in 6 months following MI in patients taking type Ia antiarrhythmics.
    - Not demonstrated with TCAs, but similar cardiac properties may warrant caution following MI.
- A few cases reported of new ventricular tachyarrhythmias with trazodone.

## HEART FAILURE

- Like other type Ia antiarrhythmics, TCAs can have a negative inotropic effect.
  - May cause decreased cardiac output or congestive heart failure.
- Pedal edema has been reported with
  - Amitriptyline
  - Trazodone

### Central Nervous System

ATAXIA

- Related to CNS depression

CONFUSION, DELIRIUM, MEMORY IMPAIRMENT

- Anticholinergic effects can cause or aggravate memory loss and confusion and induce delirium.
- If delirium is mistaken for primary psychosis, an antipsychotic drug may mistakenly be added, aggravating symptoms.
- Treatment of all anticholinergic effects is similar (see p. 35).

DEPERSONALIZATION, DEREALIZATION, "SPACINESS"

- May indicate increase of anxiety by antidepressant.
- More common with sedating antidepressants.
- Management:
  - Use slower dosage increase.
  - Change antidepressants.

EXTRAPYRAMIDAL SIDE EFFECTS (EPS)

- Most frequent with amoxapine
  - Metabolite of the neuroleptic loxapine (see p. 4)
  - May cause parkinsonism, akathisia, dystonia, occasional TD.
- SSRIs can reduce striatal dopamine release through an action on a $5HT_2$ heteroreceptor located on dopaminergic neurons.
  - Most common manifestations are emotional and cognitive blunting.
    - Can be reduced by adding a dopaminergic agent (e.g., bupropion, stimulant, pramipexole).
  - Parkinsonism and akathisia also occur with SSRIs.
    - Use SSRIs cautiously to treat depression in patients with Parkinson's disease.
  - A few cases of TD have been reported.
- Neuroleptic malignant syndrome (NMS)
  - Only reported with amoxapine.

HEADACHE

- Tension and vascular headaches are more common in depressed people than the general population.
  - Determine baseline headache frequency before concluding that headache is caused by an antidepressant.

- Serotonergic antidepressants have variable effects on migraine headaches.
  - Inhibition of platelet 5HT uptake may reduce migraine.
  - Increased circulating serotonin may exacerbate migraines.

## INCREASED ANXIETY

- Noradrenergic action of antidepressants can increase or induce anxiety as a result of activation of the locus coeruleus.
  - Serotonergic antidepressants also increase NE release.
- Anxiety may be accompanied by signs and symptoms of autonomic arousal:
  - Tremor
  - Diaphoresis
  - Palpitations
- Approaches to reducing initial jitteriness and anxiety:
  - Suppress anxiety with a benzodiazepine before starting antidepressant.
  - Increase antidepressant dose very slowly to allow time for down-regulation of noraderenrgic beta receptors.
    - For example, start with 10 mg desipramine or 1–2 mg of fluoxetine.
  - Use a beta-blocker for autonomic arousal.
  - Teach relaxation techniques.
  - Add cognitive behavior therapy (CBT)

## INSOMNIA

- Most frequent with SSRIs (especially fluoxetine), bupropion, protriptyline, venlafaxine
- Use morning dose if insomnia develops.
- If patient is otherwise tolerating and responding to antidepressant, treat insomnia with
  - Trazodone
  - Selective benzodiazepine-1 agonist (see pp. 3–62, 424–426)
  - Sedating antipsychotic drug with antidepressant properties in severe depression
    - Olanzapine
    - Quetiapine

## MANIA INDUCTION

- Treatment-emergent agitation, grossly reduced sleep, intense irritability, or psychotic symptoms may be indications of mania induction.
- Mania induction by antidepressants increases the risk of rapid cycling.

- All antidepressant treatments can induce mania/hypomania.
  - Including bright light and psychotherapy
  - Risk of mania induction is traditionally thought to be lower with SSRIs than with TCAs.
    - May reflect better screening and exclusion of bipolar patients from antidepressant trials with newer antidepressants.
    - Bupropion is probably not less likely to induce mania than other antidepressants.
- Antidepressants generally should not be prescribed for bipolar depression without co-administration of a mood stabilizer.

## MYOCLONUS, TREMORS

- More frequent with medications with antidopaminergic properties, such as
  - Amoxapine
  - SSRIs
- Nocturnal myoclonus caused by otherwise effective and well-tolerated antidepressant can be treated with dopaminergic agent (e.g., bupropion).
  - Must be taken earlier in evening to avoid causing insomnia.

## NIGHTMARES, VIVID OR STRANGE DREAMS

- Caused by REM rebound in response to REM suppression by antidepressant.
- Most frequent with SSRIs
- Very rare with nefazodone, mirtazepine, trimipramine
  - These antidepressants do not disrupt sleep architecture as much as other antidepressants.
- Management:
  - Change antidepressant.
  - Take antidepressant earlier in day.
  - Divide dose of antidepressant.
  - Add $5HT_2$ antagonist (e.g., cyproheptadine).

## PARESTHESIAS

- Rare with standard antidepressants
- More common with MAOIs
- Can sometimes be treated with pyridoxine 50–100 mg.

## SEDATION, DROWSINESS

- Can occur with any antidepressant.
- Most frequent with trazodone, nefazodone, mirtazepine, tertiary amine TCAs

- Bupropion is usually not sedating.
- Management:
  - Take entire dose at bedtime, if consistent with duration of action of antidepressant.
  - Use more frequent dosing for antidepressants requiring divided dose.
  - If mild sedation occurs, wait until it wears off before increasing dose.
    - Increase dose slowly.
    - Tolerance is more likely to develop to slight than to severe sedation.
  - Change to less sedating antidepressant.
  - If patient doing well otherwise or cannot tolerate any other antidepressant, treat sedation with
    - Modafinil
    - Stimulant
    - Bupropion

## SEIZURES

- Risk of seizures generally about 0.2–0.4% with antidepressants.
- In some cases, the dose at which seizure risk increases overlaps with the therapeutic dose:
  - Clomipramine at doses > 250 mg/day
  - Maprotiline at doses > 225 mg/day
  - Amoxapine at doses > 600 mg/day
  - Bupropion at doses > 450 mg/day, or single dose >150 mg
    - The incidence of seizures is 0.35–0.44% of patients taking bupropion in doses ≤ 450 mg/day.
- Risk of seizures is increased by
  - Seizure disorder
  - Traumatic brain injury
  - Concomitant medications that lower seizure threshold
  - Higher serum levels
- Risk of death may be greater with overdose of amoxapine than other TCAs because of intractable seizures.

## STUTTERING, PROBLEMS WITH WORD FINDING

- More common with SSRIs
- May reflect antidopaminergic effect.

## SUICIDAL IDEATION

- All antidepressants reduce suicide risk.
- Large antidepressant trials do not demonstrate new suicidal ideation > placebo with any antidepressant.

- Reports of increased suicidal ideation with fluoxetine in a small number of patients with personality disorders may have reflected discomfort caused by akathisia.
  - Since controlled studies show that SSRIs decrease suicidality, reports in the absence of controls may reflect spontaneous fluctuation of patients' clinical states, or induction of mood instability in patients with unrecognized bipolar diathesis.
- Concerns about suicidal thinking in children treated with SSRIs are probably overstated
  - May reflect failure to exclude bipolar disorder in juvenile (BDJ)
  - Suicidal thoughts fluctuate anyway
  - Autodepressant dosing more likely to be inadequate as younger patients need more frequent doses
  - No reports of actual suicides

TINNITUS

- Most common with bupropion
- Management:
  - Use more divided dose.
  - $D_2$ antagonist (e.g., quetiapine) may help.

TREMOR

- Resting tremor may occur with noradrenergic TCAs, bupropion, venlafaxine, SSRIs
- Management:
  - Give entire dose at night.
  - Reduce dose.
  - Add beta-blocker
    - Atenolol does not cross the blood–brain barrier and is less likely to affect mood adversely.

YAWNING

- Occurs without sedation.
- Occasionally occurs with SSRIs and clomipramine.

## Cancer

A critical review of research findings popularized in the press that the TCAs amoxapine, clomipramine, desipramine, doxepin, imipramine, and trimipramine, as well as paroxetine, were associated with increased risk of breast cancer 10 years after medication use (Kurdyak, Gnam, & Streiner, 2002).

- The TCA study correlated a prescription plan database with a cancer data base in Saskatchewan.
  - In 5,887 cases and 23,517 controls, 19% of breast cancer patients and 19% of controls had taken TCAs.
    - In women with > 10 years exposure to TCAs prior to breast cancer diagnosis, the relative risk for breast cancer was 1.52–2.14, with greater risk associated with higher total dose.
    - No controls for possible confounding factors, such as use of estrogen, smoking, or alcohol use.
    - The authors used at least 30 separate statistical tests, and there is a 79% chance of a spuriously significant finding with this many tests.
- The paroxetine study did attempt to control for confounding risk factors but had similar statistical flaws.
- A critical review of this research (Kurdyak et al., 2002) suggested that cancer risk is not sufficiently demonstrated to warrant changing antidepressant-prescribing practices for women.

A review of published studies of potential carcinogenicity of antidepressants found (Sternbach, 2003):

- Animal studies have contradictory results.
  - Hydrazide MAOIs (phenelzine, isocarbixazid) may be mutagenic in mice.
  - Clomipramine-potentiated antileukemia effect of vincristine and antisarcoma effect of actinomycin D.
  - Imipramine and clomipramine inhibited tumor growth.
  - Fluoxetine and citalopram reduced growth of GI tumors in rodents.
    - Serotonin can stimulate cell division.
    - Inhibiting cellular serotonin uptake may reduce mitotic activity.
  - Amitriptyline and fluoxetine stimulated growth of melanoma, mammary tumors, and fibrosarcoma in rodent models.
    - May be mediated by binding to an antiestrogen-binding site–histamine receptor involved in cellular proliferation.
  - Other studies show either no effect or promotion of carcinogenesis by fluoxetine.
- 13 epidemiological studies were identified, 3 of them prospective:
  - 3 studies found increased ovarian or breast cancer risk with chronic TCA use.
    - Other studies found no increased risk.
  - Weakness of positive studies:
    - Only assessed prescriptions, not whether patients actually took medication.

- Usually no control for health habits associated with antidepressant use (e.g., poor diet or smoking associated with depression)
  - Post hoc analysis
  - No control for family history and other risk factors
- Data do not demonstrate clear increased cancer risk with any antidepressant.

## Endocrine and Sexual Side Effects

### GYNECOMASTICA AND LACTATION

- Caused by prolactinemia induced by antidopaminergic effect of serotonergic antidepressants.
- May be accompanied by lactation.
- Can be treated with dopaminergic agent.
  - Bupropion
  - Dopamine agonist
    - Bromocriptine
    - Pramipexole

### PRIAPISM

- Caused by alpha-1 receptor blockade.
- Most common with trazodone
  - Incidence of priapism 1/6,000
    - Incidence of impotence 1/10,000
  - Not dose related
- Also can occur with chlorpromazine, thioridazine, alpha-adrenergic antagonist antihypertensives.
- Must be treated within 4–6 hours to prevent permanent impotence.
- Emergency treatment is with alpha-adrenergic agonists:
  - Neosynephrine 2 mg (supplied as 10 mg/30 mL) into corpus cavernosum every 10–15 minutes or maximum dose 6 mg
  - Metaraminol 10 mg into corpus cavernosum
  - Epinephrine for refractory priapism
  - Surgery may be necessary.
- Clitoral priapism may occur, but no long-term consequences have been identified.

### SEXUAL DYSFUNCTION

- "Organic" impotence occurs in depressed males.
- Patients may not volunteer symptoms.

- Antidepressants increase sexual function when dysfunction secondary to depression.
- Antidepressant-induced sexual dysfunction most frequent with serotonergic antidepressants, including
  - SSRIs
  - Clomipramine
  - Venlafaxine
    - Risk may be somewhat lower than with SSRIs.
  - SSRIs that are 2D6 inhibitors impair sexual dysfunction by their serotonergic action and also because nitric oxide is a 2D6 substrate.
- Incidence in postmarketing surveillance at least 35–45%
  - Prevalence of sexual dysfunction in a cross-sectional study in 1,101 U.S. primary care clinics involving 4,534 women and 1,763 men (Clayton et al., 2002):
    - SSRIs, mirtazepine, venlafaxine: 36–43%
    - Nefazodone: 28%
    - Bupropion: 22–25%
    - Odds of sexual dysfunction were four to six times higher with SSRIs and venlafaxine XR than bupropion SR.
- Manifestations of sexual dysfunction:
  - Decreased libido
    - SSRIs
  - Decreased arousal
    - SSRIs
  - Anorgasmia, decreased intensity of orgasm
    - SSRIs, venlafaxine
    - MAOIs
  - Erectile dysfunction
    - SSRIs
    - Venlafaxine
    - TCAs

Management:
- Tolerance may develop over 1–12 months.
- Reducing antidepressant dose may improve sexual side effects.
- Most treatments for antidepressant-induced sexual dysfunction are based on clinical experience.
  - Minimal data showing superiority to placebo.
- Dopaminergic medications for libido, arousal, orgasmic dysfunction

- Bupropion 75–225 mg/day
  - Of 24 patients with SSRI-induced sexual side effects, 46% of women and 75% of men had improvement of all sexual side effects with 300 mg/day bupropion SR for 7 weeks; most improvement occurred at 100–200 mg/day (Gitlin, Suri, Altshuler, Zuckerbrow-Miller, & Fairbanks, 2002).
- Amantadine 100–200 mg
  - May aggravate depression.
- Stimulant
  - For example, methylphenidate 5 mg prn or tid
- The dopaminergic agent ropinirole (starting with 0.25 mg/day and increased to 2–4 mg/day) reduced sexual dysfunction in 13 patients taking stable antidepressant doses, with 7/13 patients rated as responders (Worthington, Simon, Korbly, Perlis, & Pollack, 2002).
- Noradrenergic medications for libido, arousal, orgasmic dysfunction
  - Yohimbine 5.75 mg prn or tid
    - Can aggravate anxiety and cause insomnia.
- Ginkgo biloba (140–180 mg/day) or ginseng for libido, arousal, orgasmic dysfunction
- Serotonin receptor antagonists for libido, arousal, orgasmic dysfunction
  - $5HT_{1A}$: buspirone 20–60 mg/day
  - $5HT_2$: cyproheptadine, trazodone, nefazodone, mirtazepine
    - cyproheptadine 4–8 mg prn or tid
    - trazodone 50–200 mg
    - nefazodone 50–200 mg
    - mirtazepine 15–30 mg
  - $5HT_3$: mirtazepine, ondansetron
    - ondansetron 2–4 mg prn
- Sildenafil 50–200 mg for erectile dysfunction, anorgasmia, decreased libido, decreased lubrication in women
  - Inhibits phosphodiesterase type 5, which breaks down cGMP, which causes smooth muscle to relax and allows penis to return to flaccid state.
  - Two experimental phosphodiesterase inhibitors, tadalafil and vardenafil, seem equivalent in efficacy to sildenafil.
    - Sildenafil was found to improve orgasmic function and sexual satisfaction as well as erectile function but not desire in men also taking SSRIs (Nurnberg et al., 2001).
    - 21 men with remission of major depressive disorder on SSRI and ejaculatory delay (14 also with erectile dysfunction) had sildenafil added in doses up to 200 mg/day (Seidman, Pesce, & Roose, 2003).

At 25–100 mg, 12/14 had remission of erectile dysfunction, and 4/21 had remission of ejaculatory delay. At doses of 150–200 mg in 16 patients, 9/10 patients had improvement in ejaculatory delay, and 7 had remission. Only one patient had both ejaculatory delay and erectile dysfunction, and that patient had improvement of both side effects.

SPONTANEOUS ORGASM

- Rare side effect
- More frequent in women
- Often associated with yawning
- Reported with trazodone, clompiramine, SSRIs

TESTICULAR SWELLING

- Rare side effect of desipramine
- Indication to discontinue antidepressant.

### Eyes, Ears, Nose, and Throat Side Effects

- Anticholinergic side effects can cause
  - Blurred vision
  - Dry bronchial secretions
  - Dry eyes
  - Precipitation of narrow angle glaucoma
  - Photophobia caused by dilated pupils
- Nasal congestion
  - Most common with trazodone
    - Probably caused by alpha-adrenergic blockade.

### Falls

- Elderly patients taking antidepressants have twofold increase in risk of falls.
  - Especially if demented
- Risk with antidepressants similar to benzodiazepines.
  - Falls per dose:
    - Nortriptyline: 0.0021
    - Sertraline: 0.0012
    - Diazepam: 0.00052
- SSRIs do not have a substantially reduced risk of falls.
- Increased postural sway seen with SSRIs.

- Not only in elderly
- Risk of falls higher for women.

### Gastrointestinal Side Effects

CONSTIPATION

- Usually caused by anticholinergic side effects of TCAs.
- Paralytic ileus may occur, especially if TCA is combined with another anticholinergic medication (e.g., thioridazine).
- Management:
  - Drink plenty of water.
  - Use cholinesterase inhibitor (see Chapter 2).
  - Lactulose is sometimes helpful.

DIARRHEA

- Common (11–16%) with SSRIs
- Tolerance sometimes develops.
- Management:
  - Bismuth salicylate (Pepto Bismol)
  - Change medication.

DRY MOUTH

- Anticholinergic side effect of TCAs, and antiadrenergic side effect of trazodone
- Management (see Chapter 2):
  - Drinking fluids only helps as long as fluid is in the mouth.
  - Try sugarless hard gandy or gum.
  - Try cholinesterase inhibitor.

GLOSSITIS

- May be associated with bad taste.
- Tongue is sore or black.

HEPATOTOXICITY

A Spanish study examined the risk of hepatotoxicity with antidepressants by examining the Spanish Pharmacovigilance System database and drug sales recorded by the Spanish National Health System (Carvajal et al., 2002).

- Incidence of reported hepatotoxicity was similar for most antidepressants.
  - Risk ranged from 1.28/100,000 patient-years for sertraline to 4 for clomipramine.

- Nefazodone had the highest incidence, with 29 cases/100,000 patient-years. This may be a higher incidence than was previously suspected.
  - Has occasionally required liver transplantation or been fatal.
  - Occurs within first 18 months of treatment.
  - Routine LFTs will not identify risk.

## NAUSEA

- Common with serotonergic antidepressants, bupropion
- Caused by increased dopaminergic transmission in brainstem nausea centers.
  - Resulting either from direct effect on dopamine availability or stimulation of serotonin $5HT_3$ receptors located on dopamine neurons.
- Management:
  - Tolerance may develop over 2–4 weeks.
  - Take medication on full stomach.
  - Take ginger root capsule along with medication.
  - Take ginger root broth made by grating 2 tablespoons of fresh ginger root into a cup of hot water.
    - Can be flavored with honey.
  - Try a proton pump inhibitor.
    - For example, cisapride 5 mg bid

## WEIGHT GAIN

- Most common with antidepressants with histamine $H_1$ blockade, especially
  - Amitriptyline
  - Clomipramine
  - Doxepin
  - Trimipramine
  - Mirtazepine
- Although SSRIs are often thought to be weight neutral or promote weight loss, weight gain may be significant.
  - Paroxetine is more likely to cause weight gain than other SSRIs (Fava, 2000).
    - Fluoxetine and fluvoxamine also associated with weight gain.
  - During a 24-week double-blind study of paroxetine in social phobia (mean dose 37 mg), 23% of paroxetine patients had ≥ 7% weight gain compared to 9% of placebo patients.
    - 3% of paroxetine and 4% of placebo patients had significant weight loss (Stein, Versiani, Hair, & Kumar, 2002).
  - Weight gain usually not associated with nefazodone, venlafaxine.

- Weight gain caused primarily by stimulation of appetite.
  - Unclear whether energy production also may change.
- Management: (see pp. 57, 61–64)

WEIGHT LOSS

- Occasionally occurs with
  - Bupropion
  - Fluoxetine
  - Other SSRIs
- May be secondary to nausea or appetite suppression.
- Usually minimal, but can be problematic in elderly patients.
- Antidepressants that are often weight neutral include
  - Desipramine
  - Nefazodone
  - Trazodone
  - Bupropion
  - Sertraline
  - Citalopram, escitalopram

## Renal Side Effects

HYPONATREMIA

- Retrospective study of 199 elderly psychiatric inpatients (Kirby, Harrigan, & Ames, 2002):
  - 74 taking SSRI or venlafaxine
  - Controlled for other factors that cause hyponatremia.
    - For example, medical illness, diuretics, age, sex
  - Patients taking SSRIs or venlafaxine were 5.6 times as likely to have hyponatremia.
  - 39% of SSRI/venlafaxine patients developed hyponatremia vs. 10% of controls.
- In data on 39,000 patients over 2 years in a laboratory database, 1,391 had serum sodium concentrations ≤ 130 (Movig et al., 2002).
  - 29 of the hyponatremia patients were taking antidepressants.
    - These subjects were compared with 78 controls taking antidepressants but with normal serum sodium.
  - 76% of the hyponatremia patients taking antidepressants were on SSRIs.
  - 49% of controls were taking an SSRI.

- Comparing hyponatremia patients taking antidepressants with normal serum sodium patients taking antidepressants, the risk of hyponatremia was 3.3 times greater in those taking SSRIs.
- Hyponatremia on SSRIs is caused by SIADH.
- Hyponatremia usually develops 1 day to several months after starting antidepressant.
- Serum sodium may fall to the range of 119–125 mM.
- Risk factors:
  - Age $> 70$
  - Female gender
  - Concomitant use of diuretic
  - Past history of hyponatremia
- Sodium levels normalize when medication is withdrawn.
- Management if patient has to continue taking medication (see p. 340):
  - Water restriction
  - Add lithium 300–900 mg/day.

### Serotonin Syndrome

- Usually caused by interaction of a serotonergic antidepressant with an MAOI (Chapter 4).
- Milder forms of serotonin syndrome may occur with combinations of serotonergic antidepressants at higher doses or combinations of a serotonin reuptake inhibitor with other serotonergic agents, such as
  - L-tryptophan
  - Dextromethorphan
  - Meperidine
- Dangerous serotonin syndrome rarely occurs with a single agent.
- Mild serotonin syndrome causes
  - Headache
  - Nausea
  - Abdominal cramps, diarrhea
  - Insomnia
  - Difficulty concentrating
- More severe signs include
  - Confusion
  - Myoclonus
  - Psychosis

- Fever
- Delirium
- Coma
- Cardiotoxicity
- Management:
  - Eliminate combinations of serotonergic drugs.
  - Use less serotonergic antidepressant.
  - Administer $5HT_2$ antagonist.
    - Cyproheptadine
    - Trazodone

## Skin, Allergies, and Temperature

### ALLERGIC REACTIONS

- Can occur with any antidepressant.
- Hypersensitivity more often a response to excipients (e.g., cellulose, dyes) rather than to the active medication.
  - Tartrazine, a coloring agent, has been removed because of a high incidence of allergic reactions.
- Manifestations include
  - Rash
  - Pruritus
  - Urticaria
  - Wheezing
  - Hepatitis
  - Polyarthralgias
  - Photosensitivity
- Management of severe rash:
  - Change antidepressant.
  - Add antihistamine.
- If patient has had allergic reactions to multiple antidepressants
  - Try a medication that is available as a liquid (e.g., fluoxetine, lithium citrate) or powder (e.g., Depakote Sprinkle)
  - Start an antihistamine (e.g., ranitidine) first.
  - Desensitize patient to medication with slowly escalating doses.
  - Some cases of multiple medication allergies are conditioned responses in patients with angioneurotic edema.
    - It may be possible to demonstrate this by administering placebo and active drug in single-blind protocol.

- Patient may then be desensitized to medication with relaxation therapy, imagery, and blind reintroduction of medication.

SWEATING

Hyperhydrosis and night sweats occur in 7–12% of patients treated with noradrenergic TCAs, SSRIs, venlafaxine, or bupropion.

- Mechanism is increased adrenergic activity.
  - Can be stimulated directly by norepinephrine reuptake inhibition or indirectly by increasing serotonergic transmission.
- Management is with antiadrenergic medications:
  - Beta-adrenergic blocker (e.g., atenolol)
    - 25–50 mg hs
    - Daytime dose may be added if necessary.
  - Alpha-1 adrenergic antagonist
    - Terazosin 1 mg hs

## PREGNANCY AND LACTATION

### Teratogenicity

- TCAs have not been found to increase the risk of fetal malformations.
- SSRIs that have been studied have not had increased teratogenicity.
  - In 138 infants born to women taking SSRIs during pregnancy, the incidence of congenital anomalies (1.4%) was the same as in the general population (Hendrick et al., 2003).
    - There was an association with higher fluoxetine doses (40–80 mg) and lower birth rate, but N was too small for analysis.
- Slightly higher rate of miscarriage in patients taking fluoxetine vs. women not taking an antidepressant was not statistically significant (Chambers, Johnson, Dick, Felix, & Jones, 1996).
- 147 pregnant women in their first trimester taking trazodone or nefazodone were prospectively compared to 147 pregnant women taking other antidepressants and 147 pregnant women taking medications known not to be teratogenic (e.g., dextromethorphan, clarithromycin).
  - No differences were found 4–6 months postpartum in live births, spontaneous miscarriages, gestational age at birth, birth weight, or major malformations (Einarson et al., 2003).

Risks of prenatal exposure to antidepressants were assessed in approximately 37,000 patients enrolled in an HMO (Simon, Cunningham, & Davis, 2002).

**Table 3.7 Drug–Drug Interactions**

| DRUGS (X) INTERACT WITH: | ANTIDEPRESSANTS (A) | COMMENTS |
|---|---|---|
| Acetaminophen | X↓ A↑ | May overuse acetaminophen; increase HCA levels. |
| Acetazolamide | X↑ | Reduces HCAs' renal excretion; clinical importance unclear, hypotension increased. |
| Alcohol | X↑ A↑ | CNS depression with HCA and trazodone; not seen with SSRIs, bupropion, venlafaxine. |
| Aminopyrine | A↑? | Possible increase in HCA secondary to displaced protein-bound HCA. |
| Ammonium chloride | A↓ | May increase HCAs' excretion; clinical importance unclear. |
| Anticholinergics | X↑ | Increased anticholinergic actions with HCAs and paroxetine but not other SSRIs. |
| Antihistamines | X↑ | Increased drowsiness; use nonsedating antihistamine, such as asternizole. |
| Antipsychotics (see also phenothiazines) | X↑ A↑ | Potentiate each other; toxicity; more anticholinergic HCAs may diminish EPS; SSRIs may increase EPS and levels of thioridazine, perphenazine, clozapine, and risperidone. |
| Aspirin | A↑? | Possible increase in HCA secondary to displaced protein-bound HCA. |
| Barbiturates | X↑ A↑ | CNS depression; may decrease antidepressant plasma levels. |
| Benzodiazepines | X↑ A↑ | CNS depression. |
| Bethanidine | A↓ | Decreases HCA effect. |
| Carbamazepine | X↓ A↓ | Decreases HCA levels and effect; may lower seizure control; increased quinidine-like effect (see quinidine below). Monitor serum levels. SSRIs might decrease carbamazepine levels |
| Chloramphenicol | A↑ | Increases HCA level, effect, toxicity. |
| Chlordiazepoxide (see benzodiazepines) | | |
| Chlorothiazide | A↑ | Thiazide diuretics increase HCA actions. |
| Cholestyramine | A↓ | Decreased absorption; decreased blood levels. |
| Cimetidine | A↑ | Increased blood levels trigger toxicity; give patient less AD or substitute ranitidine or famotidine for cimetidine. |

*(continues)*

## Table 3.7 Continued

| DRUGS (X) INTERACT WITH: | ANTIDEPRESSANTS (A) | COMMENTS |
|---|---|---|
| Clonidine | X↓ | HCAs and probably venlafaxine inhibit clonidine's antihypertensive actions; trazodone, nefazodone (?), bupropion, SSRIs safer. |
| Cocaine | X↑ | Cardiac arrhythmias and increased BP with HCAs. |
| Cyclobenzaprine | A↑ | Cyclobenzaprine, which is chemically similar to HCAs, may produce cardiac problems, increased quinidine-like effects. |
| Debrisoquin | X↓ | Hypotension. |
| Dextroamphetamine | X↑ A↑ | Increase each other's effects. |
| Dicumarol | X↓ | Increased bleeding time. |
| Disopyramide (*see* quinidine) | | |
| Disulfiram | A↑ | May increase HCA level. |
| Doxycycline | A↓ | Decreased HCA level, effect. |
| Epinephrine[†] | X↑ | Increased arrhythmias, hypertension, and tachycardia. HCAs inhibit pressor effects of indirect-acting sympathomimetics (e.g., ephedrine). Because HCAs block the reuptake of direct-acting sympatho-mimetics, their concentration increases at receptor sites. Since indirect-acting sympathomimetics require uptake into the adrenergic neuron to induce their effects, HCAs block them. The cardiovascular result from the mixed-acting sympatho-mimetics depends on the % of each group. Avoid HCAs with direct-acting sympathomimetics. |
| Estrogen (*see* oral contraceptives) | | |
| Fiber, psyllium | A↓ | Decreases absorption. |
| Fluconazole (*see* imidazole antifungals) | | |
| Fluoxetine | A↑ | Increases HCA levels (300% avg.) and toxicity. |
| Griseofulvin | A↓ | Decreased HCA level, effect. |
| Guanethidine[†] | X↓ | Lose antihypertensive effect with NE uptake blockers; all HCAs and venlaflaxine, SSRIs, nefazodone, trazodone, bupropion safer. |

*(continues)*

**Table 3.7 Continued**

| DRUGS (X) INTERACT WITH: | ANTIDEPRESSANTS (A) | COMMENTS |
|---|---|---|
| Haloperidol | X↑ A↑ | Increases HCA plasma level; EPS increase with fluoxetine and possibly sertraline and paroxetine. |
| Halothane | A↑ | Increases tachyarrythmias with anticholinergic antidepressants (HCAs and possibly paroxetine); enflurane with d-turbo-curarine safer. |
| Imidazole antifungals | A↑ | Increases nortriptyline and probably other TCA levels and possibly sertraline. |
| Insulin | X↑ | HCA enhances hypoglycemia in diabetics. |
| Itraconazole (*see* imidazole antifungals) | | |
| Isoniazid | A↑ | Increases HCA level, effect, toxicity. |
| Ketoconazole (*see* imidazole antifungals) | | |
| Levodopa | X↓ A↓ | Decreases absorption of HCAs; decreases effect of levodopa. |
| Lidocaine (*see* quinidine) | | |
| Liothyronine (T$_3$) | A↑ | Potentiates antidepressant and arrhythmic effects. |
| Lithium | A↑ | Augments antidepressant effects. |
| Meperidine | X↑ A↑ | Potentiate each other; use lower doses of meperidine or another narcotic. |
| Methyldopa | X↓ | Hypotension; amitriptyline biggest problem. |
| Methylphenidate (*see* dextroamphetamine) | | |
| Miconazole (*see* imidazole antifungals) | | |
| Molindone | X↑ | Greater molindone effect. |
| MAOIs | X↑ A↑ | Adding HCAs to MAOIs can cause hypertensive crisis, mania, muscular rigidity, convulsions, high fever, coma, and death. If HCAs are to be used, first taper MAOI, keep patient off MAOI for 10–14 days, maintain MAOI diet during this interval, and then slowly begin HCA. If HCAs are combined with MAOIs, start both drugs together or add the MAOI to the HCA; do not use imipramine or clomipramine. Start with low doses of both classes. Trazodone can be combined with MAOI, but may increase hypotension. |

(*continues*)

## Table 3.7 Continued

| DRUGS (X) INTERACT WITH: | ANTIDEPRESSANTS (A) | COMMENTS |
|---|---|---|
| Morphine | X↑ A↓ | CNS depression; may decrease HCA levels; common with amitriptyline and desipramine; HCA may augment opiate analgesia. |
| Oral contraceptives | A↑ | Increased HCA level, effect, toxicity; inhibits HCA metabolism; higher estrogen doses may decrease HCA effect. |
| Pancuronium | A↑ | Increased tachyarrythmias with anticholinergic antidepressants; all HCAs; enflurane with d-tubocurine safer. |
| Paroxetine | X↑ A↑ | Increases HCA level (avg. 200%) and effects of both drugs. |
| Phenothiazines (*see also* antipsychotics) | X↑ A? | Increases neuroleptic and HCA plasma levels; increased cardiac arrythmias with thioridazine, clozapine, pimozide; increased anticholinergic and hypertensive effects but decreased EPS. |
| Phenylbutazone | X↓ A↑ | HCAs may delay absorption of phenylbutazone; increases HCA due to displaced protein-bound HCA. |
| Phenytoin | X↓ A↑? | Lower seizure control; may decrease antidepressant plasma levels due to induced metabolism; may increase antidepressant plasma level due to displaced protein-bound HCA and with SSRI; venlafaxine may be safest alternative. Paroxetine levels decrease. |
| Prazosin | X↓ | Hypertension; safer to use bupropion, fluoxetine, desipramine, protriptyline. |
| Procainamide (*see* quinidine) | | |
| Propranolol | X↓↑ A↓ | Patients may become more depressed on β-blockers; venlafaxine may reverse β-blocker effects; HCAs may exaggerate hypotension. |
| Quinidine | X↑ A↑ | Because of HCAs' quinidine-like effects, possible myocardial depression, diminished contractility, and dysrhythmias, which can lead to congestive heart failure and heart block. Quinidine and HCAs may yield irregular heartbeat early on. |
| Reserpine | X↑ A↑ | Patients may develop increased hypotension. |
| Scopolamine | A↑? | Possible increased antidepressant levels secondary to displaced protein-bound antidepressant. |

*(continues)*

**Table 3.7  Continued**

| DRUGS (X) INTERACT WITH: | ANTIDEPRESSANTS (A) | COMMENTS |
|---|---|---|
| Sertraline | X↑ A↑ | Increases HCA level (~30%) and effects of both drugs. |
| Sulfonylureas | X↑ | HCA enhances hypoglycemia in diabetics. |
| Thiazide diuretics | X↑ A↑ | Increased hypotension with HCAs. |
| Thioridazine | A↑ | Increased HCA arrythmias. |
| Tobacco smoking | A↓ | Smoking may lower HCA plasma levels; importance unclear. |

| DRUGS (X) INTERACT WITH: | AMITRIPTYLINE (A) | COMMENTS |
|---|---|---|
| Disulfiram | X↑ | Two cases of organic brain syndrome; cleared when both drugs stopped. |
| Ethchlorvynol | X↑ | Transient delirium. |
| Valproic acid | X↑ A↑ | Increased plasma levels of both drugs. |

| DRUGS (X) INTERACT WITH: | DESIPRAMINE (D) | COMMENTS |
|---|---|---|
| Methadone | D↑ | Desipramine reported to increase by 108%; use together carefully. |

| DRUGS (X) INTERACT WITH: | DOXEPIN (D) | COMMENTS |
|---|---|---|
| Propoxyphene | D↑ | Propoxyphene doubles doxepin levels, inducing lethargy; five days after stopping propoxyphene, patient's mental status returns to normal. |

| DRUGS (X) INTERACT WITH: | FLUOXETINE (F) | COMMENTS |
|---|---|---|
| Alprazolam | X↑ | Increased plasma level, confusion. Not seen with clonazepam or triazolam. |
| Diazepam | X↑ | Confusion. Not seen with clonazepam or triazolam. |
| Trazodone | X↑ | Increased plasma level. |
| Valproic Acid | X↑ | Increased plasma level. |
| Methadone | X↑ | Increased plasma level. |

*(continues)*

## Table 3.7  Continued

| DRUGS (X) INTERACT WITH: | FLUOXAMINE (F)† | COMMENTS |
|---|---|---|
| Theophylline | X↑ | Toxic plasma levels. P4501A2 inhibited by fluvoxamine but not other SSRIs. |
| Tacrine | X↑ | Fluvoxamine but not other SSRIs. |

†P4501A2 and 3A4 inhibitor

| DRUGS (X) INTERACT WITH: | SSRIs (s): FLUOXETINE FLUVOXAMINE* PAROXETINE SERTRALINE** | COMMENTS |
|---|---|---|
| Buspirone | S↑ | May augment antidepressant effect. |
| *Calcium channel-blockers* Nifedipine Verapamil | X↑ | Enhanced effect. |
| Dextromethorphan | X↑ S↑ | Hallucinogen-type reaction reported with fluoxetine—bright colors, distorted shapes; similar serotonergic effects possible with all SSRIs. |
| Carbamazepine (*see* P4502D6) | | |
| Cyproheptadine (*see* seratonin 5HT$_2$ receptor antagonists) | | |
| Digitoxin, digoxin | X↑ | Two cases of organic brain syndrome; cleared when both drugs stopped. SSRIs can free protein-bound digitoxin; no effect seen in healthy people. Increased plasma levels. |
| Furosemide | X↑ S↑ | Rarely SSRIs cause SIADH; additive hypo-natremia result. |
| Lithium | X↑↓ | Lithium neurotoxicity may occur at normal levels. |
| L-tryptophan | X↑ | Serotonin syndrome. |
| MAOI* | X↑ S↑ | Prompt serotonin syndrome. |
| Metroprolol, propranolol | X↑ | Bradycardia and heart block seen; other 2D6 metabolized include timolol and bufarol; consider atenolol as alternative. Probably increased levels of metoprolol and propranolol. |
| *P4502D6 and 3A4 enzyme metabolized drugs* | X↑ | All SSRIs inhibit 2D6 enzyme system; but fluvoxamine only 5%, and setraline only 15–30% at starting dose. |

(*continues*)

**Table 3.7  Continued**

| DRUGS (x) INTERACT WITH: | SSRIs (s): FLUOXETINE FLUVOXAMINE* PAROXETINE SERTRALINE** | COMMENTS |
|---|---|---|
| Narrow therapeutic index— HCAs, carbamazepine, vinblastine, encainide flecainide, dextromethorphan. | | Fluvoxamine does increases imipramine, amitriptyline, and clomipramine by 1A2 path. Fluoxetine and fluvoxamine inhibit 3A4, thereby raising carbamazepine levels. |
| Neuroleptics | X↑ | Increased risk for EPS. Increased level for P4502D6 neuroleptics, haloperidol, perphenazine, thioridazine. Fluvoxamine least risk. |
| Procyclidine | X↑ | Paroxetine increases procyclidine levels (avg. ~35%); may occur with other SSRIs. |
| *Serotonin 5HT$_2$ receptor antagonists*(cyproheptadine, risperidone, clozapine) | S↓ | Potentially reverses antidepressant effect. |
| Tryptophan | S↑ | Prompts agitation, restlessness, and GI distress. |
| Venlafaxine | X↑ | SSRIs potentially inhibit metabolism of venlafaxine. |
| Warfarin | X↑ | Increased bleeding time possibly due to anticoagulant effects of SSRIs. Displacement of protein-bound warfarin may sometimes occur. |

β-blockers (*see* metoprolol)

\* Fluvoxamine's effects on P4502D6 are usually negligible.

\*\* Sertraline's effects by 2D6 path, or P4502D6, are small at 50 mg but increase with dose.

| DRUGS (x) INTERACT WITH: | MAPROTILINE (M) | COMMENTS |
|---|---|---|
| Propranolol | M↑ | Maprotiline toxicity. |

| DRUGS (x) INTERACT WITH: | TRAZODONE (T) | COMMENTS |
|---|---|---|
| Barbiturates | T↑ | BP drops; avoid. |
| Digitalis | X↑ | Increases digitalis. |
| Clonidine, other antihypertensives | X↑ | May exaggerate hypotensive effects. Alpha drugs may increase priapism risk. |

↑ Increases; ↓ Decreases; ↑↓ Increases and decreases; ? Unsure.

**Table 3.8 Effects on Laboratory Tests**

| GENERIC NAMES | BLOOD/SERUM TESTS* | URINE TESTS |
|---|---|---|
| Amoxapine | WBC ↓, LFT ↑** | None |
| Fluoxetine | ESR ↑, bleeding time ↑<br>Glucose ↓<br>Cholesterol ↑, lipids ↑<br>Potassium ↓, sodium ↑<br>Iron ↓<br>LFT ↑↓ | Albumin ↑ |
| Nefazodone | Hematocrit (hemodilution) ↓ | |
| Paroxetine | Sodium ↓ | |
| Sertraline | Bleeding time ↑<br>ALT ↑<br>Cholesterol ↑<br>Triglycerides ↑<br>Uric acid ↓ | |
| Trazodone | WBC ↓, LFT ↑ | None |
| Venlafaxine | Cholesterol ↑ | |

\* ↑ Increases; ↓ Decreases
\*\* LFT are liver function tests; AST (SGOT), ALT (SGPT), LDH, bilirubin, alkaline phosphatase.

- All live births between January 1, 1986 and December 31, 1998 were reviewed.
- 209 infants were exposed to a TCA during gestation.
- 185 infants were exposed to an SSRI during gestation.
- Comparing infants exposed to either class of antidepressant and matched nonexposed controls revealed the following:
  - Infants exposed to TCAs did not differ in gestational age, birth weight, or head circumference on Apgar scores.
    - Also no difference in weight or head circumference at any point from birth to age 2.
  - Infants exposed to SSRIs had significantly lower gestational age (i.e., they were more likely to be born prematurely), birth weight, and Apgar scores.
    - Absolute rate of prematurity was 10%.
    - Differences in premature birth and birth weight were similar with exposure in the first or second trimester and exposure in the third trimester only.
    - Lower Apgar scores were seen only with third-trimester exposure.
    - From 6 months of age on, there were no differences in these parameters.

- Infants exposed to any of the antidepressants did not have an increased rate of major or minor malformations, developmental delays, or neurological disorders.

## Direct Effect on Newborn of Prenatal Antidepressant Exposure

- Anticholinergic effects can cause tachycardia.
- Neonatal antidepressant withdrawal sometimes causes jitteriness, myoclonus, colic, and poor feeding.

## Behavioral Teratogenicity

- There were no differences in IQ, language development, or behavioral development of 55 preschool children exposed to fluoxetine in utero compared with 84 children without antidepressant exposure (Nulman et al., 1997)
- A comparison using the Bayley Scales of Infant Development of 31 children ages 6–40 months of depressed mothers who took SSRIs during pregnancy and 13 age-matched children of depressed mothers who did not take SSRIs during pregnancy found that
  - Mental development was similar but psychomotor development was slower in children exposed to SSRIs during pregnancy (Casper et al., 2003).

## Lactation

- Breast milk medication concentrations = 50–100% of serum concentration.
- Actual dose received by infant is very low.
- A comparison of 11 mothers taking citalopram 20–40 mg/day and their infants with 10 women and their infants not taking any medication examined plasma and breast milk concentrations of the antidepressant for 2 months postpartum (Heikkinen, Ekblad, Kero, Ekblad, & Laine, 2002):
  - Mean trough maternal plasma levels were 46–214 nmol/L.
  - Citalopram and citalopram metabolite levels in milk were two or three times higher in milk than in maternal plasma.
  - Infant citalopram and metabolite levels were low or undetectable.
  - Even though infant levels were about 60% of maternal levels at birth, there were no effects of the medication on delivery or subsequent infant development followed up to 1 year of age.

- Blood levels in the mother and infant and breast milk levels of antidepressant were measured in 10 postpartum women taking a mean dose of 34 mg/day of fluoxetine (Suri et al., 2002).
  - Fluoxetine and norfluoxetine were detectable in breast milk.
  - Total daily volume of breast feeding was 700–840 mL/day, with one infant getting 1680 mL.
  - Total daily dose of fluoxetine received by infants was 0.004–0.085 mg/day.
  - Total daily dose of norfluoxetine received by infants was 0.01–0.09 mg/day.
- Study of nursing mothers taking 50–200 mg of sertraline and their infants Epperson et al., 2001 found:
  - 70–90% reduction of maternal platelet serotonin levels.
  - No change in infant platelet serotonin.
  - Maternal levels of sertraline and desmethyl-sertraline 31 and 45 ng/mL.
  - Infant levels undetectable.
- Occasional case reports of adverse reactions of nursing infants to antidepressants taken by mother.
  - TCAs
    - Respiratory depression, urinary retention
    - Especially doxepin
  - SSRIs
    - Colic, sleep myoclonus, sedation, activation
- Lower milk:serum ratio with drugs that are
  - Less lipid soluble
  - More protein bound (higher binding protein concentration in serum than milk)
- Milk:plasma ratio low for sertraline and paroxetine.
  - Higher with fluoxetine.
- Prescribing guidelines during lactation:
  - Obtain pediatric assessment of infant.
  - Use a single medication at the lowest possible dose.
  - Medications with shorter half-lives may be preferable.
  - Instruct mother to breast-feed before taking the medication.
  - Monitor infant serum levels for first 10 weeks.
  - Do not use doxepin or long half-life benzodiazepines.
  - Use lithium or divalproex only if absolutely necessary.

## WITHDRAWAL

Antidepressants do not cause dependence or addiction. Tolerance to the antidepressant effect occurs rarely. However, discontinuation syndromes occur with some regularity.

- Cholinergic rebound can occur with rapid discontinuation of all anticholinergic antidepressants, especially TCAs and paroxetine.
  - Influenza-like syndrome
  - Abdominal cramps, nausea, diarrhea
  - Increased salivation
  - Headache
  - Rhinorrhea, dizziness, coryza
  - Can be treated by slower drug discontinuation or addition of an anticholinergic agent.
- Antidepressant withdrawal produces a stress response resulting in excessive activity of glucocorticoids, glutamate, nitric oxide, and NMDA receptors (Harvey, McEwen, & Stein, 2003).
  - These changes exacerbate the pathophysiology of depression.
- Rebound depression is common with rapid withdrawal of any antidepressant, even if it does not seem to have been helpful.
  - More common with shorter-acting antidepressants, especially paroxetine and venlafaxine.
    - Depression or withdrawal symptoms may appear between doses.
    - May occur even with extended-release preparations.
  - Preventing rebound depression:
    - If severe interactions are not anticipated, add a new antidepressant before withdrawing the existing one.
    - Decrease dose very slowly
    - For example, 37.5 mg venlafaxine q 2–3 weeks
    - Give venlafaxine more frequently if interdose rebound depression or withdrawal occurs.
- Withdrawal dyskinesias occasionally occur with amoxapine.

## TOXICITY AND OVERDOSE

- Antidepressant overdose accounts for 4–7% of all suicides.
- TCAs are most dangerous in overdose.
  - $LD_{50}$ is about a 1-week supply.

- In a study of deaths in England, Scotland, and Wales from poisoning by a single medication, with or without alcohol, during the years 1993–1999 (Buckley & McManus 2002), deaths/million prescriptions were:
  - Desipramine: 201
  - Amoxapine: 94
  - Amitryptiline: 38
  - Lithium: 37
  - Venlafaxine: 34
  - Imipramine: 33
  - Fluoxetine: 18
  - Trimipramine: 17
  - Tranylcypromine: 16
  - Trazodone: 11
  - Paroxetine: 11
  - Sertraline: 7
  - Phenelzine: 6
  - Citalopram: 5
  - Fluvoxamine: 2
  - Mirtazepine: 1
  - Nefazodone: 0
  - Isocarboxazid: 0
  - Reboxetine: 0
- In a review of 256 consecutive admissions to a hospital toxicology service, patients who took overdoses of TCAs had significantly longer lengths of stay, a greater need for intubation, a higher incidence of seizures, longer QRS intervals, and longer stays on the ICU (Graudins, Dowsett, & Liddle, 2002).
  - Serotonin syndrome was only seen with SSRIs.
    - Patients with serotonin syndrome had lengths of stay three times as long as patients taking SSRIs who did not have serotonin syndrome.
- Management of overdose:
  - Maintain airway and oxygenation.
  - Activated charcoal, which may be used with sorbitol, is as or more effective than emesis/lavage.
  - Monitor EKG.
  - Consider anticonvulsant for overdose with amoxapine, maprotiline, clomipramine, bupropion.
  - Dialysis does not help because serum drug concentrations are low.

## PRECAUTIONS

- Be careful using TCAs in patients with
  - Recent myocardial infarction
  - Narrow angle glaucoma or significantly increased intraocular pressure
  - Hypersensitivity to TCAs
  - Use of an MAOI within 2 weeks
    - MAOIs can be added to TCAs other than imipramine and clomipramine, but the reverse order can cause life-threatening interactions (see pp. 226–227).
- SSRIs
  - CYP2D6 inhibitors (e.g., fluoxetine and paroxetine) can increase TCA levels substantially.
  - CYP3A4 inhibitors (e.g., fluvoxamine, nefazodone) can elevate levels of digoxin, cyclosporine, triazolobenzodiazepines, and many other medications.
  - Do not combine any SSRI, nefazodone, bupropion, duloxetine, or venlafaxine with MAOIs.
    - Trazodone does not inhibit serotonin reuptake significantly and can be combined with MAOIs.
- Seizure disorders
  - Avoid amoxapine, clomipramine, maprotiline, bupropion.
  - Secondary amine TCAs and SSRIs do not lower seizure threshold significantly.
- Precipitation of mania:
  - Any antidepressant can induce mania and rapid cycling.
  - The higher risk of antidepressant-induced mania that is usually quoted with TCAs is probably a historical artifact.
    - Virtually all figures on risk of mania in large populations come from phase-III efficacy trials.
    - These trials attempt to exclude bipolar patients.
    - Because TCA trials were conducted a decade or more before phase-III studies of newer antidepressants, investigators were not as good at identifying bipolar risk before enrolling patients in the trials. Inclusion of more unrecognized bipolar patients probably accounts for increased rate of manic switching.

## ADVICE FOR CARETAKERS

Patients often need encouragement to continue antidepressant until it takes effect. Benefit may not be apparent for up to 2–3 months in more persistent depression.

The risk of suicide is 5–15% in depressed patients.

- No antidepressant has been found to increase the risk of suicide unless it precipitates manic or mixed states in bipolar patients.
- Taken in adequate doses, antidepressants reduce suicide risk.
- Sudden, unexplained improvement may be an indication that patient has formulated a suicide plan.
- If concern is high that patient may overdose on an antidepressant, it is probably safer to hospitalize the patient and treat more aggressively than to dole out small amounts of medication, which will increase noncompliance.

Nonadherence

- At least 50% of depressed patients do not take antidepressants as prescribed.
- Common reasons for nonadherence include
  - Cost of medication
  - Adverse effects
  - Complicated dosing
  - Interactions with other treatments
  - Discouragement with slow onset of action
  - Misconception that antidepressants are only needed on days when person feels more depressed.
  - Belief that it is shameful to take antidepressants.
  - Discouragement of adherence by family members.
  - Fear of becoming dependent on medication.
    - This fear often symbolizes fear of becoming dependent on the person prescribing the medication.
    - All-or-nothing thinking leads patient to believe that accepting any help at all is equivalent to being completely helpless.
- Those involved with patient, as well as those prescribing medications, should discuss treatment adherence regularly.
- Rapid abatement of a troublesome side effect may indicate that patient has stopped the medication.

## NOTES FOR PATIENT AND FAMILY

Patients should understand that antidepressants are not "uppers" and are not addicting.

- Patients who are afraid of becoming dependent on an antidepressant may take the lowest possible dose and skip doses when they feel better.

- Fear of dependence on an antidepressant often symbolizes fear of becoming dependent on the person prescribing the medication.
  - Can be addressed by discussing the common but false depressive belief that to depend on anyone for anything means total dependency.

Antidepressants must be taken for 1–3 months to be fully effective.
- Some patients can be reassured that early side effects are an indication that the medication is beginning to work.
- Patients should also be told that antidepressants do not work when they are taken prn—regular administration is necessary for a therapeutic effect.

Most antidepressants can be taken with or without meals.
- Trazodone absorption is increased by food, but peak plasma levels are lower and occur later.
- Sertraline absorption is increased about 25% by food.
  - Taking this medication with meals may allow use of a lower dose.

TCAs other than protriptyline, which is very activating, can usually be taken in a single bedtime dose to maximize compliance and reduce side effects.

If a dose is missed, patient should take it within 3 hours if a bedtime dose or 8 hours if taken during the day.
- If a longer period of time has elapsed, wait for the next dose.
  - Do not double the dose.

After a first episode of major depression, the antidepressant should be continued for 6–12 months.
- Antidepressants speed up symptomatic but not physiological recovery.
- If the episode was not associated with psychosis, suicidality, severe impairment, or very poor decisions, the antidepressant might be withdrawn over 2–3 months.
  - More rapid withdrawal may produce rebound depression and withdrawal symptoms such as gastrointestinal distress, malaise, and an influenza-like syndrome.
    - If withdrawal occurs and the physician is not available, take one dose and locate the physician.
  - If symptoms start to return as the antidepressant is being discontinued, the medication can be gradually reinstituted.
    - However, if rebound depression occurs, the patient may no longer respond to or tolerate a previously effective antidepressant.

- Following a third episode of major depression of any severity, or a single severe or dangerous episode, it is safest to continue an antidepressant indefinitely.
  - Antidepressants substantially reduce the risk of relapse and recurrence in unipolar depression.
    - 20% relapse with maintenance antidepressant vs. 90% after 3–4 major depressive episodes without maintenance treatment.

# CHAPTER FOUR

# Monoamine Oxidase Inhibitors

Monoamine oxidase inhibitors (MAOIs) were introduced as antidepressants in the 1960s after observations of an antidepressant effect of the antitubercular MAOI clorgyline. These medications still have an important role in the treatment of many disorders. This chapter addresses use of MAOIs in

- Major depressive disorder
- Atypical depression
- Personality disorders
- Mixed anxiety and depression

Conditions treated with MAOIs discussed elsewhere include:

- Dysthymia (Antidepressants, Chapter 3)
- Dementia (p. 162)
- Bipolar depression (Chapter 5)
- Bulimia (Antidepressants, pp. 131–132)
- Cataplexy (Chapter 9)
- Irritable bowel syndrome (p. 130)
- Migraine headaches (Antidepressants, p. 130)
- Narcolepsy (Chapter 9)
- OCD (Chapter 7)
- Panic disorder (Antianxiety, Chapter 7)
- Refractory depression (pp. 165–174)
- Social phobia (Chapter 7)

Table 4.1 provides a basic overview of the drugs addressed in this chapter.

**Table 4.1  Names, Dose Forms, Colors**

| GENERIC NAME | BRAND NAME | DOSE FORMS (MG)* | COLORS |
|---|---|---|---|
| | HYDRAZINES | | |
| isocarboxazid | Marplan | t: 10 | t: peach |
| phenelzine | Nardil | t: 15 | t: orange |
| | NONHYDRAZINE | | |
| tranylcypromine | Parnate | t: 10 | t: rose-red |
| | OTHERS | | |
| selegiline (L-deprenyl) | Eldepryl | c: 5 | c: blue |

\* t = tablets; c = capsules

## PHARMACOLOGY

Monoamine oxidase (MAO) is an intracellular enzyme that oxidizes monoamines such as norepinephrine, serotonin, and dopamine. Currently available MAOIs irreversibly inhibit two major forms of monoamine oxidase:

- MAO-A preferentially metabolizes tyramine, dopamine, and phenylalanine.
  - Located primarily in the gut, lungs, and brain.
- MAO-B preferentially metabolizes noerepinephrine and serotonin.
  - Located primarily in the brain and blood platelets.
- An antidepressant effect of the MAOIs is associated with about 80% inhibition of platelet MAO.
  - Brain and platelets are related
    - Both come from the same embryonic precursor.
    - Both have serotonin uptake pumps and $5HT_2$ receptors.
  - However, no correlation between platelet and brain MAO inhibition.
  - Platelet MAO inhibition may be a marker of another action that is more relevant to therapeutic efficacy.
- Inhibition of MAO-A is responsible for hypertensive reactions.
  - Tyramine, a naturally occurring pressor amine found in cheese, soy, and certain aged foods, is metabolized in the gut by intestinal MAO-A.
    - Limits the extent to which dietary tyramine is absorbed.
  - Inhibition of intestinal MAO results in increased absorption of tyramine, which elevates blood pressure.

- MAO inhibition in sympathetic nerve ganglia further increases hypertension.
- Since MAO-A also metabolizes serotonin, ingesting substances containing this monoamine when MAO is inhibited results in excessive circulating serotonin levels, which are toxic to the brain and heart.

Strategies for preventing dietary interactions with MAOIs
- Selective MAO-B inhibitors
  - Selegiline (L-deprenyl) is selective for MAO-B at doses ≤ 10 mg/day.
    - No dietary restrictions at these doses.
    - However, antidepressant effect not reliable at doses < 20 mg/day.
    - Dietary restrictions necessary for use of selegiline as antidepressant because it is no longer selective for MAO-B at these doses.
- Reversible inhibitors of MAO-A (RIMAs)
  - Bind weakly to MAO-A and can be displaced by tyramine.
  - When foods containing tyramine or serotonin are ingested, the monoamine displaces the MAOI from the enzyme, which is then available to metabolize the monoamine normally and prevent excessive absorption.
  - Moclobemide (Mannerix) is a RIMA available in many countries outside of the United States (Bonnet, 2003).
    - No dietary restrictions at moderate doses.
    - Effective for depression and anxiety.
    - More effective than placebo and equivalent to TCAs and SSRIs for major depression.
    - Equivalent to fluoxetine and clomipramine for panic disorder in open trials.
    - Not consistently effective for social phobia in controlled studies.
    - Risk of mania induction about the same as other antidepressants.
    - Therapeutic dose usually 300–900 mg/day in bid or tid schedule.
    - No dietary restrictions at these doses, but dietary interactions may occur at higher doses.
    - No weight gain.
    - Fewer GI and sexual side effects than SSRIs.
    - U.S. patent expired before phase-III trials were completed, making it unlikely that any manufacturer will complete studies necessary for United States release.
  - Befloxatone
    - No psychomotor or memory impairment
    - No sedation
    - Most likely candidate for United States release.

Three MAOI classes are currently available in the United States:

- Hydrazines (phenelzine, isocarboxazid)
  - Resynthesis of MAO after inhibition takes 10–20 days.
- Non-hydrazines (tranylcypromine)
  - Resynthesis of MAO begins sooner than with hydrazines (6 hours to 5 days).
- Propargylamines (selegiline)
- Combining MAOIs from different classes can cause fatal interactions.

Elimination half-lives of MAOIs are relatively short, but pharmacodynamic half-lives (i.e., duration of inhibition of MAO) are longer. Short half-lives require divided doses, with the last dose being given early enough to reduce the risk of insomnia. Elimination half-lives (hours) are

- Phenelzine: 2.8
- Isocarboxazid: 2.8
- Tranylcypromine: 2.4
- Selegiline: 1.9

Features of MAOIs
- Probably more effective than TCAs for
  - Atypical depression
    - SSRIs almost as effective for atypical depression.
  - Depression with anxiety
  - Panic disorder
  - Bipolar depression
    - More data on tranylcypromine than other antidepressants.
- Women respond more frequently than men.
- Effective for geriatric depression.
  - Better tolerated than TCAs because they are less anticholinergic.
  - However, hypotensive side effects are poorly tolerated by elderly.
  - Demented patients may not remember dietary restrictions.

## CLINICAL INDICATIONS AND USE

### Choosing an MAOI

As is true of other antidepressants, patients may respond to, or tolerate, one MAOI much better than the others.

PHENELZINE

- More controlled studies in depression with panic attacks and social phobia.

- Less likely to disrupt sleep or cause spontaneous hypertension than tranylcypromine.
- Often more sedating.
- More weight gain and anticholinergic effects.
- May aggravate hypoglycemia in diabetic patients.

## Isocarboxazid

- Less sedation and weight gain than phenelzine.
- Less activation than tranylcypromine.
- May be difficult to obtain in some regions.

## Tranylcypromine

- Weight gain not as common as with phenelzine.
- More activating than phenelzine and isocarboxazid.
  - Useful for anergic, hypersomnic, depression
- More published experience than other MAOIs in bipolar depression.
- Amphetamine-like metabolite improves attention but occasionally interacts with parent compound to produce spontaneous hypertensive reactions.

## Selegiline

- Has stimulant properties that make the medication very activating.
- Antioxidant effect may slow deterioration of the nervous system.
- Limited research in mood disorders.
- Less weight gain and sedation than other MAOIs.
- First choice for depressed patient with Parkinson's disease.
- May also be useful for depression associated with Alzheimer's disease.
  - If patient can remember dietary restrictions.
- Selegiline transdermal patch:
  - Appears not to inhibit intestinal MAO-A at antidepressant doses because it is not administered through GI tract.
  - Avoids first-pass metabolism, resulting in higher selegiline levels and lower levels of amphetamine-like metabolites than with oral preparation.
  - In an animal study, transdermal selegiline at doses that produced maximal inhibition of MAO-B and of brain MAO-A inhibited GI MAO-A by just 30–40% (Wecker, James, Copeland, & Pacheco, 2003).
  - Usual dose is 20 mg.
  - Patch changed daily.
  - A randomized, double-blind controlled study in 152 of 177 depressed outpatients who completed the trial found significantly greater

reduction with selegiline than placebo in depressive symptoms, more responders, and higher remission rate (Bodkin & Amsterdam, 2002).

- In an 8-week double-blind placebo-controlled study of selegiline transdermal patch 20 mg/20 cm$^2$ in 289 patients with major depression (Amsterdam, 2003):
  - Patients did not follow the MAOI diet.
  - They did avoid proscribed medications.
  - Selegiline was superior to placebo beginning at week 4.
  - Side effects mainly involved rash, itching, erythema, irritation, or swelling at patch site.
  - No hypertensive reactions.
  - No difference between selegiline and placebo in sexual side effects.

## Using MAOIs

Table 4.2 provides basic dosing information for MAOIs.

- Start with one tablet.
  - Initial dose in morning for more activating preparations (e.g., tranylcypromine, selegiline).
- Increase dose slowly, as tolerated.
  - One tablet every few days, to one tablet every 1–2 weeks.
- Give in divided dose.
- Assess response at daily dose of
  - 45–60 mg phenelzine
  - 40–60 mg tranylcypromine
  - 20–40 mg isocarboxazid
  - 20–40 mg selegiline

**Table 4.2  Doses**

| GENERIC NAMES | EQUIVALENT DOSES (MG) | USUAL DOSES (MG/DAY) | HIGH/LOW RANGE (MG/DAY) | STARTING DOSES (MG/DAY) | GERIATRIC DOSES (MG/DAY) |
|---|---|---|---|---|---|
| isocarboxazid | 10 | 10–30 | 10–50 | 30 | 5–15 |
| phenelzine | 15 | 45–60 | 30–145 | 15 | 15–45 |
| tranylcypromine | 10 | 20–40 | 10–150 | 10 | 10–30 |
| selegiline* | 5 | 20–40 | 10–50 | 5 | 10–20 |

\* Antiparkinsonian dose 5–10 mg/day.

- If patient not well after 1–2 months, increase dose, if tolerated, to
  - 90 mg phenelzine
  - 80 mg tranylcypromine
  - 60 mg isocarboxazid
  - 50 mg selegiline
- Further dosage increments may be effective for some patients.
  - 50% of Caucasians are rapid acetylators of tranylcypromine and require high doses.
  - Older studies that suggested low efficacy of MAOIs were the result of inadequate doses.
  - Case reports exist of response at 150–200 mg tranylcypromine and 105–135 mg phenelzine.
- Serum levels are not correlated with clinical response.
- Response may be most reliable at 80% platelet MAO inhibition.
  - Requires comparing platelet MAO at therapeutic dose to baseline level.
  - Measures are difficult to obtain and not entirely reliable.
- Insomnia in a patient who is otherwise responding to an MAOI can be treated with trazodone, a benzodiazepine, or a selective benzodiazepine receptor agonist (e.g., zolpidem).
- Tolerance to MAOIs seems to develop more frequently than with other antidepressants. Tolerance may be
  - Pharmacokinetic
    - Due to medication inducing its own metabolism.
    - Responds to increased antidepressant dose.
    - Repeated dosage increases may be necessary before patient has complete response.
  - Pharmacodynamic
    - Caused by loss of receptor responsiveness to antidepressant.
    - Increasing dose results in brief improvement followed by loss of response again.
    - The medication usually will not produce a sustained response.
    - Tolerance is often specific to one MAOI.
    - The patient may respond to a second trial a few months later.
- Augmentation for partial response (see pp. 165–174):
  - MAOIs can be safely combined with augmenting agents (listed in Chapter 3) *except* for buspirone, pindolol, and other serotonergic agents.
  - Interactions with anesthesia used during ECT are probably not dangerous, but continuing an MAOI during ECT may inhibit therapeutic response.

**Table 4.3  Adding or Replacing MAOIs, TCAs, and SSRIs**

| START WITH | ADD/SUBSTITUTE | RISKS AND INSTRUCTIONS |
|---|---|---|
| TCA | MAOI | Lower risk of interaction; reduce TCA dose by 50%, slowly add MAOI. If patient recovers, slowly taper TCA. If not, carefully increase doses of both medications. |
| MAOI | TCA | High risk of interaction; wait 2–4 weeks for phenelzine and 7–10 days for tranylcypromine between stopping MAOI and starting TCA. |
| MAOI + TCA together | | Lower risk of interaction; raise doses slowly. |
| venlafaxine/duloxetine/ SSRI/clomipramine/ imipramine/ nefazodone | MAOI | High risk of serotonin syndrome. Wait at least 2 weeks after stopping antidepressant (6–8 weeks for fluoxetine) before starting MAOI. |
| MAOI | Venlafaxine/duloxetine/ SSRI/clomipramine/ imipramine/nefazodone | High risk of serotonin syndrome when these drugs are combined in any manner. Wait at least 2 weeks between stopping MAOI and starting new antidepressant. |
| MAOI | Mirtazapine | Risk of hypertensive reaction or serotonin syndrome. Wait 2 weeks between medications. |
| MAOI hydrazine (phenelzine) | MAOI nonhydrazine (tranylcypromine) | Subarachnoid hemorrhage reported with this combination. Wait 2–4 weeks before changing MAOI classes. |
| MAOI | Epinephrine/norepinephrine | Peripheral epinephrine metabolism is mainly dependent on catechol-O-methyltransferase (COMT), which is diffusely found in all extraneuronal tissues. There are no reports of hypertensive crisis with epinephrine because MAOIs do not block its metabolism. However, norepinephrine is mainly degraded by MAO localized to nerve terminals and risks hypertensive crisis. |

## COMBINING AN MAOI WITH A TCA

- Most studies suggest no superiority of the combination to either one alone.
  - Most of these observations are based on assignment of nonrefractory patients to a TCA, an MAOI, or both.
    - Outcome is the same with all three treatments.
    - This approach does not address whether the combination is more effective in patients who have failed to respond to each medication by itself.
    - Some reports suggest that MAOI–TCA combinations are more effective than monotherapy in refractory depression.
- Principles of combining medication classes:
  - The MAOI must be added to the TCA.
    - Fatal interactions have occurred with the opposite sequence.
    - Both may be started in low doses at the same time.
  - MAOIs can be added to TCAs *except* imipramine and clomipramine.
    - Primary risk is of serotonin syndrome.
    - Even amitriptyline is not sufficiently serotonergic to cause dangerous interactions.
  - MAOIs cannot be combined with any of the newer antidepressants except trazodone.
  - When combining an MAOI and a TCA:
  - Start with the TCA or start both medications together.
  - Consider a trial of a therapeutic dose of the TCA first, with or without augmentation.
  - If no response, reduce the TCA dose to 25–50 mg of desipramine equivalent.
  - Add a single MAOI tablet.
  - Increase the MAOI dose to a moderate level (e.g., 30 mg phenelzine).
  - Then alternate increases of each medication to therapeutic doses.
  - If patient has full response, a decrease in the dose of the TCA can be considered to see if the patient needs both medications.
- In patients with a history of treatment resistance, augmenting a new antidepressant with a TCA can be followed by a trial of the TCA and then a TCA–MAOI combination.
  - If the combination is tried after failure on an MAOI, it will be necessary to withdraw the MAOI, wait, start a TCA, and then add the MAOI.
- MAOIs and MAOI–TCA combinations can be augmented with stimulants.

- Methylphenidate probably safer than Dexedrine.
- Most other agents used to augment MAOIs can augment MAOI–TCA combinations.
- Some clinicians think that a TCA might reduce the risk of a hypertensive reaction by inhibiting GI tyramine uptake, but this has not been proven, and dietary restrictions should still be followed.

## Atypical Depression

MAOIs may be effective more frequently than other antidepressants for major depression with atypical features.
- Atypical depression is characterized by
  - Increased appetite, craving carbohydrates or sweets, weight gain
  - Hypersomnia
  - Initial insomnia
  - Reverse diurnal mood swing (feeling worse as the day goes on)
  - Rejection sensitivity
  - Mood reactivity (feeling better temporarily in response to positive interactions or events)
  - Phobic anxiety
  - Panic attacks
  - Somatization
- Of these features, anxiety is the best predictor of a response to an MAOI.
- SSRIs almost as effective as MAOIs for atypical depression.

## Borderline Personality Disorder

Drug treatment of personality disorders is usually targeted toward specific symptoms rather than the overall disorder, which is treated with psychotherapy (e.g., dialectic behavior therapy). For example:
- Low doses of atypical antipsychotics for cognitive disorganization and paranoia, which usually represents psychotic transference
- Lithium, anticonvulsants, or SSRIs for affective lability and impulsivity
- Naltrexone for parasuicidal behavior such as cutting or burning
- Antidepressants for comorbid depression

Whereas MAOIs may be more effective for depression accompanying personality disorders SSRIs are also helpful, especially for depression and impulsivity. Patients who use self-destructive behavior to defeat the practitioner may ignore dietary restrictions (consciously or unconsciously) and experience dangerous interactions with prohibited foods, despite (or perhaps because of) being repeatedly warned about them.

## INTERACTIONS

### Drug Interactions

MAOIs inhibit metabolism of monoamines, including serotonin, norepinephrine and dopamine. Inhibition of serotonin breakdown can result in serotonin syndrome, which is a manifestation of the neurotoxicity and cardiotoxicity of high serotonin levels. Reduced norepinephrine and dopamine metabolism can result in sympathetic overstimulation and hypertension. Excessive accumulation of dopamine can cause activation and hypertension.

SEROTONIN SYNDROME

- Occurs when MAOIs are combined with highly serotonergic medications, such as
  - SSRIs
  - Imipramine
  - Clomipramine
  - Nefazodone
  - Venlafazine
  - Duloxetine
  - Possibly mirtazepine
  - Buspirone
  - Meperidine
  - Dextromethorphan
  - Tryptophan
- Features of serotonin syndrome can include
  - Fever
  - Myoclonus
  - Muscle fasciculations
  - Shivering
  - Hyperreflexia
  - Hypotension
  - Agitation, anxiety
  - Confusion
  - Delirium
  - Cardiac arrhythmias
  - Seizures
  - Coma
  - Death

- There is no definitive treatment for serotonin syndrome. However, since this reaction is mediated by $5HT_2$ receptors, $5HT_2$ antagonists may be helpful.
  - Cyproheptadine 4–8 mg tid
  - Trazodone 50–100 mg one to four times/day

## HYPERTENSIVE INTERACTIONS

- Occur with tyramine-containing foods (see pp. 230–237) and with highly noradrenergic or dopaminergic agents:
  - Bupropion
  - Mirtazepine
  - Venlafaxine
  - Dextroamphetamine
  - Ephedrine
  - Pseudoephedrine
  - Isometheptine
  - Phenylephrine
  - Phenylpropanolamine
  - Pramipexole
  - L-dopa in higher doses
  - Dopamine
  - Cyclobenzaprine (Flexeril)
  - Metaproterenol
  - Norepinephrine
    - Epinephrine is not metabolized by MAO (metabolism is not intracellular).
    - Epinephrine can be used to treat allergic reactions in patients taking MAOIs.
  - Illicit drugs that can cause hypertensive crisis with MAOIs include
    - Cocaine
    - Stimulants
    - Methamphetamine

Features of hypertensive reactions
- Hypertension
- Tachycardia
- Severe occipital headache
- Retrobulbar pain
- Stiff neck
- Flushing, sweating, cold, clammy skin

- Nosebleeds
- Dilated pupils
- Photophobia
- Chest pain
- Coronary artery vasospasm
- Stroke

Treatment of hypertensive reactions

- Patient should be certain that a hypertensive reaction is occurring, because treatments for hypertensive crisis can cause dangerous hypotension.
  - Patient should be given
    - Wallet card describing MAOI regimen (may be obtained from Pfizer/Roerig at 800-223-0432).
    - List of contraindicated foods and medicines.
    - Bracelet or letter instructing ER physician not to administer meperidine for headache.
  - Teach patients to take their own blood pressures.
  - Seek emergency treatment if
    - Headache is the worst headache the patient has ever had.
    - Systolic blood pressure > 170 or diastolic > 110
    - Other symptoms of hypertensive reaction are occurring.
    - Any doubt about whether a severe reaction has developed.
- Chewing a 10 mg nifedipine tablet and placing contents under tongue has been recommended, but nifedipine is poorly absorbed from buccal mucosa.
  - Taking 10–20 mg nifedipine orally may be more reliable, but onset of antihypertensive effect takes longer.
  - Nifedipine occasionally causes significant hypotension.
- Definitive treatment is with
  - Phentolamine 2–10 mg IV slowly
  - IV sodium nitroprusside

## Combining MAOIs with Other Medications

- MAOIs can have dangerous interactions with the newer antidepressants and with very serotonergic TCAs, especially imipramine and clomipramine.
- TCAs that have been combined safely with MAOIs include
  - Amitriptyline
  - Nortriptyline

- Doxepin
- Trimipramine
- Maprotiline
- Trazodone does not have SRI properties and can be added to MAOIs.
  - Most frequent use is for insomnia.
  - MAOI-induced insomnia also can be treated with zolpidem, zaleplon, or a benzodiazepine.
- Although dopamine-releasing stimulants such as dextroamphetamine can be risky combined with MAOIs, methylphenidate is safer, and stimulants can be added cautiously to MAOIs to treat
  - Refractory depression
  - MAOI-induced hypotension in a patient who is responding to the antidepressant
- Modafinil is not a stimulant and can be used to treat sedation caused by MAOIs.
- Because carbamazepine has a tricyclic structure, it is sometimes recommended that it not be combined with MAOIs.
  - However, carbamazepine is not noradrenergic or serotonergic, and no adverse interactions have been reported.
- Hydrazine (e.g., phenelzine) and non-hydrazine MAOIs (e.g., tranylcypromine) should not be combined with each other because of reports of cerebral hemorrhage with the combination.
  - Do not overlap these medications when changing from one to the other.
- MAOIs may prolong sedative and hypotensive effects of general anesthetics, but MAOIs have been used safely with anesthesia.
- The only narcotic analgesic that is clearly contraindicated with MAOIs is meperidine, which is serotonergic.
- Triptans such as sumitriptan are supposed to be avoided by patients taking MAOIs.
  - These medications reduce rather than increase serotonin release and therefore do not cause serotonergic interactions.
  - The primary interaction is an increase in the sumitriptan AUC (area under time-concentration curve) by the MAOI.

### MAOIs in Patients with Asthma

- Beta-adrenergic bronchodilators may cause hypertensive reactions.
  - For example
    - Metaproterenol
    - Albuterol

- Beclomethasone inhaler is safer.
- Ephedrine should be avoided.
- In office monitor blood pressure after patient has used bronchodilator.

## MAOIs and Dental Anesthesia

- Avoid local anesthetics with norepinephrine (used to keep lidocaine from diffusing away from local site).
- Plain lidocaine or lidocaine with epinephrine is safe.

## Food Interactions

At least 6 mg of tyramine/serving is usually necessary to precipitate a hypertensive crisis with phenelzine; less with tranylcypromine.

- For many people ≥ 10 mg tyramine in 4 hours is dangerous for patients taking phenelzine.
  - ≥ 4–5 mg/serving is risky with tranylcypromine.
- Because tyramine content increases with the time food ages, no reaction may occur on one occasion when a tyramine-containing food is ingested, whereas the same product on a different day with a longer shelf life may produce a severe hypertensive reaction.
  - Cheese from the center of a cheese wheel has higher tyramine content than cheese from the outside of the wheel.
  - Warn patients who feel they have gotten away with "experimenting" with a particular food that this does not mean that all samples of the food are safe.

Foods that should definitely be avoided include

- All cheese except cottage cheese, ricotta, processed cheese slices, and cream cheese
- Fava bean pods (contain dopamine)
- Pure soy products (e.g., soy sauce, tofu)
- Dark, fermented beer
  - Includes fermented alcohol-free beers
    - Some microbrews may be risky because of coarse filters that allow bacterial contamination, producing further fermentation after brewing.
    - Other beers are safe.
- Air-dried sausage, salami
- Chicken liver > 5 days old
  - Fresh chicken liver is safe.
- Sauerkraut

- Concentrated yeast extract (especially Marmite)
  - Some powdered protein diet supplements contain yeast extracts.
  - Brewer's yeast is safe.
  - Yeast used for baking is safe.
- Pickled herring in brine

Foods that are safe include

- Bologna
- Pepperoni
- Summer sausage
- Corned beef
- Liverwurst
- Chocolate in moderate amounts
- Figs, raisins, avocados
- Overripe fruit
- Bananas
  - Overripe banana *peels* contain tyramine.
- Caffeine-containing beverages
- White and red wines
- Yogurt
- Caviar, escargot, tinned fish
- Tinned and packet soup
  - Large amounts of bouillon or meat extract can be risky.

The following tables (4.4–4.13) present average tyramine content of common beverages and foods. Remember that actual values vary and that people differ in their sensitivity to tyramine reactions. *Less tyramine is necessary to produce hypertensive reactions with tranylcypromine than with phenelzine.*

## SIDE EFFECTS

### Cardiovascular Side Effects

HYPOTENSION

- Despite hypertensive interactions, MAOIs are primarily antihypertensive.
- Resting and orthostatic hypotension with phenelzine equivalent to TCAs.
- Manifestations of hypotension include
  - Dizziness
    - Occurs in 20–50% of patients.
    - About the same as for nortriptyline

Table 4.4 Tyramine Content of Beers

| BEER | BREWER | TYRAMINE CONCENTRATION µG/ML | TYRAMIN CONTENT (MG) PER SERVING* |
|---|---|---|---|
| **BEERS WITH ALCOHOL** | | | |
| Amstel | Amstel | 4.52 | 1.54 |
| Export Draft | Molson | 3.79 | 1.29 |
| Blue Light | Labatts | 3.42 | 1.16 |
| Guinness Extra Stout | Labatts | 3.37 | 1.15 |
| Old Vienna | Carling | 3.32 | 1.13 |
| Canadian | Molson | 3.01 | 1.03 |
| Miller Light | Carling | 2.91 | 0.99 |
| Export | Molson | 2.78 | 0.95 |
| Heineken | Holland | 1.81 | 0.62 |
| Blue | Labatts | 1.80 | 0.61 |
| Coors Light | Molson | 1.45 | 0.49 |
| Carlsberg Light | Carling | 1.15 | 0.39 |
| Michelob | Anheuser-Busch | 0.98 | 0.33 |
| Beck's | Braueri Beck | 0.90 | 0.30 |
| Genesee Cream | Genesee | 0.86 | 0.29 |
| Stroh's | Stroh's | 0.78 | 0.27 |
| Old Milwaukee | Pacific Western | 0.34 | 0.11 |
| **DEALCOHOLIZED BEERS** | | | |
| O'Douls Malt Beverage | Anheuser-Busch | 2.25 | 0.68 |
| Labatts | Labatts Brewing Co. | 1.18 | 0.36 |
| Buckler | Heineken | 1.08 | 0.32 |
| Special Light Swan | Special Light Swan Lager | 0.97 | 0.29 |
| Texas Select | San Antonio Beverage Co. | 0.82 | 0.25 |
| Sharp's | Miller Brewing Co. | 0.37 | 0.11 |
| Molson Excel | Molson Breweries | 0.00 | 0.00 |
| Tourtel | Kronenbourg | 0.00 | 0.00 |
| Upper Canada Point Nine | Upper Canada Brewery | 0.00 | 0.00 |
| **PARTICULARLY RISKY TAP BEERS** | | | |
| Upper Canada Lager | Sleeman | 112.91 | 37.62 |
| Kronenbourg | Kronenbourg | 37.85 | 15.94 |
| Rotterdam's Pilsner | Rotterdam | 29.47 | 9.82 |
| Rotterdam's Lager | Rotterdam | 27.05 | 9.00 |

Generally U.S. and Canadian canned and bottled beers are safe if ≤ 4 servings consumed; all Canadian beers (Labatts, Molson, Upper Canada, Pacific Western) < 3 µg/ml.

\* Based on a 341 ml serving (one bottle).

### Table 4.5  Tyramine Content of Wines

| WINE | COLOR | TYPE | COUNTRY | TYRAMINE CONCENTRATION (μG/ML) | TYRAMINE CONTENT (MG) PER SERVING* |
|---|---|---|---|---|---|
| Rioja (Siglo) | Red | | Spain | 4.41 | 0.53 |
| sherry | Red | | | 3.60 | 0.43 |
| Ruffino | Red | Chianti | Italy | 3.04 | 0.36 |
| Blue Nun | White | | Germany | 2.70 | 0.32 |
| retsina | White | | Greece | 1.79 | 0.21 |
| La Colombaia | Red | Chianti | Italy | 0.63 | 0.08 |
| riesling | | | | 0.60 | 0.07 |
| Brolio | Red | Chianti | Italy | 0.44 | 0.05 |
| sauterne | White | | | 0.40 | 0.05 |
| Beau-Rivage | White | Bordeaux | France | 0.39 | 0.05 |
| Beau-Rivage | Red | Bordeaux | France | 0.35 | 0.04 |
| Maria Christina | Red | | Canada | 0.20 | 0.20 |
| port | Red | | | 0.20 | 0.02 |
| Cinzano | Red | Vermouth | Italy | † | † |
| LePiazze** | Red | Chianti | Italy | † | † |

\* Based on a 120 ml (4 ounce) serving.
\*\* Other Chianti sampled also with no tyramine.
† Nil.

### Table 4.6  Tyramine Content of Other Alcohol

| TYPE | TYRAMINE CONCENTRATION (μG/ML) | TYRAMINE CONTENT (MG) PER SERVING |
|---|---|---|
| ale | 8.8 | 3.0/341 ml |
| Harvey's Bristol Cream | 2.65 | 0.32 mg/4 ounces |
| Dubonnet | 1.59 | 0.19 mg/4 ounces |
| vermouth | high | high |
| bourbon | † | † |
| London distilled dry gin (Beefeater) | † | † |
| gin | † | † |
| vodka | † | † |
| rum | † | † |
| scotch | † | † |

† Nil.

**Table 4.7 Tyramine Content of Cheeses**

| TYPE | TYRAMINE CONCENTRATION (μ/G) | TYRAMINE CONTENT (MG) PER SERVING* |
|---|---|---|
| liederkranz | 1454.50 | 21.8 |
| cheddar (New York State) | 1416.00 | 21.2 |
| English stilton | 1156.91 | 17.3 |
| cheddar, old center (Canadian) | 1013.95 | 16.4 |
| blue cheese | 997.79 | 15.0 |
| Swiss | 925.00 | 13.9 |
| white (3-year-old) | 779.74 | 11.7 |
| camembert (Danish) | 681.50 | 10.2 |
| emmentaler | 612.50 | 9.2 |
| extra-old | 608.19 | 9.1 |
| gruyère (British) | 597.50 | 9.0 |
| brick (Canadian) | 524.00 | 7.9 |
| gruyère (American) | 516.00 | 7.7 |
| cheddar (25 samples) | 384.00 | 5.8 |
| gouda | 345.00 | 5.2 |
| edam | 310.00 | 4.7 |
| colby | 285.00 | 4.3 |
| mozzarella | 284.04 | 4.2 |
| roquefort (French) | 273.50 | 4.1 |
| Danish blue | 256.48 | 4.1 |
| d'Oka (imported) | 234.00 | 3.5 |
| limberger | 204.00 | 3.1 |
| cheddar, center cut (Canadian) | 192.00 | 2.9 |
| Argenti (imported) | 168.00 | 2.5 |
| Romano | 159.0 | 2.4 |
| cheese spread, Handisnack | 133.81 | 2.0 |
| gruyère (Swiss) | 125.17 | 1.9 |
| cheddar, fresh (Canadian) | 120.00 | 1.8 |
| muenster | 101.69 | 1.5 |
| provolone | 94.00 | 1.4 |
| camembert (American) | 86.00 | 1.3 |

*(continues)*

**Table 4.7　Continued**

| TYPE | TYRAMINE CONCENTRATION (μ/G) | TYRAMINE CONTENT (MG) PER SERVING* |
|---|---|---|
| parmesan, grated (Kraft) | 81.08 | 1.3 |
| old coloured, Canadian | 77.47 | 1.2 |
| feta | 75.78 | 1.1 |
| parmesan, grated (Italian) | 69.79 | 1.1 |
| gorgonzola | 55.94 | 0.8 |
| processed (American) | 50.00 | 0.8 |
| blue cheese dressing | 39.20 | 0.6 |
| mozzarella cheese | 36.32 | 0.5** |
| medium (Black Diamond) | 34.75 | 0.5 |
| processed (Canadian) | 26.00 | 0.4 |
| Swiss Emmentaler | 23.99 | 0.4 |
| brie (M-C) with rind | 21.19 | 0.3 |
| cambozola Blue Vein (germ) | 18.31 | 0.3 |
| brie (d'Oka) without rind | 14.65 | 0.2 |
| farmers, Canadian plain | 11.05 | 0.2 |
| cheez whiz (Kraft) | 8.46 | 0.1 |
| brie (d'Oka) with rind | 5.71 | 0.1 |
| cream cheese (plain) | 9.04 | 0.1 |
| brie (M-C) without rind | 2.82 | <0.1 |
| sour cream (Astro) | 1.23 | <0.1 |
| boursin | 0.98 | <0.1 |
| cottage cheese | <0.20 | † |
| cream cheese | <0.20 | † |
| cheese powder (for macaroni) | † | † |
| havarti (Canadian) | † | † |
| ricotta | † | † |
| bonbel | † | † |

\* Based on a 15-gram (single slice) serving.
\*\* Range 0.15–2.4 mg/15 gm
† Nil.

**Table 4.8 Tyramine Content in Fish**

| TYPE | TYRAMINE CONCENTRATION (μG/G) | TYRAMINE CONTENT (MG) PER SERVING* |
|---|---|---|
| pickled herring* | up to 3030 | — |
| pickled herring brine | 15.1/ml | — |
| lump fish roe | 4.4 | 0.2/50 g |
| sliced schmaltz herring in oil | 4.0 | 0.2/50 g |
| smoked carp | † | † |
| smoked salmon | † | † |
| smoked white fish | † | † |

\* Other reports indicate that the tyramine content of pickled herring is nil.
† Nil.

**Table 4.9 Tyramine Content in Meat and Sausage\***

| TYPE | TYRAMINE CONCENTRATION (μG/G) | TYRAMINE CONTENT (MG) PER SERVING* |
|---|---|---|
| sausage, Belgian, dry-fermented | 803.9 | 24.1 |
| liver, beef, spoiled | 274 | 8.2 |
| sausage, dry-fermented | 244 | 7.3 |
| salami | 188 | 5.6 |
| mortadella | 184 | 5.5 |
| air-dried sausage | 125 | 3.8** |
| sausage, semi-dried fermented | 85.5 | 2.6 |
| chicken liver (day 5) | 77.25 | 1.5 |
| bologna | 33 | 1.0 |
| aged sausage | 29 | 0.9 |
| smoked meat | 18 | 0.5 |
| corned beef | 11 | 0.3 |
| kolbasa sausage | 6 | 0.2 |
| liver, beef, fresh | 5.4 | 0.2 |
| liverwurst | 2 | 0.1 |
| smoked sausage | 1 | <0.1 |
| sweet Italian sausage | 1 | <0.1 |
| pepperoni sausage | † | † |
| chicken liver (day 1) | † | † |

\* Based on 30 g serving.
\*\* 2 of 10 > 6 mg, 2 of 10 4–6 mg.
†Nil.

### Table 4.10 Tyramine Content in Paté*

| TYPE | TYRAMINE CONCENTRATION (μG/G) | TYRAMINE CONTENT (MG) PER SERVING* |
|---|---|---|
| salmon mousse paté | 22 | 0.7 |
| country style paté | 3 | 0.1 |
| peppercorn paté | 2 | 0.1 |

\* Based on 30 g serving.

### Table 4.11 Tyramine Content in Fruits and Vegetables

| TYPE | TYRAMINE CONCENTRATION (μG/G) | TYRAMINE CONTENT (MG) PER SERVING* |
|---|---|---|
| banana peel* (blackened) | 81.62 | 2.58/peel |
| banana peel* (fresh) | 58.35 | 1.424/peel |
| raspberries | † | † |
| raspberry jam | <38.0 | — |
| avocado, fresh** | 23.0 | † |
| orange | 10.0 | — |
| plum (red) | 6.0 | — |
| tomato | 4.0 | — |
| eggplant | 3.0 | — |
| potato | 1.0 | — |
| spinach | 1.0 | — |
| banana (fresh pulp) | † | † |
| grapes | † | † |
| figs, California-Blue Ribbon | † | † |
| raisins (California seedless) | † | † |
| fava (Italian) (broad) bean pods¥ | † | † |

\* The peel of the banana and the pod of the fava bean contain considerable dopamine; the banana pulp and the actual fava bean carry no risk.
\*\* Some claim fresh avocado is nil.
¥ Dopamine = 700 μg/g.
† Nil.

**Table 4.12 Tyramine Content in Yeast Extracts**

| TYPE | TYRAMINE CONCENTRATION (μG/G) | TYRAMINE CONTENT (MG) PER SERVING* |
|---|---|---|
| Marmite concentrated yeast extract | 1184 | 6.45/10 g |
| Yeast extracts | 2156 | — |
| Brewer's yeast tablets (Drug Trade Co.) | — | 191.27 g/400 mg |
| Brewer's yeast tablets (Jamieson) | — | 66.72 g/400 mg |
| Brewer's yeast flakes (Vegetrates) | — | 9.36 g/15 g |
| Brewer's yeast debittered (Maximum Nutrition) | — | † |

† Nil.

**Table 4.13 Tyramine Content in Other Foods**

| TYPE | TYRAMINE CONCENTRATION (μG/G) | TYRAMINE CONTENT (MG) PER SERVING* |
|---|---|---|
| soy sauce (Japanese) | 509.30 | — |
| soy sauce (Tamari) | 466.00 | — |
| meat extracts (soup, gravy, bases) | 199.50 | — |
| soybean paste | 84.85 | — |
| beef bouillon mix (Bovril) | — | 231.25 |
| sauerkraut (Krakus) | 56.49 | 13.84 |
| beef bouillon (Oetker) | — | 0.102/cube |
| fermented soybean curd | — | 3–11/1–2 cubes |
| tofu (Vita) (7 days in refrigerator) | — | 4.8 |
| fresh tofu (Vita) | — | 0.2 |
| soy sauce (Pearl River Bridge) | — | 3.4/15 ml |
| soy sauce (Kimlan) | — | 0.5/15 ml |
| soy sauce (Kikkoman) | — | 0.4/15 ml |
| soy sauce (generic) | 18.72 μg/ml | 0.2/10 ml |
| soy sauce (Wing's) | — | 0.15/15 ml |
| soy sauce (chemically hydrolized) | 1.8 | — |
| worcester sauce (Lea & Perrins, Sharwood, no name) | | ≤0.12/15 ml |
| veggie burger (soybean curd) (9 days in refrigerator) | | 0.6/g |
| ½ medium double cheese, double pepperoni Pizza Hut* | 136 g | 0.06 |

*(continues)*

**Table 4.13 Continued**

| TYPE | TYRAMINE CONCENTRATION (μG/G) | TYRAMINE CONTENT (MG) PER SERVING* |
|---|---|---|
| ½ medium double cheese Pizza Pizza* | 133 g | 0.17 |
| ½ medium double cheese, double pepperoni Domino's Pizza* | 104 g | 0.38 |
| 1 deluxe or pepperoni pizza McDonald's* | 80 g | 0.04 |
| cocoa powder | 1.45 | — |
| beef gravy (Franco American) | 0.858/ml | <0.1/30 ml |
| chicken gravy (Franco American) | 0.46/ml | <0.1/30 ml |
| chicken bouillon mix (Maggi) | † | † |
| vegetable bouillon mix | † | † |
| yogurt | <0.2 | † |

\* Large chain pizza might be relatively safe, but smaller outlets or gourmet pizza may contain aged cheese; Kosher pizzas do not generally have aged cheese and are more likely to be safe.
† Nil.

- Coldness
- Headaches
- Fainting
- Falls may occur in the elderly.
- Management:
  - Avoid adding other medications with hypotensive properties.
  - Avoid fluid restriction.
  - Salt tablets
  - Fludrocortisone if severe
  - Dextroamphetamine is sometimes effective.
  - General measures are summarized on page 38.

HYPERTENSION

- Spontaneous hypertension has occasionally been reported, primarily with tranylcypromine.
  - Probably the result of an interaction between tranylcypromine and an amphetamine-like metabolite.
- Treatment is same as for hypertensive crisis; then withdraw the medication.

PERIPHERAL EDEMA

- Reported in 5–19% on phenelzine.
- Less edema seen with tranylcypromine.
- Management:
  - Use support hose.
  - Decrease dose.
  - Add diuretic.

## Central Nervous System Side Effects

INSOMNIA

- All MAOIs are activating and can cause insomnia.
  - Most frequent with tranylcypromine and selegiline.
  - Nocturnal myoclonus (see below) can disrupt sleep.
- Management:
  - Take all doses earlier in day.
    - Some patients develop insomnia if MAOI is taken after noon.
  - Add hypnotic.
    - Trazodone
    - Zolpidem or zaleplon
    - Benzodiazepine
  - Use less-activating MAOI.

MYOCLONUS

- Nocturnal myoclonus is common with MAOIs.
  - May disrupt sleep.
  - SSRIs also can cause myoclonus.
- Management:
  - Reduce dose of MAOI.
  - Change MAOI.
  - Have patient take medication more frequently.
  - Add clonazepam, other benzodiazepine, carbamazepine, or valproate.
    - Zolpidem may be helpful.

PROBLEMS WITH WORD FINDING

- May occur with any MAOI, especially phenelzine.
- Management:
  - Reduce dose.
  - Change medications.

- Cholinesterase inhibitor if MAOI is the only antidepressant that has worked.

## PERIPHERAL NEUROPATHY

- Most common with hydrazine MAOIs.
- Manifestations include
  - Paresthesias and numbness
  - Muscle spasm
  - Pain
  - Abnormal deep-tendon reflexes
- Two possible causes:
  - Direct toxicity of MAOI
  - Interference with pyridoxine (vitamin B6) absorption
    - Differentiate between these etiologies by treating with pyridoxine.
- Pyridoxine deficiency
  - Signs and symptoms include
    - Neuropathy
    - Stomatitis
    - Anemia
    - Hyperacusis
    - Buzzing in ears
    - Irritability
    - Depression
    - Carpal tunnel syndrome
    - Ataxia
    - Clonus
    - Seizures (very rare)
  - Treatment:
    - Pyridoxine 100 mg/day
    - Somewhat higher doses sometimes necessary.
    - Response occurs in 2–10 weeks.
    - Excessive pyridoxine replacement may cause peripheral neuropathy.

## SEDATION

- Sedation is most common with phenelzine, but isocarboxazid and tranylcypromine also can be sedating.
- Insomnia caused by MAOI can contribute to daytime sleepiness.
- Management:
  - Treat insomnia.
  - Take modafinil in morning.

NIGHTMARES

- MAOIs are potent REM suppressors.
- This effect can be useful for patients with nightmares related to PTSD.
- Some patients experience REM rebound.
  - REM rebound with vivid dreams may persist up to 6 weeks after rapid discontinuation of MAOI.

OVERSTIMULATION

- Tranylcypromine and selegiline are most activating.
- May be manifested by jitteriness, agitation, insomnia.
- Some patients develop hypomanic features that do not necessarily indicate a primary bipolar mood disorder.
  - Seen in 7% taking phenelzine and 10% taking tranylcypromine.
- Paranoia occasionally develops.
- Management:
  - Decreasing MAOI dose often results in remission of hypomanic and paranoid symptoms.
  - Change antidepressant.
  - Add mood stabilizer.

## Endocrine and Sexual Side Effects

- Sexual side effects occur most frequently with phenelzine but may occur with any MAOI.
- Types of sexual dysfunction with MAOIs
  - Anorgasmia
    - In 22% on phenelzine and 2% on tranylcypromine
  - Erectile dysfunction
  - Decreased libido
  - Retarded ejaculation
- Management:
  - Antidepressant-induced sexual dysfunction discussed in Chapter 3.
    - Do not combine yohimbine with an MAOI.
  - Reduce dose of MAOI.
  - Cyproheptadine 2–4 mg as needed or tid.
  - Bethanechol 10 mg tid sometimes improves erectile function.
    - Sildenafil is more effective but also much more expensive.
  - Add trazodone.

CARBOHYDRATE CRAVING

- Most common with phenelzine, least with selegiline.

## Hypoglycemia

- MAOIs can potentiate hypoglycemic action of lithium.
- Occurs more commonly with hydrazines.

## Lymphadenopathy

- Reported occasionally with phenelzine and tranylcypromine.
- Resolves without treatment when medication withdrawn.

### Eyes, Ears, Nose, and Throat Side Effects

## Anticholinergic Side Effects

- Most common with phenelzine
- Blurred vision
- Dry mouth
- Dry eyes
- Precipitation of narrow angle glaucoma
- Constipation
- Urinary hesitency

## Meniere's-like Syndrome

- Manifests as vertigo, tinnitus, nystagmus.
- Remits when MAOI discontinued.

### Gastrointestinal Side Effects

## Hepatotoxicity

- Extremely rare
  - Primarily reported with isoniazid
- Frequency: isocarboxazid > phenelzine > tranylcypromine
- Signs and symptoms:
  - Weakness, malaise
  - Rash
  - Nausea, anorexia
  - Jaundice
  - Eosinophilia
  - Elevated LFTs
- Tranylcypromine and selegiline preferred for patients with liver disease.

FLATUS

- Rare
- May respond to oral lactose.

WEIGHT GAIN

- Most frequent with phenelzine but can occur with tranylcypromine.
  - Up to 70% taking phenelzine gain weight.
  - Typical weight gain 5–10 pounds.

### Skin, Allergies, and Temperature Side Effects

DECREASED SWEATING

- May be anticholinergic side effect.

FEVER, CHILLS

- Exclude serotonin syndrome or hypertensive reaction before attributing to primary medication side effect.

## WITHDRAWAL

MAOIs do not cause dependence or addiction.

- Tolerance develops to antidepressant effect more frequently than with other antidepressants.

Abrupt withdrawal of MAOIs may cause

- Agitation
- Nightmares and other symptoms of REM rebound
  - For example, hypnogogic hallucinations
- Insomnia
- Hypersomnia
- Mania
- Psychosis
- Anxiety
- Rebound depression
- Headache
- Diarrhea
- Tremulousness
- Hot and cold feelings
- Muscle weakness
- Confusion

## Table 4.14  Drug–Drug Interactions

| DRUGS (X)<br>INTERACT WITH: | MONOAMINE-OXIDASE<br>INHIBITORS (M) | COMMENTS |
|---|---|---|
| acetabutolol (*see* β-blockers)<br>albuterol | X↑ | Palpitations, tachycardia, anxiety, increased BP. |
| alcohol | M↑ | May trigger hypertensive crisis (*see* pp. 225–227). |
| anesthetics | X↑ | Potentiate CNS depression or excitement, muscle (general) stiffness or hyperpyrexia. |
| anticholinergics | X↑ | Increased atropine-like effects. |
| antihypertensives | X↑ | Hypotension. |
| antipsychotics | X↑ M↑ | Hypotension; may increase EPS, particularly in typical agents and in risperidone at higher doses (5 mg or more). |
| atenolol (*see* beta-blockers) | | |
| barbiturates | X↑ | Additive CNS depression. |
| benzodiazepines | X↑ | Increased benzodiazepine effect; disinhibition, edema. |
| beta-blockers<br>  acetabutolol (CS)<br>  atenolol (CS)<br>  betaxolol (CS)<br>  labetolol (CS)<br>  nadolol (CS)<br>  penbutalol (NCS)<br>  pindolol (NCS)<br>  propranolol (NCS)<br>  timolol (NCS) | X↑ M↑ | Hypotension, bradycardia, and rebound BP increase if quickly stopped. |
| betaxolol (*see* β-blockers) | | |
| bupropion | X↑ | Hypertension; psychosis possible. |
| buspirone | X↑ | Possible serotonin syndrome |
| caffeine | X↑ | Irregular heartbeat or high BP; reports of hypertensive crisis; avoid in high quantities. |
| carbamazepine | X↓ | Seizures in epileptics; monitor levels. |
| clomipramine | X↑ | Serotonin syndrome: Do not combine. |
| clonidine | M↑ | May potentiate MAOIs. |
| cocaine | M↑ | Hypertensive crisis (*see* sympathomimetics). |
| cyclobenzaprine | X↑ M↑ | Fever, seizures, and death reported |

(*continues*)

**Table 4.14 Continued**

| DRUGS (X) INTERACT WITH: | MONOAMINE-OXIDASE INHIBITORS (M) | COMMENTS |
|---|---|---|
| dextroamphetamine | M↑ | Hypertensive crisis, especially with tranylcypromine. Combination may be used cautiously to treat hypotension |
| dextromethorphan | M↑ | A few reports of serotonergic crisis. |
| disulfiram | X↑ | Severe CNS reactions; unclear. |
| diuretics (thiazides) | X↑ | BP drop. |
| doxapram | X↑ | CNS stimulation, agitation, and hypertension; MAOI may lower doxapram's cardiovascular effect; until more evidence exists, *avoid combination.* |
| enflurane | X↑ | *See* anesthetics (general). |
| ephedrine | M↑ | Hypertensive crisis (*see* sympathomimetics). |
| fenfluramine | M↑ | Serotonin syndrome |
| fluoxetine (*see* SSRIs) | | |
| fluvoxamine (*see* SSRIs) | | |
| guanadrel | X↑ | Initial hypertension followed by hypotension; wait 10–14 days between drugs. |
| guanethidine | X↑ | Initial hypertension followed by hypotension; wait 10–14 days between drugs. |
| halothane | X↑ | *See* anesthetics (general). |
| hydralazine | X↑ | Tachycardia; may increase BP. |
| hypoglycemics (oral) | X↑ | May lower blood sugar. |
| insulin | X↑ | May lower blood sugar. |
| labetolol (*see* β-blockers) | | |
| levodopa (L-dopa) | X↑ M↑ | Hypertensive crisis and CNS stimulation possible. |
| MAOIs | M↑ | Hypertension with phenelzine to tranylcypromine; not reported in other direction. |
| meperidine | M↑ | Severe serotonin syndrome. Most other opiates (e.g., morphine, methadone) safe. |
| metaraminol | M↑ | Hypertensive crisis (*see* sympathomimetics). |

(*continues*)

## Table 4.14 Continued

| DRUGS (X) INTERACT WITH: | MONOAMINE-OXIDASE INHIBITORS (M) | COMMENTS |
|---|---|---|
| methyldopa | M↑ | Hypertensive reaction could occur because of increased stored norepinephrine, but not reported. |
| methylphenidate | M↑ | Hypertensive crisis (*see* sympathomimetics). |
| nadolol (*see* β-blockers) | | |
| paroxetine (*see* SSRIs) | | |
| phenothiazines | X↑ M↑ | Increased hypotension and anticholinergic effects. |
| phenylephrine | M↑ | Hypertensive crisis (*see* sympathomimetics). |
| phenylpropanolamine | M↑ | Hypertensive crisis (*see* sympathomimetics). |
| pseudoephedrine | M↑ | Hypertensive crisis (*see* sympathomimetics). |
| reserpine | X↑ | Initial hypertension followed by hypotension; wait 10–14 days between drugs. |
| sertraline (*see* SSRIs) | | |
| SSRIs | X↑ | Serotonergic crisis some deaths; wait at least 2 weeks after stopping MAOI before starting SSRI; wait at least 5 weeks after stopping sertraline, paroxetine, or fluvoxamine before starting MAOI. |
| succinylcholine | X↑ | Prolonged muscle relaxation or paralysis only by phenelzine. |
| sumitriptan | X↑ | Increased sumitriptan AUC |
| sympathomimetics (indirect): appetite suppressants amphetamines cocaine cyclopentamine ephedrine isoproterenol levodopa metaraminol methylphenidate pemoline phentermine phenylephrine phenylpropanolamine pseudoephedrine sumatriptan tyramine | M↑ | Hypertensive crisis generated with indirect-acting sympathomimetics but not by direct-acting sympathomimemtics (e.g., epinephrine does not cause this reaction). Most common with more stimulating tranylcypromine. |

(*continues*)

**Table 4.14 Continued**

| DRUGS (X) INTERACT WITH: | MONOAMINE-OXIDASE INHIBITORS (M) | COMMENTS |
|---|---|---|
| terfenadine | M↑ | Increased MAOI side effects. |
| thiazide diuretics | X↑ M↑ | Hypotension. |
| TCAs | M↑ | See Table xxx |
| theophylline | X↑ | Palpitations, tachycardia, anxiety. |
| tryptophan | X↑ | Serotonin syndrome; tryptophan off American market, but old bottles exist and is available in Canada. |
| tubocurarine | X↑ | Prolonged muscle relaxation or paralysis. |
| tyramine | M↑ | Hypertensive crisis (*see* sympathomimetics). |

↑ Increases; ↓ Decreases.

- Delirium
- Withdrawal symptoms more common with higher doses.
- However, MAOI withdrawal is not life threatening.

  MAOI diet should be continued for 2 weeks after last medication dose.

- MAO may regenerate faster after discontinuation of tranylcypromine.

## TOXICITY AND OVERDOSE

MAOI overdose can be lethal

- $LD_{50}$ is a 10-day supply.
- Toxicity develops in 4–12 hours and is maximal at 24–48 hours.
- Toxicity usually resolves in 3–4 days but may persist 12–14 days.
- Manifestations of overdose:
  - Hypotension
    - May be complicated by cardiovascular insufficiency, shock, myocardial infarction.
  - Drowsiness
  - Dizziness
  - Headache
  - Insomnia
  - Restlessness, anxiety, irritability, hyperactivity

**Table 4.15  Potentially Dangerous Prescription and Nonprescription Medicines**

### EPHEDRINE

| | | |
|---|---|---|
| Broncholate CS, softgels, syrup | Marax | Quadrinal tablets |
| Bronkaid | Mudrane tablets, gel, G elixer | Rynatuss tablets and suspension |
| Bronkolixer | Pazo hemorrhoid oitment | Vicks Vatronel nose drops |
| | Primatene | |

### PHENYLEPHRINE

| | | |
|---|---|---|
| Atrohist suspension and plus tablets | Duratex | Prefrin liquifilm |
| Cerose-DM | Dura-vent | Protid |
| Codimal | Endel-HD | R-Tannate tablets and suspension |
| Congespirin for children | Entex capsules and liquid | Relief eye drops |
| Comhist LA capsules | Extendryl chewable tablets, Jr. and Sr. T.D. capsules and 4-Way fast-acting nasal spray—new formula | Robitussin night relief |
| D.A. chewable tablets | | Ru-Tuss |
| Dallergy caplets, tablets | | Ryanatan tablets and suspension |
| Deconasal sprinkle capsules | Histussin | Rynatus tablets |
| Despec liquid | Hycomine compound | St. Joseph's nasal congestant |
| Donatussin DC and drops | Neo-Synephrine nasal spray and nose drops | Triotann suspension and tablets |
| Dimetane decongestant | Nostril nasal decongestant | Vanex forte and HD |
| Dristan decongestant | Novahistine elixir and DMX | Vicks sinex decongestant nasal spray and ultra fine mist |
| Dristan nasal spray | Pediacof cough syrup | |
| Duo-medihaler | Phenergan | |
| Dura-gest | | |

### PHENYLPROPANOLAMINE

| | | |
|---|---|---|
| Atrohist plus tablets | Dimetapp | Poly-Histine |
| Alka-Seltzer plus cold and nighttime cold medicine | Duadacin cold and allergy | Propagest tablets |
| A.R.M. allergy relief | Dura-Gest | Robitussin-CF |
| Acutrim appetite pills | Duratex | Ru-Tuss II caps |
| Allerest allergy, headache | Dura-Vent | Ru-Tuss with hydrocodone |
| BC cold powder | E.M.T. | Sinarest |
| Bayer children's cough and cold remedies | Entex capsules and liquid | Sine-off sinus |
| Cheracol plus head cold/cough formula | Entex LA capsules | Simulin tablets |
| | Exgest LA tablets | Snaplets-DM, EX |
| Comtrex multi-symptom cold reliever | 4-Way cold tablets | St. Joseph's cold tablets |
| | Gelpirin | Triaminic |
| Contact decongestants | Hycomine syrup | Triaminicin |
| Coricidin "D" decongestants | Naldecon CX, DX, EX | Triaminicol |
| Coricidin maximum strength | Nolamine timed-release tablets | Tylenol cold medication |
| Despec caps, liquid | Nolex LA tablets | Vanex-forte |
| Dexatrim appetite pills | Ornade spansule caps | |
| Dimetane-DC cough syrup | Phenylpropanolamine HCL and guaifenesin | |

*(continues)*

**Table 4.15  Continued**

## PSEUDOEPHEDRINE

Actified
AllerAct
Allerest no drowsy formula
Anatuss LA tablets
Anatuss DM
Atrohist sprinkle capsules
Benadryl combinations
Bomarest DX cough syrup
Brexin LA capsules
Bromfed capsules (timed
    release)
Bromfed DM cough syrup
Bromfed tablets
Bromfed-PD capsules
CoAdvil
Codimal LA capsules
Comtrex allergy sinus
Comtrex cough formula
Comtrex multi-symptom
Congress Jr. TD capsules
Congress Sr. TD capsules
Contact cold and sinus
Dallergy Jr. capsules
Deconsal II Tablets
Dimacol
Dimetane DX cough syrup
Dorcol cough and
    decongestant
Dristan maximum strength
Dura-Tap/PD capsules
Duatuss HD

Duratuss tablets
Entex PSE tablets
Excedrin sinus
Fedahist
Guaifed capsules
Guaifed PD capsules
Guaimax D tablets
Isoclor
Kronofed A Jr.
Lodrane LD capsules
Nasabid capsules
Novafed A capsules
Novafed capsules
Novahistine DMX
Nucofed expectorant
Ornex
P.V. Tussin syrup
Pediacare
Pediacare cold-allergy
    chewable tablets
Pediacare cough-cold
    chewable tablets
Pediacare Infants
    decongestant drops
Pediacare nightrest
Pseudoephedrine
    hydrochloride tablets
Robitussin DAC syrup
Robitussin PE
Rondec
Ru-Tuss DE tablets

Ryna, C, CX
Seldane D tablets
Sinarest no drowsiness
Sine-aid IB caplets
Sine-aid maximum strength
Sine-Off, no drowsiness
Sinatub
Sudafed
Toura LA caplets
Touro A&H capsules
Triaminic night light
Trinalin tablets
Tuss DA RX
Tussafed drops and syrup
Tussar DM
Tussar SF
Tussar-2
Tylenol allergy sinus
    medicated gelcaps
Tylenol allergy sinus nighttime
    caplets
Tylenol cold
Tylenol cold and flu
Tylenol cough
Tylenol flu
Tylenol med
Tylenol sinus
Vick's 44-D, 44-M
Vick's Daycare daytime cold
Vick's NyQuil

## DEXTROMETHORPHAN
### (ALSO ANY DRUG NAME WITH DM OR TUSS IN IT)

Anatuss DM syrup and tablets
Bromarest DM
Bromarest DX
Bromfed DM
Cerose DM
Cheracol
Cheracol plus
Codimal DM
Comtrex multi-symptom cold
    reliever
Comtrex day and night
Comtrex non-drowsy
Dimetane DX cough syrup
Dristan cold and flu
Dristan juice mix-in

Humibid DM sprinkle and
    tablets
Iodur DM
Iotuss DM
Par-glycerol DM
Pedia care cough-cold
Pedia care night rest
Phenergan with
    dextromethorphan
Poly-histine DM
Quelidine poly-histine DM
Rescon DM
Robitussin DM
Rondec DM
Safe tussin 30

Touro DM
Tusibron DM
Tuss DA
Tussafed drops and syrup
Tussar DM
Tussi-organidin DM
Tylenol children's cold plus
    cough liquid formula
Tylenol cold and flu no drowsi-
    ness and hot medicine
Tylenol cold medication
Tylenol cough medication
Tylenol flu maximum

**Table 4.16 Effects on Laboratory Tests**

| GENERIC NAMES | BLOOD/SERUM TESTS* |
|---|---|
| Isocarboxazid | LFT ↑** |
| Phenelzine | Glucose ↓ LFT ↑ |
| Tranylcypromine | Glucose ↓ |

\* ↑ Increases; ↓ Decreases; ? Undetermined.
\*\* LFT = SGOT, SGPT, LDH, alkaline phosphatase, bilirubin.

- Ataxia
- Confusion
- Tachycardia
- Seizures
- Hallucinations
- Hyperreflexia
- Fever
- Respiratory depression
- Spasm of masticatory muscles
- Rigidity
- Coma
- Management of overdose:
  - Hypotension
    - Give fluids.
    - Use pressor amines (e.g., norepinephrine) very cautiously, because effect will be amplified by MAOI.
  - Avoid CNS stimulants.
  - Give anticonvulsants for seizures.
  - Obtain LFTs to assess for hepatotoxicity.
  - Observe patient for 1 week after overdose.

## PRECAUTIONS

MAOIs are contraindicated in the presence of
- Inability to remember or adhere to diet
- Pheochromocytoma
- Carcinoid
- Medications listed on pages 224–225.
- Hypersensitivity to MAOIs
- Myelography

Do not give MAOIs to children under age 16.

MAOIs should be used cautiously in patients with

- Coronary heart disease
  - MAOIs may suppress pain of angina.
- Diabetes mellitus
  - MAOIs may enhance hypoglycemic effect of insulin.
- Renal impairment
- Hepatic disease
- Hypertension
  - MAOIs may have additive hypotensive effect with antihypertensives.
- Asthma
  - Steroids and chromalyn do not interact with MAOIs.
- Allergic reactions with need for epinephrine
  - Test dose of epinephrine in office is advisable.

## ADVICE FOR CARETAKERS

Patients may feel overwhelmed by conflicting dietary recommendations. Discuss meaningful restrictions and review patient's use of favorite foods, over-the-counter medications, and nonprescription substances.

- Remind patient that heavily caffeinated beverages may produce anxiety, insomnia, or overstimulation.
- Be sure that patient understands manifestation of hypertensive crisis.
- Explain how to use medications for hypertensive crisis (e.g., nifedipine).

## NOTES FOR PATIENT AND FAMILY

MAOIs may be taken with meals.

- If patient forgets a dose, it can be taken within 4 hours.
- Otherwise, wait for the next dose.
- Do not double the dose.

Be careful about operating heavy machinery or driving, especially with sedating MAOIs such as phenelzine.

Wear a bracelet or carry a Medic Alert card or physician's letter informing ER and other medical staff about MAOI use.

- Inform all physicians, dentists, and pharmacists about MAOI use.
- Check label of any over-the-counter substance.
- Ask about use of soy and other products in restaurant food.

- A hypertensive crisis is associated with an excruciating headache, often with severe neck pain.
- Check blood pressure, if possible, before taking nifedipine.
- If blood pressure is severely elevated, go to the ER immediately, even if nifedipine has been used.
- Inform ER staff that severe headache is a common symptom of hypertensive crisis.
  - Do NOT take meperidine.
  - Brain imaging is rarely necessary.
  - Definitive treatment is with phentolamine.
- Remain on the MAOI diet 10–14 days after discontinuing the MAOI.
- MAOIs should be discontinued gradually to avoid withdrawal symptoms.

# CHAPTER FIVE

# Lithium

Lithium was introduced as a treatment for mania by J. F. G. Cade in 1949. Cade was studying uric acid and found that lithium urate had a calming effect, first in animals and then in a group of manic patients. He realized that improvement of the mania was due to the lithium and not the urate. Lithium chloride was used widely as a salt substitute until a number of deaths were reported in patients also taking diuretics for hypertension. The drug was withdrawn from the market until researchers realized that it was the *combination* of the diuretic and a low-salt diet that was producing the lithium toxicity. Lithium was reintroduced in the 1970s as an antimanic drug, with the recommendation that concomitant use of salt-free diets and diuretics be minimized.

Lithium remains the "gold standard" mood stabilizer. It is clearly effective acutely for mania and for prevention of manic recurrences. Lithium is probably better at preventing recurrences of bipolar depression than unipolar depression. Medications that reduce affective recurrences are referred to as *mood stabilizers.*

- Medications with mood-stabilizing properties include:
  - Lithium
  - Some anticonvulsants
  - Some calcium channel-blockers
  - Atypical antipsychotics are all effective for mania
    - Less support for their use as mood stabilizers.

This chapter reviews the use of lithium for
- Bipolar disorder
  - Mania
  - Bipolar depression
- Postpartum psychosis
- Cyclothymia
- Personality disorders

- Unipolar depression
- Schizoaffective disorder
- Medical disorders
  - Neutropenia
  - Syndrome of inappropriate antidiuretic hormone secretion (SIADH)

Conditions treated with lithium discussed elsewhere include:

- Aggression (Anticonvulsants, Chapter 6)
- Alcoholism (pp. 452–457)
- Premenstrual dysphoric disorder (pp. 135–136)
- Use of anticonvulsants and antipsychotics in bipolar disorder are discussed in detail in Chapter 6.

Table 5.1 provides a basic overview of the drugs discussed in this chapter.

## PHARMACOLOGY

Lithium has multiple actions, including

- Increased serotonin release
- Attenuation of hyperactive intracellular calcium signaling
- Antagonism of magnesium ions that activate breakdown of G-proteins into active components
- Inhibition of inositol-1-phosphatase, an important (but not the rate-limiting) enzyme in phosphoinositide turnover
- Alteration of activity of the membrane Na-K pump
- Increased nitric oxide (NO) production, resulting in decreased NMDA receptor activity and reduced excitotoxicity
- Increased activity of a neuroprotective variant of bcl-2

**Table 5.1  Names, Dose Forms, Colors**

| GENERIC NAMES | BRAND NAMES | DOSE FORMS (MG)* | COLORS |
|---|---|---|---|
| lithium carbonate | Eskalith | t: 300<br>c: 300 | t: gray<br>c: gray-yellow |
| | Eskalith CR[†] | t: 450 | t: yellow |
| | Lithane | t: 300 | t: green |
| | Lithobid | t: 300 | t: |
| lithium citrate | Cibalith-S | s: 8 mEq/5 ml | s: raspberry |

* c = capsules; s = syrup; [†] = sustained release; t = tablets.

- Decreased activity of glycogen synthase kinase-β, resulting in decreased susceptibility to apoptosis

Lithium is completely absorbed 6 hours after oral administration.
- Bioavailability is 100%.
- Peak serum levels occur in ⅓–2 hours.
- Elimination half-life with chronic treatment takes around 24 hours.
  - Steady state achieved in 4–7 days.
- Ratio of brain:serum levels (Moore, Demopulos, & Henry, 2002):
  - 0.92 in bipolar adults.
  - 0.58 in bipolar children.
    - Children may need higher serum levels to attain brain levels equivalent to adults.
- Lithium is excreted without being metabolized.
  - 95% of excretion is renal.
  - 1% excreted in feces.
    - Diarrhea does not significantly affect lithium levels.
  - 4–5% of lithium excreted in sweat.
    - Loss of lithium during heavy sweating is offset by increased renal conservation of lithium.
  - ⅓–⅔ of lithium is excreted in 6–12 hours.
    - The remainder is excreted over 10–14 days.
- 70–80% of lithium is reabsorbed in the proximal tubules.
  - Kidneys cannot distinguish between lithium and sodium.
  - If sodium is lost (e.g., sweating, salt-free diet, sodium-wasting diuretic), kidneys also conserve lithium, resulting in increased lithium levels.

Lithium preparations include:
- Lithium carbonate (generic)
- Sustained-release lithium: Lithobid (300 mg) and Eskalith-CR (450 mg)
  - GI absorption is slower, resulting in fewer fluctuations of serum level.
  - Peak level occurs 3.5–12 hours after oral administration.
  - Trough levels may be higher than with immediate-release lithium.
  - Levels do not fluctuate as much with sustained-release preparations.
  - Because less lithium is released in the stomach, gastric side effects may be reduced.
  - Because more lithium is delivered to the small intestine, diarrhea may be increased.
  - Breaking sustained-released pills converts them to immediate-release pills.

- Lithium citrate (liquid)
  - Absorbed within 0.5–1 hour after oral administration.
  - May have fewer GI side effects.
  - Useful alternative when very small dosage increments are needed or when patients have allergic reactions to pills.

## LABORATORY INVESTIGATIONS

Chronic lithium therapy requires regular monitoring of
- Thyroid function
  - Every 6–12 months in adults
  - Every 3–6 months in children
- Serum calcium
  - Lithium causes mild hyperparathyroidism in most patients.
    - Often not clinically significant
    - Consider if patient develops potential complications of hypercalcemia, such as depression, cataracts, or polyuria.
- Usually not necessary to follow CBC.
  - Mild increase in neutrophil count is not clinically important.
    - May treat neutropenia associated with other medications (e.g., cancer chemotherapy).
- Effect of chronic lithium therapy on renal function is controversial.
  - Ideally, 24-hour urine volume should be monitored once a year.
  - Serum creatinine is easier to obtain.
  - If either increases significantly, measure creatinine clearance.
  - If creatinine clearance decreases significantly, obtain renal consultation.
- Obtain EKG in older patients and children.
  - Lithium slows rate of depolarization of sinus node and conduction through AV node.

Table 5.2 lists tests that should be obtained at baseline and then every 6–12 months.

## DOSING

Clinical response to lithium in bipolar disorder is correlated with 12-hour serum level.
- Red cell lithium levels may correlate better with toxicity and clinical response, but insufficient data to use clinically.

**Table 5.2  Lithium Monitoring**

| TEST | RATIONALE | FREQUENCY |
|---|---|---|
| EKG | Lithium decreases rate of depolarization of SA node and slows conduction through the AV node. | In patients > 40 or with history of heart disease; repeat if heart rate slows or patient develops cardiac symptoms |
| Free $T_4$, TSH | Lithium causes hypothyroidism by interfering with TSH signaling in thyroid; risk greater in children. | Every 6 months for 1 year, then yearly; every 3 months in children |
| BUN, creatinine | Lithium impairs renal water conservation by interfering with antidiuretic hormone signaling in renal tubule; lithium also may be nephrotoxic. | Yearly; more frequently if previous levels were higher than baseline |
| Urine volume | May increase substantially if impaired renal function; also increase in polydipsia and impaired water excretion. | Yearly |
| Creatinine clearance | More reliable measure of impaired renal function | If urine volume increases significantly or there is other evidence of impaired renal function |
| Electrolytes | Hypernatremia may be an early indication of nephrogenic diabetes insipidus; electrolyte abnormalities may predispose to dysrhythmias with lithium. | With BUN |
| Urinalysis | Low specific gravity in first voided specimen may indicate nephrogenic diabetes inspidus; follow with serum and urine osmolality obtained at same time. | If patient develops polyuria or polydipsia |
| Total calcium | Lithium causes hyperparathyroidism by interfering with parathyroid hormone signaling. Occasionally, parathyroid adenomas may occur. If serum total calcium is increased, obtain ionized calcium and PTH. | Yearly, or if patient develops possible evidence of hypercalcemia, such as lethargy, depression, impaired vision, or polyuria |
| Pregnancy test | Lithium increases risk of Ebstein's anomaly and may complicate management of delivery. | At baseline in women at risk |

- African Americans may have higher intracellular lithium levels than Caucasians with similar serum levels.
  - These patients may have similar response to lower serum levels.
- Lithium dose should be adjusted according to clinical response as well as serum level.

Peak and trough serum levels are important in dosing.
- Peak levels occur 1.5–2 hours after dosing.
- Steady state occurs in 4–7 days.
- Higher peak levels during the day are more likely to produce nausea, GI distress, tremor, dazed feeling, lethargy, urinary frequency.
- Side effects associated with peak levels can be reduced by
  - Giving entire dose at bedtime.
  - Using sustained-release preparation.
  - Reducing dose.
  - Using more frequent dosing.

In adults, 12-hour lithium levels above 0.8 have been found to be more effective but produce more side effects (Gelenberg et al., 1989). However, this finding was contradicted by a finding that lower levels worked as well. Prepubertal children and younger adolescents may need higher serum levels to achieve the same brain level (see p. 282). The recommendation that maintenance levels can be lower than levels for the acute treatment of mania has not been substantiated by controlled research.

- The number of manic patients responding to lithium increases with the serum level, although some patients respond to lower levels.
- No correlation has been found between blood level and response in bipolar depression (Sproule, 2002).
- Several methods have been suggested for calculating the initial dose of lithium.
  - None of these is valid in the presence of medications (e.g., NSAIDs) or disorders (e.g., kidney disease) that alter lithium levels.
  - Check lithium level 24 hours after a single 600 mg dose of lithium, then prescribe the corresponding dose in Table 5.3.
  - Check lithium level 12 hours after a single 900 mg dose of lithium, then use the equation:

$$d = \frac{2700}{5.61x - 0.21} \qquad \begin{aligned} d &= \text{daily total dose} \\ x &= \text{12 hour lithium level} \end{aligned}$$

  - Use the following formula if no test dose available.

Daily dose in mg = $486.8 + 746.83 \times$ (desired lithium level, mmol/l) $- (10.08 \times$ age in years) $+ 5.95 \times$ weight in kg $+ (92.01 \times$ outpatient

Table 5.3  Lithium Level and Dose

| 24-HOUR LITHIUM LEVEL (mM) | INITIAL DAILY DOSE (mg) |
|---|---|
| 0.05–0.09 | 3600 |
| 0.10–0.14 | 2700 |
| 0.15–0.19 | 1800 |
| 0.20–0.23 | 900 |
| 0.24–0.3 | 600 |
| > 0.30 | 300 |

or inpatient status) + (147.8 × gender) − (74.73 × presence or absence of antidepressant)

Inpatient status = 1, outpatient status = 0
Female = 0, male = 1
Antidepressant present = 1, absent = 0

These calculations are approximations; most practitioners simply adjust the dose empirically.

Gradually adjusting the lithium dose according to tolerance and response has several advantages:

- More accurate final levels
- Greater patient acceptance
  - More side effects occur when dose is increased rapidly.
- Fewer adverse effects on mood
  - Mood-stabilizing medications work faster against mania and cycling than depression, especially when dose is escalated quickly.
    - Symptoms such as agitation, insomnia, irritability, and increased energy remit rapidly, but patient feels more acutely sluggish or depressed because mixed depressive symptoms are no longer counteracted by elevated mood and energy.
- Patient reaches steady state before dose is changed.
- Patient and doctor have opportunity to form therapeutic alliance.
- Alternative methods for measuring lithium levels:
  - For patients who are squeamish about having blood drawn, enough blood may be obtained from a finger stick.
  - Saliva lithium levels are usually two to three times the serum levels.
    - The specific ratio for an individual patient can be calculated by comparing a few simultaneously obtained serum and saliva levels and then using saliva levels.

Higher lithium levels will occur on the same dose in the presence of sodium depletion (e.g., use of thiazide diuretics, low-salt diet).

- Use lower doses and increase dose more cautiously.

The elimination half-life of lithium (~24 hours with chronic administration) permits once daily dosing (usually at bedtime).

- Peak levels are higher, but these occur when patient is asleep and side effects associated with peak levels (e.g., nausea, cognitive dysfunction) are usually not as bothersome.
  - Diarrhea may be a little more frequent with once daily dosing.
  - Risk of impaired renal function may be lower with less frequent dosing because there are fewer peak levels over the course of the day.
- A single daily dose is easier to remember.
- Efficacy of once daily and every other day dosing (with lower daily doses) equivalent to divided daily dosing.
  - Some patients tolerate one schedule better than another.
  - Every third day dosing is not reliably effective.

## CLINICAL INDICATIONS AND USE

Lithium is approved for the treatment of mania and the prevention of recurrences of mania. Predictors of a good response to lithium include

- Past history of response to lithium
- First-degree relative with a positive response to lithium
- Classic mania or hypomania with elation and/or grandiosity
- Typical bipolar depression (i.e., bipolar depression with hypersomnia, mental slowing, and anergia)
- Absence of rapid cycling, psychosis, and mixed mania
- Sequence of mania followed by depression rather than depression followed by mania
- History of treatment adherence
- Manic switch on antidepressant

Lithium may be less effective in the presence of

- Rapid/ultradian cycling
- Mixed mania
- Dementia or other neurological syndromes
  - Adverse neurological and cognitive effects are more troublesome than neuroprotective action is helpful.
- Lithium-resistant mania is discussed in Chapter 6.

### Initiating Therapy

MANIA AND HYPOMANIA

Response rates to lithium in classic mania are
- Remission: 70%
- Partial initial response: 20%
- No initial response: 10%

Lithium is most effective for features of mania such as
- Elation
- Grandiosity
- Flight of ideas
- Irritability
- Anxiety
- Pressured speech
- Paranoia
- Agitation
- Assaultive behavior
- Insomnia
- Hypersexuality
- Distractibility

Amelioration of acute symptoms with lithium generally takes 10–30 days; complete resolution of a manic episode can take months.
- Because of its slow onset of action, lithium is usually not used as initial monotherapy for hospitalized manic patients.
- If rapid antimanic effect or control of agitation is needed, begin treatment with an antipsychotic drug and/or a benzodiazepine.
  - Neuroleptics such as haloperidol are effective for mania but have high rates (70%) of EPS, especially when combined with lithium.
  - Antipsychotic drugs are effective in mania whether or not psychosis is present.
  - All atypical antipsychotics have been found to have antimanic effects as monotherapy or combined with lithium or divalproex (see pp. 320–325).
  - Clonazepam and lorazepam are the most frequently used benzodiazepines in mania.
  - Clonzazepam is more sedating and may promote sleep better than lorazepam, which has a shorter half-life but is more useful acutely for agitation.

- Benzodiazepines can be combined with antipsychotic drugs.
  - Clonazepam may increase risk of lithium-induced EPS.
- Any benzodiazepine other than alprazolam should be effective.
  - Alprazolam has antidepressant properties that can be troublesome in mania.

If an antipsychotic drug and/or a benzodiazepine is used for rapid symptomatic control

- Start with olanzapine in doses up to 20 mg, or
- Quetiapine in doses up to 500–600 mg if patient exhibits significant insomnia or
- Risperidone in doses up to 4–6 mg if patient is more psychotic.
  - All other atypical antipsychotics are also effective for mania.
  - If patient refuses oral medication and requires emergency medication, use haloperidol 2.5–5 mg IM or IV.
  - Haloperidol 5–15 mg PO can be considered if other medications are not working.
    - Lithium has had occasional severe neurotoxic interactions with neuroleptics and clonazepam

If a benzodiazepine is used for agitation

- Begin with lorazepam 1–2 mg tid–qid or
- Clonazepam 0.5–1 mg bid
  - If patient needs parenteral treatment, use lorazepam 0.5–2 mg IM or IV.
- Add lithium gradually as agitation and psychosis decrease.
- The dose required for a therapeutic lithium level in mania is often higher than the dose required for the same level when mania has remitted.
  - Mania is associated with a state-dependent defect in a lithium–sodium countertransport pump, resulting in intracellular accumulation of lithium and lower serum levels.
  - With remission of mania, the cellular defect reverses itself and lithium leaves cells and enters the bloodstream, followed within 24 hours by a lithium diuresis.

Prevention of recurrence is at least as important as treating any acute episode of mania.

- Treatment adherence is one of the most reliable predictors of long-term mood stabilization.
- Maximizing long-term outcome involves balancing the need for rapid symptom control with minimizing adverse effects (including acute depression) that will make the patient less likely to keep taking the medication.

Lithium can be started at 300 mg as patient begins to stabilize.

- Increase the dose by 300 mg every 4–7 days to 300 mg tid.
- Then obtain 12-hour level.
- Adjust subsequent dose to level around 1–1.2 mM unless patient has limiting side effects or full response at lower dose.
- Obtain level after each dosage increase > 900 mg/day.

Older patients should have slower dosage escalation, checking lithium level after each dosage increase.

- Start with no more than 300 mg.
- Wait longer before checking level.
  - Time to steady state may be twice as long (1–2 weeks) as in younger patients.
- Increase dose by 150–300 mg every 2–3 weeks.
- Dose needed for therapeutic level may or may not be lower than for younger patients.
  - Some older patients respond to lithium levels around 0.3–0.6 mM.
- Older patients are more sensitive to lithium side effects, which may last longer than in younger patients.

Children often need more frequent dosing than adults because they eliminate lithium (as well as other medications) more rapidly.

- Even with sustained-release preparations, divided doses may be necessary.
- An open trial in 100 acutely manic adolescents ages 12–18 treated for 1 month with lithium found that 63 responded (mania reduced by one-third) and 26 remitted (Young Mania Rating Scale [YMRS] score ≤ 6; Kafantaris, Coletti, Dicker, Padula, & Kane, 2003).
  - Comorbid ADHD, prominent depressive features, severity of mania, and age at illness onset did not predict response.
  - Nonpsychotic patients responded as well as psychotic patients to adjunctive antipsychotic medication.
- Some younger children also may require higher serum levels (although not necessarily higher doses) than adults.
  - Lithium-7 magnetic resonance spectroscopy, used to measure in vivo brain levels in 9 children and adolescents (mean age 13) and 18 adults (mean age 37 years), demonstrated that the younger patients had lower brain-to-serum ratios (0.58) than adults (0.92; Moore et al., 2002).
    - Suggests either increased lithium efflux or decreased entry across the blood–brain barrier.
    - Some younger patients may need higher serum levels to get the same brain concentration.

Gradually withdraw neuroleptic/benzodiazepine as therapeutic lithium level is achieved and patient's clinical state stabilizes.

- When patient is stable, gradually move entire dose to bedtime.
  - If patient has more difficulty with this schedule, continue divided dosing.
- Once lithium level is therapeutic and patient is stable clinically (or maximal benefit has been achieved), recheck level every 2–3 weeks to look for increased level as acute physiology of illness remits.
- Once lithium level remains consistent, recheck level monthly for 3–6 months, then every 6 months.

Although rapid increases in the lithium dose can produce response in mania in 10 days, this duration of treatment is difficult to justify in modern inpatient settings where short lengths of stay and adjunctive treatment with an antipsychotic drug (a benzodiazepine or divalproex) is often necessary.

- ECT is at least as effective as lithium for mania and has a faster onset of action.
- Lithium monotherapy is useful for hypomania, manic episodes that do not require hospitalization, and other situations in which a very rapid response is not required.

Dosing process:
- Start lithium at 300 mg hs.
- Increase the dose by 150–300 mg q 1–3 weeks, depending on side effects and clinical response.
  - Alternate between 300 mg (Lithobid) and 450 mg (Eskalith CR) preparations to increase dose by 150 mg at a time.
- Follow levels, as noted above.

BIPOLAR DEPRESSION

Lithium improves as many as two-thirds of cases of pure bipolar depression (i.e., depression without mixed dysphoric hypomania).

- Response may take 2 months.
- Usual therapeutic levels are effective.
- Lithium is more reliable as augmenting agent.
  - More effective for augmenting antidepressants in bipolar than in unipolar depression.
- Lithium is rarely effective as monotherapy for unipolar depression.
- Lamotrigine is effective as monotherapy for bipolar depression (see pp. 306–307).

- In an 8-week industry-sponsored multicenter comparison of olanazpine, a combination of olanzapine and fluoxetine, and placebo (Tohen et al., 2003):
    - 833 patients with bipolar I depression were randomized to placebo (N = 377), olanzapine 5–20 mg (N = 370), or olanzapine–fluoxetine combinations in doses of 6/25, 6/50 or 12/50 mg.
    - About half the patients in each active treatment group and two-thirds in the placebo group did not complete the study.
    - From weeks 4–8, combination treatment was significantly more effective than olanzapine alone.
        - Effect size 0.68 for combination
        - 0.32 for olanzapine
        - Combination twice as effective as olanzapine alone, but an effect size similar to that seen with 20 mg of fluoxetine in unipolar depression.
    - Response rates (≥ 50% reduction in depression scores)
        - Placebo: 30%
        - Olanzapine: 39%
        - Olanzapine + fluoxetine: 56%
    - Remission (defined as depression score about one-third that of the initial score):
        - Placebo: 25%
        - Olanzapine: 33%
        - Combination: 49%
    - Increases in mania scores did not differ between groups.
    - In both groups taking olanzapine, clinically significant weight gain (at least 7% increase) occurred in 19%.

There are few controlled studies of the treatment of bipolar depression. One protocol (see Figure 5.1) follows.

- Start with a mood stabilizer.
    - Lithium and carbamazepine are more likely to treat depression than valproate or a calcium channel-blocker.
- If depression is complicated by mood cycling or is mixed with hypomanic symptoms such as insomnia, racing thoughts, decreased sleep, extreme interpersonal sensitivity, or hallucinations that do not remit with a single mood stabilizer, then add a second mood stabilizer.
    - If mood cycling or mixed hypomanic symptoms are still present, add another mood stabilizer or an antipsychotic drug.
        - Antipsychotic drugs may help to eliminate mixed symptoms and cycling even if psychotic symptoms are absent.

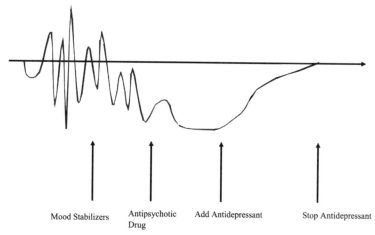

Mood Stabilizers    Antipsychotic    Add Antidepressant    Stop Antidepressant
                    Drug

**Figure 5.1  Treatment of Bipolar Depression**

Uncomplicated bipolar depression that is present initially or that emerges with combinations of mood stabilizers is associated with anergia, hypersomnia, and mental slowing.

- Depression may cycle away without an antidepressant.
- If it does not, add an antidepressant.
  - Lamotrigine may be safest (see pp. 306–308).
  - Stimulants have the advantage of rapid onset of action and rapid termination of action when medication withdrawn in case antidepressant induces hypomania or mood cycling.
    - Methylphenidate or dextroamphetamine 15–30 mg/day
  - Artificial bright light in the morning can be useful even in nonseasonal bipolar depression.
    - "Dose" can be titrated precisely by adjusting duration of exposure to light.
    - 15–30 minutes is often sufficient.
    - Treatment can be withdrawn rapidly or dose reduced if patient becomes overstimulated.
    - Useful for hypersomnia.
    - May normalize sleep–wake cycle.
  - Bupropion was thought to be less likely than other antidepressants to induce mania and rapid cycling, but this has not been confirmed.
  - Short-acting SSRI or venlafaxine is effective.
  - Extensive experience with tranylcypromine has been published.
    - Activating effect useful for anergic bipolar depression.

- Selegiline also can be useful, although no research with this medication.
- MAOIs are not more likely to induce mania than other antidepressants.
- TCAs are often not first choices for bipolar depression because of their reputation for being more likely to induce mania.
  - Data on mania induction by TCAs come from earlier studies of unipolar depression, in which more conversions to mania were observed because investigators were not as accurate in excluding bipolar patients.
- Sleep deprivation is associated with a higher response rate in bipolar than unipolar depression (75% vs. 50%).
  - Even a single night of sleep deprivation can induce mania.
- Antidepressants should rarely be used for bipolar depression without concomitant use of a mood stabilizer.

An attempt should be made to withdraw the antidepressant slowly once the depression has remitted fully.
- Continuing the antidepressant for too long may induce mania/hypomania or mood cycling.
- A study of refractory bipolar disorder, using very stringent criteria for antidepressant-induced mania (first episode of mania occurring for the first time within 8 weeks of starting antidepressant), suggested that 50% of risk of mania while taking an antidepressant is attributable to the antidepressant and 50% to natural history of the illness (Altshuler et al., 1995).
  - This method ignored hypomania and subsyndromal symptoms developing on antidepressants.
- An open life-charting study of patients with bipolar depression found no difference between SSRIs and bupropion in the risk of antidepressant-induced mania or cycle acceleration (Joffe et al., 2002).
- Analysis of 155 trials of different antidepressant classes (TCAs, SSRIs, bupropion, other new antidepressants) in 41 bipolar patients (Rosenquist, Ghaemi, Ko, Goodwin, & Baldessarini, 2003) found
  - Risk of mania: 35% with concurrent mood stabilizer; 66% without concurrent mood stabilizer
  - No difference between antidepressants in risk of mania induction
- Chart review of 78 outpatients receiving 228 antidepressant trials (Ghaemi et al., 2004):
  - 41 bipolar, 37 unipolar
  - Nonresponse to antidepressant after 4 weeks 1.6 times as common in bipolar vs. unipolar depression.
    - No difference found between antidepressant classes.

- Manic switch (new manic episode within 8 weeks of starting anti-depressant) occurred in 49% of bipolar patients.
- Manic switch 4.3 times as likely in patients not also taking mood stabilizers.
  - No difference found between antidepressants in risk of mania induction.
  - Including TCAs, bupropion, MAOIs.
- Antidepressant-induced cycle acceleration (at least two DSM-IV episodes more than in comparable period before taking antidepressant) in 26% of bipolar patients.
  - Not prevented by mood stabilizers
  - No difference between antidepressants
- DSM-IV rapid cycling seen in 32% of bipolar patients taking anti-depressants for at least 1 year.
  - Risk not reduced by mood stabilizers.
- Loss of response (relapse after 1 month or more of remission) to anti-depressant 3.4 times as common in bipolar vs. unipolar depression.
  - No difference between antidepressants.
  - Not prevented by mood stabilizers.
- Relapse after antidepressant discontinuation 4.7 times as likely in unipolar vs. bipolar depression.
- Mood-stabilizing medications are often more effective at preventing recurrence of depression than at treating it acutely.
- Reduce the dose of antidepressant by one dose every few weeks.
  - Rapid antidepressant withdrawal can result in rebound depression or rebound mania.

Study of antidepressant discontinuation after treatment of bipolar depression (Altshuler et al., 2003):
- Of 549 patients in Stanley Foundation Bipolar Network who took an antidepressant, 189 took an antidepressant for at least 2 months.
  - All patients were taking multiple mood stabilizers.
  - 84 (44%) of the 189 patients responded.
  - Of these 84 patients
    - 43 discontinued antidepressant in a mean of 74 days after re-sponse (defined as within 6 months).
    - 41 continued antidepressant for a mean of 484 days (defined as > 6 months).
  - Risk of depressive relapse 4.1 times greater for those who dis-continued antidepressant in < 6 months.
  - A total of 36 patients (43%) had a depressive relapse.

- 15 patients (18%) had a manic relapse.
- Depression, mania, and relapse were defined by a single global assessment on CGI-Bipolar Scale.
    - Outcome measure was a single nonblind global assessment.
    - Patients who developed mood cycling were excluded from study, and hypomania was ignored.
- Speed of antidepressant withdrawal was not considered.
- No random assignment used.
- Best interpretation of results is that
    - Only 189/549 bipolar depressed patients were able to continue an antidepressant for 6 weeks.
    - If the other two-thirds stopped the antidepressant because of manic symptoms, the actual rate of manic switch was 68% ([549 − 189 + 15]/549).
    - Early antidepressant discontinuation was within 2 months, which may not have reflected stable antidepressant response and may have indicated rapid antidepressant withdrawal resulting in rebound depression.
    - Patients who do well for at least 6 months with an antidepressant added to a mood stabilizer may continue to do well for another 6 months.

A review of 18 patients with bipolar II major depressive episodes in a day hospital (Perugi, Toni, Ruffolo, Frare, & Akiskal, 2001):
- Dopamine agonists pramipexole or ropinirole added to antidepressants and mood stabilizers
    - To which patients had not responded after 8 weeks.
- After an average of 18 weeks and mean doses of 1.23 mg of pramipexole and 2.97 mg of ropinirole
    - Five patients had marked improvement.
    - Three had moderate improvement.
    - Five had just transient improvement.

### CYCLOTHYMIA

Cyclothymia consists of mood swings not severe enough to meet criteria for mania, hypomania, or depression, but still causing suffering or impairment of functioning.
- Considered a mild form of bipolar disorder.
- Antidepressants often induce hypomania.
- Lithium reduces affective recurrences.

## RAPID CYCLING

The classical definition of rapid cycling is four affective episodes/year, with 2 weeks of euthymia between episodes, or a direct switch from one pole to the other. Ultra-rapid cycling refers to at least one affective recurrence per day. Ultradian cycling involves brief episodes of dysphoric hypomania and depression that recur multiple times over the course of the day. It can be difficult to distinguish between ultradian cycling and fluctuating chronic mixed states, but treatment of the two is similar.

- Classic rapid cycling and ultradian cycling may be different stages in the evolution of bipolar mood disorders.
  - Ultradian cycling is the more refractory form.
- Most published reports do not differentiate between subtypes of rapid cycling.
- Lithium is traditionally believed to be less effective than anticonvulsants in the treatment of rapid cycling.
  - This impression comes from studies of lithium-refractory patients who later responded to anticonvulsants.
  - A direct comparison of lithium and carbamazepine found them to be equally effective for rapid cycling (Okuma, 1993).
- As many as 70% of patients with rapid cycling have subclinical hypothyroidism (Bauer, Whybrow, & Winokur, 1990).
  - Correcting hypothyroidism is often necessary for a treatment response.
  - Adjunctive treatment with suprametabolic doses of thyroxine (0.075–0.4 mg/day) improved response to mood stabilizers in a small series of patients with refractory rapid cycling (Afflelou, Auriacombe, Cazenave, Chartres, & Tignol, 1997; Bauer & Whybrow, 1990).
    - Has been used in initially euthyroid patients as well as those who are euthyroid after thyroid replacement.
    - Thyroid replacement induces hyperthyroidism.
    - Risks of excessive thyroid replacement include anxiety, insomnia, tremor, osteoporosis, atrial fibrillation.
- Rapid cycling, and especially ultradian cycling, are physiologically complex forms of bipolar illness and require more aggressive treatment.
  - Combinations of two or three mood stabilizers may be necessary.
  - Anticonvulsants may be combined with each other or with lithium (see Chapter 6).
  - Start with one mood stabilizer and add the next one if mixed symptoms or cycling persist.
  - Continue the protocol noted for bipolar depression (see p. 265).

POSTPARTUM PSYCHOSIS

As discussed on pages 127–128, incidence of postpartum psychosis is 0.1–0.4%.

- The majority of cases are bipolar psychoses.
- There is a high rate of recurrence with subsequent pregnancies.
- Lithium is effective for treatment and prophylaxis of recurrence.

SUICIDALITY

- Lithium reduces suicide risk 5–7-fold (Tondo et al., 1998).
  - Reduction of suicide attempts and successful suicide in patients with or without mood disorders.
    - Possibly related to nonspecific reduction of impulsivity and aggression.
    - Separate from prophylactic effect.
- A meta-analysis of 33 studies of lithium in bipolar disorder found that the annual rate of attempted or completed suicide was 0.197% during lithium treatment vs. 2.57% without lithium (Baldessarini, Tondo, & Hennen, 2001).
- Suicide risk without lithium is 8–9 times higher.
- A retrospective cohort study of 20,638 patients who received outpatient treatment between 1994 and 2001 for bipolar disorder in two managed care health plans found that the risk of attempted or successful suicide was 1.5–3 times higher during treatment with divalproex than during treatment with lithium (Goodwin et al., 2003).
  - The same proportional superiority of lithium was found when compared with carbamazepine, but the N taking carbamazepine was too small to be reliable.
- However, lithium is lethal in overdose.

## Maintenance Therapy

Bipolar disorder is highly recurrent.

- Recurrence rate is substantially reduced by lithium and other mood stabilizers.
- Lithium is prophylactic in two-thirds of patients and reduces the suicide rate eight-fold.
- Lithium seems to be more effective in patients with fully remitting courses than in mixed states or rapid cycling.
- A naturalistic 5-year prospective follow-up of patients on lithium prophylaxis found that lithium significantly reduced rehospitalization rates in patients with and without mood-incongruent psychotic features (Maj, Pirozzi, Bartoli, & Magliano, 2002).
  - The latter patients did not do as well.

- A review of nine randomized placebo-controlled trials of lithium prophylaxis in a total of 825 patients with bipolar and unipolar mood disorders found that lithium was > placebo for preventing relapse (Burgess et al., 2002).
  - The most consistent prophylactic effect was in bipolar disorder (risk of relapse 0.29 of risk on placebo).
- Prophylactic efficacy of lithium may be reduced over time.
- Patients who are euthymic on lithium and discontinue it after long-term treatment have earlier recurrences of mania and bipolar depression than would be predicted from the natural history of the illness if it had been untreated (Baldessarini et al., 1996).
  - Rebound of the mood disorder is most likely if lithium is discontinued rapidly.
  - Patients may become refractory to lithium if it is discontinued and then restarted later (Tondo, Baldessarini, Floris, & Rudas, 1997).
  - No data on rebound and discontinuation-induced refractoriness with other mood stabilizers, but this probably occurs.
- There is no evidence that the effective maintenance lithium level is lower than the therapeutic level.
  - Lithium levels $\geq 0.8$ mM appear to be more effective in preventing recurrence than levels $< 0.6$, but other studies contradict this finding.

Following a single manic episode, lithium should be maintained for at least a year.

- In view of the high rate of recurrence and increasing complexity of illness with each recurrence, it is most prudent to continue maintenance treatment indefinitely.
- Many patients discontinue mood stabilizers even when they understand intellectually that this may result in deterioration of the mood disorder because of
  - Denial
  - Intolerance of side effects
  - Dislike of laboratory monitoring
  - Uncertainty about whether medication is still necessary
  - Contemplation of pregnancy
  - Emerging hypomania
- It is useful to discuss these issues once acute symptoms have remitted.
  - Patient should then be followed regularly even if asymptomatic.
  - If family is supportive and can help monitor symptoms, medication withdrawal is safer.
  - Inform patient and family about subtle symptoms of emerging recurrence.

- If patient decides to discontinue medication, advise that this be done over 3–6 months to reduce risk of rebound symptoms.
- For example, decrease dose by 300 mg every 1–2 months.
    - This pace will reduce risk of rebound and facilitate restarting treatment if symptoms reemerge.
- If patient develops recurrence after discontinuing lithium, restart it gradually, if possible.
    - Medication may not be as well tolerated when reintroduced.
    - Rapid dosage escalation may result in treatment-emergent depression.

Long-term maintenance therapy should be encouraged in patients with
- Severe manic or depressive episode
- Two or more previous episodes
- Inadequate social supports
- First-degree relatives with bipolar disorder

Management of manic recurrence
- Check lithium level.
    - Level may have decreased with activation of physiology of the mood disorder or with nonadherence.
    - Add a second antimanic drug (e.g., divalproex).
        - If episode remits, cautiously reduce lithium dose to see if patient needs both medications.
    - Add an atypical antipsychotic if no response.
    - Addition of a benzodiazepine (e.g., lorazepam, clonazepam) may result in remission of emerging hypomanic recurrence on lithium.
        - Can be slowly withdrawn once acute symptoms remit.

Management of depressive recurrence:
- Check lithium level, serum calcium, and thyroid function.
- Wait a few weeks if depression not severe to see if it cycles away spontaneously.
- Add carbamazepine, oxcarbazepine, or lamotrigine.
- If antidepressant is necessary, follow protocol on pages 264–268.

Unipolar Depression

Lithium is more effective for bipolar than for unipolar depression.
- Lithium has been found to reduce recurrence rates in unipolar depression somewhat less effectively than antidepressants.
- Augmentation with lithium improves response to antidepressants in unipolar depression.

- Overall response rate about two-thirds.
- Response to lithium augmentation more likely in bipolar depression and possibly in depression with family history of bipolar disorder.
- Some patients respond to 300–600 mg/day.
  - Response usually occurs in 2–4 weeks.
  - If no response and patient tolerates lithium, increase dose to achieve usual therapeutic levels.
- Lithium has been found to be superior to antidepressants in preventing recurrences in recurrent brief depression (Angst & Hochstrasser, 1994).

## SCHIZOAFFECTIVE DISORDER

Schizoaffective disorder is diagnosed in DSM-IV-TR when psychotic symptoms have been present during at least 2 weeks of euthymia.

- Mood incongruent psychotic symptoms and formal thought disorder, which are used to diagnose schizoaffective disorder in the Research Diagnostic Criteria, have not been shown to predict course or treatment response because they also occur in bipolar disorder.
- Affective symptoms in schizoaffective disorder may be predominantly depressive (schizodepressive), in which case the disorder is closer to schizophrenia in treatment response, or predominantly bipolar (schizomanic), in which case course and treatment response are not significantly different from bipolar disorder.
- Lithium is most useful for affective symptoms.
  - Usually combined with an antipsychotic drug in schizoaffective disorder.
- Schizodepressive subtype is treated with antidepressants plus antipsychotics.

## PERSONALITY DISORDERS WITH EMOTIONAL INSTABILITY

"Emotionally unstable character disorder" (not a DSM-IV-TR diagnosis) is characterized by mood swings, impulsivity, depression, antisocial behavior, and promiscuity. In some cases this disorder may represent a subsyndromal form of bipolar mood disorder. Borderline personality disorder is often accompanied by affective lability, which may improve with lithium.

- No medication can treat the entire disorder.
- Antipsychotic drugs can be useful on a prn basis for disorganization and transference psychosis.
- Lithium or anticonvulsants may improve mood swings, impulsivity, aggression, and self-destructive behavior.
- MAOIs and SSRIs are useful for comorbid depression.

- Patients with severe personality disorders may overdose on potentially dangerous medications such as lithium in order to defeat the clinician and undo the benefits of treatment (negative therapeutic reaction).

MEDICAL DISORDERS

- Lithium can increase neutrophil count and reduce recurrences of cyclic neutropenia.
- Because lithium increases release of neutrophils into circulation, it can be used to treat neutropenia caused by cancer chemotherapy or blood dyscrasias.
- Interference of lithium with vasopressin signaling may be useful in treatment of SIADH.
- Lithium has been found to have possible neuroprotective actions.
    - Lithium increases N-acetyl-aspartate, a marker of neuronal viability.
    - An MRI study of 12 untreated bipolar patients, 17 lithium-treated bipolar patients, and 46 controls found that total gray matter volumes were significantly greater in lithium-treated patients than the other groups.
        - Possibly reflects a neurotrophic effect of lithium (Sassi et al., 2002).
    - Such findings suggest that lithium may counteract loss of neurons in the hippocampus and elsewhere with progression of mood disorders.
    - Could be beneficial in brain injury, although lithium can acutely impair memory.

## SIDE EFFECTS

Sodium depletion can elevate lithium levels and increase toxicity. Side effects at therapeutic doses may be intensified by hypokalemia.

### Cardiovascular Side Effects

EKG CHANGES

- Lithium slows the rate of depolarization of the SA node and slows conduction through the AV node.
    - May result in bradycardia.
    - Additive effects occur with other medications that cause cardiac slowing.
        - Beta-adrenergic blockers
        - Calcium channel-blockers
        - Cholinesterase inhibitors

- Lithium also may cause
  - Nonspecific T-wave changes in 20% of patients.
    - Similar to changes associated with hypokalemia.
  - QRS widening.
  - These changes are benign and not correlated with lithium level.
- Lithium toxicity can cause
  - ST depression
  - QT prolongation

ARRHYTHMIAS

- Bradycardia can cause dizziness, fainting, and palpitations.
  - More common in the presence of lithium-induced hyperparathyroidism.
    - Probably reflects more substantial interference with calcium signaling in SA node as well as parathyroid gland.
- Most arrhythmias are supraventricular.

## Central Nervous System Side Effects

AFFECTIVE BLUNTING

Dulling of emotional responsiveness is a common lithium side effect most noticeable when acute symptoms resolve.

- Loss of hypomanic intensity may make everything dull by comparison.
- Subsyndromal depression may present as affective blunting.

COGNITIVE IMPAIRMENT

As many as 50% of patients develop impaired memory, difficulty with word finding, or cognitive dulling.

- More likely at higher levels
- A direct effect of the drug, or secondary to
  - Hypothyroidism
  - Hypercalcemia
  - Subclinical depression
  - Absence of feeling the intense mental clarity associated with mania
- Management:
  - Exclude causes listed above.
  - Give entire dose at bedtime.
  - Decrease dose if possible.
  - Add cholinesterase inhibitor (see Chapter 2).
  - Change mood stabilizer.

### Parkinsonism

- EPS occasionally occurs with lithium alone.
- More likely when lithium combined with antipsychotic drugs.
- Antiparkinsonian drugs are poorly tolerated.

### Pseudotumor Cerebri

- Presents with blurred vision.
- Headache is not always present.
- Papilledema
  - Remits a few months after lithium withdrawn.
- Elevated CSF pressure
  - Does not always resolve when lithium discontinued.

### Tremor

- Two kinds of tremor may occur:
  - Fine dose-related benign tremor
  - Coarse tremor indicating lithium toxicity

Benign tremor
- Usually involves fingers.
  - If severe, may involve hands and wrists.
- Rapid
- Irregular
- Variable severity throughout day
- Present at rest; worse with intention
- Increased by anxiety
- More likely in patients with essential tremor
- May interfere with writing or eating
- Most marked at peak lithium level
- Differences from parkinsonian tremor
  - Not pill rolling
  - No micrographia
  - Fingers, hand, and wrists do not move as a unit.
- Tremor can be reduced by several interventions.
  - Use sustained-release preparation.
  - Give medication in one bedtime dose.
    - Peak level occurs while patient is asleep.
  - Reduce level.
  - Propranolol 10–80 mg/day in divided dose may be helpful.

- Lithium and propranolol may cause additive cardiac slowing.
  - Atenolol may not be as helpful because tremor thought to be a central effect.
  - Antiparkinsonian drugs are not helpful.

## Endocrine and Sexual Side Effects

IMPAIRED THYROID FUNCTION

- Interference with thyroid function occurs in 20% of patients.
- Risk of hypothyroidism is 30% in children.
- Lithium interferes with TSH signaling in thyroid gland and with conversion of $T_4$ to $T_3$.
- Clinical indications of hypothyroidism may occur:
  - Fatigue
  - Weakness
  - Weight gain
  - Dry skin
  - Cold intolerance
  - Cognitive impairment
  - Depression
  - Menstrual abnormalities
- Chemical hypothyroidism can occur in the absence of signs or symptoms.
  - Marginally decreased $T_4$ with elevated TSH
  - Normal $T_4$ with elevated TSH indicates initial compensation for decreased thyroid function.
    - May be associated with euthyroid goiter.
  - Normal $T_4$ and normal TSH with hyperactive TSH response to TRH (increase over baseline $> 30$ IU/L after 500 $\mu$g of TRH) is not medically important but can affect response of mood disorder.
    - Onset of hypothyroidism usually occurs within 6–18 months of starting lithium.
- Even in absence of clinical hypothyroidism, marginal decrements in thyroid function can affect mood disorder.
  - Treatment resistance is associated with subclinical hypothyroidism in 40% of patients.
  - 70% of women with rapid cycling have one or another form of hypothyroidism.
  - Correcting hypothyroidism improves treatment response.

Management:

- Patients taking lithium require regular monitoring of TSH and $T_4$ in unclear cases.
  - Every 6–12 months in adult
  - Every 3 months in children
    - Taking iodine-containing cold preparations increases the risk of hypothyroidism in children on lithium.
  - Isolated moderate elevation of TSH (e.g., 5–10 IU/L) is not medically important.
    - Initiate treatment if mood disorder does not respond well to treatment.
  - Add thyroid replacement for higher TSH or impaired treatment response with mild TSH elevation.
    - Starting dose 0.05–0.1 mg/day thyroxine
    - Improved sense of well-being reported when thyroid replacement is given as 75% $T_4$ and 25% $T_3$.
    - Some patients with mood disorders and some patients with hypothyroidism may have incomplete conversion of $T_4$ to $T_3$ in brain.

## Glucose Intolerance

Lithium interferes with insulin signaling.

- Does not usually cause diabetes mellitus.
- May impair response to treatment of diabetes.
- Lithium also causes carbohydrate craving.
- In a group of 38 patients with type I or type II diabetes without mood disorders, fasting blood glucose and 1-hour postprandial glucose levels decreased significantly after treatment with lithium (Hu, Wu, & Chao, 1997).
- In a group of bipolar patients followed before starting lithium and for up to 6 years after (total exposure time to lithium = 495.5 years), mean blood sugar did not change, and only one patient developed diabetes (Vestergaard & Schou, 1987).

## Hyperparathyroidism

The majority of patients taking lithium long term develop increases in serum calcium and higher PTH levels than would be predicted from serum calcium, indicating hyperparathyroidism.

- Caused by interference with calcium signaling in parathyroid gland, so that PTH production is not normally suppressed by increasing calcium levels.

- Changes usually are not clinically important.
- Some patients develop clinically meaningful hyperparathyroidism, causing
  - Depression
  - Mania
  - Fatigue, lassitude
  - Cognitive impairment
  - Cataracts
  - Decreased renal concentrating ability
  - Increased bond resorption
- Parathyroid adenomas occasionally occur.
- Hyperparathyroidism remits when lithium discontinued.
- Parathyroid adenoma does not disappear when lithium withdrawn.
- No specific treatment, other than withdrawing lithium, if hyper-parathyroidism is medically important or interferes with mood stabilizer.

## Gastrointestinal Side Effects

### Nausea

- Often occurs early in treatment.
- More frequent with rapid lithium dosage increase.
- Associated with peak serum levels.
- Usually dose related, but may occur with low doses.
- Vomiting may cause dehydration, which increases lithium levels.
- Management:
  - Increase dose slowly.
  - Use sustained-release preparation.
  - Give entire dose at bedtime.
  - Take with meals.
  - Use ginger root capsules or fresh ginger root (see cholinesterase inhibitors, Chapter 2).
  - If changing mood stabilizers is not practical, consider adding ondansetron 2–4 mg once to three times/day or granisetron 1 mg bid–tid.

### Diarrhea

Marker of toxicity, but also may occur with therapeutic doses.
- More common with sustained-release and once daily dosing.

- Management:
  - Reduce dose.
  - Give lithium more frequently.
  - Take medication with meals.
  - Switch to immediate-release lithium or lithium citrate (absorbed more rapidly).
  - Add antidiarrheal medication (e.g., loperimides).

## Weight Gain, Edema

- Overall risk of weight gain about 25–40%.
- Caused by increased food intake and possibly alteration of insulin action.
- When weight gain does occur:
  - Weight gain > 10 pounds not caused by fluid retention: 25%.
- Edema can occur without changes in renal or cardiac function.
  - May cause 5–7 pounds of weight gain.
- Management:
  - Decrease lithium dose if possible.
  - Recommend low-calorie diet with normal sodium intake.
    - Crash diets can result in lithium toxicity.
  - Change mood stabilizer.
  - Topiramate 50–400 mg/day produced average weight loss 6.2 kg at 1 year in patients who remained on drug that long, but last observation carried forward (LOCF) average weight loss for all patients was 4.5 kg (McElroy & Keck, 2000).
    - Mood-stabilizing effects of topiramate not clearly demonstrated.
    - Some patients may become too activated.
  - Zonisamide (mean dose 427 mg/day) produced mean weight loss of 5.9 kg versus 0.9 kg on placebo in a 16-week double-blind study of obese adults (Gadde et al., 2003).
    - Almost 50% of zonesamide patients and no placebo patients lost 10% of their body weight by 32 weeks.
    - Zonisamide does not appear to be effective for bipolar disorder, but it may not make it worse.
  - Treat edema cautiously with potassium-sparing diuretics.
    - Amiloride 5–10 mg/day
    - Spironolactone 50 mg bid
    - Furosemide 20–80 mg/day

## Hematologic Side Effects

### LEUKOCYTOSIS

Lithium shifts neutrophils into circulation.

- Average 35% increase in neutrophil count shortly after starting medication.
- Total white blood count may increase to 12,000–15,000/mm$^3$.
- Increase is benign.
- May be used to treat leukopenia caused by other medications.

## Renal Side Effects

Lithium impairs renal tubule response to vasopressin (antidiuretic hormone or ADH), resulting in increased renal water loss.

- Some degree of polyuria occurs in 50–70% of patients taking lithium chronically.
  - Urine volume > 3 liters in 10%
- May be more frequent with sustained-release lithium and with divided dosing.
- Features:
  - Increased urine volume
    - > 3 liters/day
    - May reach 4–8 liters.
  - Increased frequency of urination
  - Nocturia
  - Polydipsia
    - Usually secondary to polyuria, but lithium can primarily increase thirst.
  - Dehydration
  - Increased serum sodium
  - Decreased serum potassium
- Management:
  - Give one daily dose of lithium.
  - Decrease lithium dose.
  - Increase noncaloric fluid intake.
  - Sodium-sparing diuretics (e.g., amiloride 5–10 mg bid):
    - Have minimal effect on lithium level.
    - Monitor serum lithium and electrolytes.
  - Hydrochlorothiazide may be helpful.

- Can increase lithium levels by 30–50%.
- May reduce potassium levels.
- Indomethacin
  - Multiple reports of efficacy in nephrogenic diabetes insipidus.
  - The usual dose is 50 mg once or twice per day.
  - Indomethacin can raise serum lithium levels by interfering with renal lithium excretion.
- Carbamazepine
  - May increase ADH secretion and counteract reduced ADH effect.
- However, arginine vasopressin (DDAVP) not effective for nephrogenic diabetes insipidus.

## TUBULO-INTERSTITIAL NEPHROPATHY

- Renal changes reported on lithium include
  - Interstitial nephrosis
  - Tubular atrophy
  - Glomerular atrophy
- Not clear if these changes are caused by lithium or by bipolar disorder itself.
- Medically important nephrotoxicity with chronic lithium therapy is rare.
- Obtain nephrology consultation if
  - Creatinine increases > 1.6 mg/dL.
  - Creatinine clearance decreases.
  - 24-hour urine volume increases substantially.

## Skin, Allergies, and Temperature Side Effects

### ACNE

- May appear or worsen with lithium.
- May be limiting side effect, especially for adolescents.
- Management:
  - Topical tretinoin
  - Erythromycin
    - Tetracycline can have toxic interactions with lithium.

### PSORIASIS

- Usually exacerbation of preexisting psoriasis.
- Dry, noninflamed papular eruption is common.
- Reducing lithium dose may help.

RASH

- Allergic rash not common.
  - When it does occur, allergy is usually to excipients in the pill.
  - Change preparation or use lithium citrate.
- Maculopapular rash
  - Not severe
  - Ameliorated by 50:50 zinc ointment
- Alopecia
  - May be caused by hypothyroidism.
  - Occurs in 12% of women.
    - Rare in men
  - Hair may lose its curl.
  - Hair may grow back on or off lithium.
- Mycosis fungoides
  - Rarely occurs with chronic lithium treatment.
  - Pruritic, erythematous, hyperkeratotic lesions
  - No systemic signs
  - Lithium should be discontinued.

## PREGNANCY AND LACTATION

### Teratogenicity and Other Issues in First-Trimester Use

- Lithium increases the risk of Ebstein's anomaly (abnormal placement of tricuspid valve) about 10-fold over general population.
  - Risk in general population: 1/1000–1/10,000 live births
  - Can be identified by ultrasound.
- Lithium clearance increases during pregnancy because of increased blood volume.
  - Lithium dose may have to be increased by 40%.
  - Level decreases with parturition.
  - Monitor levels every 2–4 weeks during pregnancy.
- Alternatives to lithium that are safer during pregnancy:
  - Verapamil
  - Antipsychotic drugs
  - ECT
- Avoid NSAIDs because they increase lithium levels 30–60%.

### Prenatal and Neonatal Effects

- Lithium levels increase rapidly postpartum because of decrease in total maternal blood volume.
  - Reduce dose in anticipation of delivery.
  - Obtain weekly lithium levels during last month of pregnancy.
- Nephrogenic diabetes in fetus rarely causes polyhydramnios, which can restrict the mother's respiration.
- Lithium occasionally associated with preterm labor.
- Neonatal goiter sometimes occurs.
  - May compromise breathing.
  - No long-term sequelae.
- Newborns exposed to lithium in utero may develop hypotonia, cyanosis, and decreased feeding.
- Neonatal lithium toxicity occasionally occurs even if mother's lithium level is normal.

### Lactation

- Lithium is excreted in breast milk.
- Level in breast milk about 40% of serum level, but dose to infant is low (0.41 mg/kg/day).
- Infant lithium level usually 20–60% of maternal level.
- Minimize exposure to infant by using immediate-release lithium and nursing before each dose.
- Case reports of infants nursing from mothers taking lithium have described occasional
  - Cyanosis
  - Hypotonia
  - EKG changes
  - Lithium toxicity

## DRUG–DRUG INTERACTIONS

Table 5.4 summarizes lithium interactions with other drugs.

## EFFECTS ON LABORATORY TESTS

Table 5.5 lists the effects of lithium on laboratory tests.

## Table 5.4 Drug–Drug Interactions

| DRUGS (X) INTERACT WITH: | LITHIUM (L) | COMMENTS |
| --- | --- | --- |
| ACE (angiotensin-converting enzyme) inhibitors: benazepril captopril enalapril fosinopril lisinopril quinapril ramipril | L↑ | Increases serum lithium. Lithium toxicity and impaired kidney function may occur; may need to stop lithium or ACE inhibitor. |
| acetazolamide | L↓ | Reduces serum lithium and efficacy; sometimes used for detoxification in lithium overdose. |
| alcohol | L↑ | Alcohol may increase serum lithium. |
| albuterol (*see* bronchodilators) | | |
| amiloride | L↑ | Potassium-sparing diuretic occasionally increases lithium concentration and toxicity. |
| aminophylline (*see* bronchodilators) | | |
| ampicillin | L↑ | Increased lithium effect and toxicity. |
| antipsychotics: haloperidol thioridazine others | X↑ L↑ | Occasionally increased neurotoxicity. May rarely be irreversible. Reported most frequently with haloperidol, probably because haloperidol used more frequently in mania before introduction of atypicals. NMS may occur. Lower lithium levels seen when liquid lithium citrate given with liquid neuroleptic (i.e., chlorpromazine or trifluoperazine) secondary to lithium precipitate being formed. |
| antithyroids: carbimazole methimazole radioactive iodine | X↑ | Lithium increases thyroid suppression; may be clinically useful when β-blocker contraindicated for hyperthyroidism. |
| baclofen | X↓ | Increases hyperkinetic symptoms when lithium added. |
| bronchodilators: albuterol aminophylline theophylline | L↓ | Theophylline, aminophylline, and possibly albuterol increase lithium clearance and decrease lithium levels; chromolyn and nonsystemic steroids safer. |
| caffeine | L↓ | Increases lithium excretion; heavy coffee drinkers have trouble reaching therapeutic levels on even 2400 mg/day. Stopping caffeine when patient has therapeutic lithium level risks too high lithium. Increases lithium tremor. |

(*continues*)

**Table 5.4 Continued**

| DRUGS (X) INTERACT WITH: | LITHIUM (L) | COMMENTS |
|---|---|---|
| calcium channel-blockers:<br>diltiazem<br>nifedipine<br>verapamil | L↑ | Additive effects on SA node cause increased cardiac slowing. Risk of lithium neurotoxicity may be increased by verapamil. |
| captopril (*see* ACE inhibitors) | | |
| carbamazepine | X↑ L↑ | Additive risk of neurotoxicity. Increased therapeutic effect of both drugs. |
| carbonic anhydrase inhibitors | L↓ | Increases lithium clearance. |
| corticosteroids:<br>hydrocortisone<br>methylprednisolone | L↓ | Increase lithium clearance; monitor lithium closely. |
| decamethonium | X↑ | Prolonged muscle paralysis. |
| dehydroepiandrosterone (DHEA) | L↓ | DHEA-associated mania may occur with or without lithium. |
| dextroamphetamine | X↓ | Lithium may inhibit dextroamphetamine's euphoria. |
| digitalis | X↑↓ | May cause cardiac arrhythmias, particularly bradyarrhythmias; occasionally lithium reduces effects. |
| diuretics (*see* indoline, loop, osmotic, thiazide, xanthine) | | |
| diltiazem (*see* calcium channel-blockers) | | |
| enalapril (*see* ACE inhibitors) | | |
| HCAs (*see* TCAs) | | |
| hydroxyzine | L↑ | Cardiac conduction disturbances. |
| indoline (indapamide) | L↑ | Increases lithium level. |
| ketamine | L↑ | Increased lithium toxicity from sodium depletion. |
| loop diuretics:<br>ethacrynic acid<br>furosemide | L↑↓ | May increase or decrease lithium slightly; decreased lithium levels not as significant as with thiazides. Potassium-sparing diuretics safest (amiloride, spironolatone). |
| marijuana | L↑ | Increased absorption of lithium; importance unclear. |
| mazindol | L↑ | A few cases of lithium toxicity after 3 days of mazindol; worse with inadequate salt intake. |

*(continues)*

## Table 5.4  Continued

| DRUGS (X) INTERACT WITH: | LITHIUM (L) | COMMENTS |
|---|---|---|
| methyldopa | L↑ | Lithium toxicity may develop with a normal lithium level; toxicity ends 1–9 days after stopping methyldopa. |
| metronidazole | L↑ | Increased lithium level; toxicity. |
| NSAIDs:<br>  diclofenac<br>  ibuprofen<br>  indomethacin<br>  ketoprofen<br>  ketorolac<br>  mefenamic acid<br>  naproxen<br>  piroxicam<br>  phenylbutazone | L↑ | Listed NSAIDs increase plasma lithium 30–61% in 3–10 days. Sulindac, naproxen sodium, aspirin, and acetaminophen do not appear to change levels, and phenylbutazone averages only 11% increase. |
| osmotic diuretics | L↑ | Decreases lithium level and efficacy. |
| pancuronium | X↑ | Prolonged muscle paralysis. |
| phenytoin | L↑ | A few cases of lithium toxicity. |
| physostigmine | L↓ | May reduce efficacy of lithium. |
| potassium iodide | L↑ | Sometimes produces hypothyroidism and goiter, which is no reason to halt lithium; treat thyroid instead. |
| sodium bicarbonate | L↓ | Decreases lithium level. |
| sodium chloride | L↓↑ | High sodium decreases lithium level; low sodium intake may increase serum lithium and toxicity. |
| spectinomycin | L↑ | Increased lithium effect and toxicity. |
| spironolactone | L↑ | Potassium-saving diuretic may occasionally increase lithium concentration and toxicity. |
| succinylcholine | X↑ | Prolonged neuromuscular blockade. |
| sympathomimetics:<br>  dobutamine<br>  epinephrine<br>  norepinephrine | X↓ | Lithium decreases pressor actions of norepinephrine and other direct-acting sympathomimetics. |
| tetracyclines | L↑ | Tetracycline and doxycycline moderately increase lithium levels and may have neurotoxic interactions. Unclear if other tetracyclines affect lithium. |
| theophylline (*see* bronchodilators) | | |
| thiazide diuretics:<br>  chlorothiazide<br>  hydrochlorothiazide | L↑ | Any diuretic that promotes sodium and potassium excretion can increase lithium levels substantially; monitor levels if |

*(continues)*

**Table 5.4 Continued**

| DRUGS (X) INTERACT WITH: | LITHIUM (L) | COMMENTS |
|---|---|---|
| | | lithium is prescribed with one of these. Potassium-sparing diuretics are safer but may increase lithium levels. Watch for hypercalcemia. |
| TCAs | L↑ | Increased tremor. |
| ticarcillin | X↑ | Hypernatremia. |
| triamterene | L↑ | Potassium-saving diuretic may increase lithium concentration and toxicity. |
| tryptophan | L↑ | Increases lithium efficacy; tryptophan off American market. |
| urea | L↓ | Urea may reduce lithium but no clinical evidence that this occurs. |
| valproic acid | L↑ | Increased neurotoxicity and anticycling effect. |
| verapamil | L↑↓ | Lithium-induced neurotoxicity, nausea, weakness, ataxia, and tinnitus. Rarely, decreased lithium levels. |
| xanthine diuretics | L↓ | Increased lithium excretion and decreased plasma levels. |

↑ Increases; ↓ Decreases; ↑↓ Increases and decreases.

## WITHDRAWAL

Lithium is not associated with tolerance, dependence, or withdrawal. However, rapid discontinuation can result in three undesirable conditions:

- Rebound of the mood disorder
  - Meta-analysis of controlled trials in which lithium was discontinued, for whatever reason, after extended remission found that both mania and depression recurred sooner than would have been predicted from the natural history of the disorder (Baldessarini et al., 1996).
    - Rapid discontinuation ($< 6$ weeks) was most likely to result in rebound.
    - Slower discontinuation (over months) resulted in less rebound.
- Discontinuation-induced refractoriness
  - Lithium has been noted to be ineffective or less tolerated when reintroduced for symptom rebound after it was discontinued (Tondo et al., 1997).

**Table 5.5  Lithium Effects on Laboratory Tests**

| BLOOD TESTS* | URINE TESTS |
|---|---|
| $^{131}I$ uptake ↑ | Glucose ↑ |
| $T_3$ ↓ | Albumin ↑ |
| $T_4$ ↓** | VMA ↑ |
| Leukocytes ↑ | Renal concentrating |
| | Ability ↓ |
| Eosinophils ↑ | Calcium ↑ |
| Platelets ↑ | |
| Lymphocytes ↓ | |
| $Ca^{++}$, $Mg^{++}$ ↑↑ | |
| Serum phosphate ↓ | |
| Serum Calcium ↑ | |
| Parathyroid hormone ↑ | |
| Glucose tolerance ↓ | |
| Creatinine ↑ | |
| Lithium ↑*** | |

* ↑ Increases; ↓ Decreases; ↑↓ Increases and decreases; r = rarely.
** Mania itself may transiently increase TSH and $T_4$.
*** Atomic absorption spectrophotometry most accurate assay for lithium. Ion-selective
electrode method can give falsely higher lithium levels of 0.2–0.4 mEq/l
increase probably secondary to aging electrodes.

▪ Unless rapid discontinuation is indicated for medical reasons, lithium
(and probably any other mood stabilizer) should be withdrawn over
3–6 months.
  ▪ Reduces risk of rebound.
  ▪ Increases likelihood that reinstituting previous dose in the event of
  relapse or recurrence will be effective.

Table 5.6 summarizes the side effects of lithium in relation to lithium
carbonate levels.

## TOXICITY AND OVERDOSE

Lithium has a low therapeutic index (ratio of toxic:therapeutic dose)
compared to other psychiatric drugs.
▪ Therapeutic indexes of
  ▪ Antipsychotics: 100
  ▪ TCAs: 10
  ▪ Lithium: 3

**Table 5.6  Side Effects at Different Lithium Levels**

| THERAPEUTIC LITHIUM LEVELS (0.6–1.5 mEq/L) | MILD TO MODERATE TOXICITY (1.5–2.0 mEq/L) | MODERATE TO SEVERE TOXICITY (2.0–2.5 mEq/L) |
|---|---|---|
| *Central Nervous System*<br>  Hand tremor<br>  Memory Impairment | *Central Nervous System*<br>  Dizziness<br>  Drowsiness<br>  Dysarthria<br>  Excitement<br>  Hand tremor (coarse)<br>  Lethargy<br>  Muscle weakness<br>  Sluggishness | *Cardiovascular*<br>  Cardiac arrhythmia<br>  Pulse irregularities |
| *Endocrine*<br>  Goiter<br>  Hypothyroidism | | *Central Nervous System*<br>  Choreoathetoid movements<br>  Clonic limb movements<br>  Coma<br>  Convulsions<br>  Delirium<br>  EEG changes<br>  Fainting<br>  Hyperreflexia<br>  Leg tremor<br>  Muscle fasciculations |
| *Gastrointestinal*<br>  Diarrhea (mild)<br>  Edema<br>  Nausea<br>  Weight gain | *Eyes, Ears, Nose, Throat*<br>  Vertigo<br><br>*Gastrointestinal*<br>  Abdominal pain<br>  Diarrhea<br>  Dry mouth<br>  Vomiting | |
| *Renal*<br>  Polydipsia<br>  Polyuria | | *Eyes, Ears, Nose, Throat*<br>  Nystagmus<br>  Vision blurred<br><br>*Gastrointestinal*<br>  Anorexia<br>  Nausea (chronic)<br>  Vomiting (chronic) |

- Lithium toxicity is much more likely at higher levels.
    - More likely with
        - Dehydration
        - Decreased fluid intake (e.g., during acute affective episode)
        - Fever
        - Electrolyte loss (e.g., during vomiting)
        - Renal insufficiency
        - Water loss caused by lithium-induced nephrogenic diabetes insipidus
        - Concomitant use of diuretics, NSAIDs, tetracycline
    - Levels > 2 mM frequently associated with toxicity.
- Features
    - New onset of diarrhea after chronic treatment may be first sign of toxicity.
    - Coarse tremor
    - Myoclonus

- Confusion
- Cardiotoxicity
- Seizures
- Delirium
  - Accompanied by EEG slowing.
- CNS toxicity may persist for a week in younger patients and months in older patients after lithium has been eliminated.
  - Lithium toxicity poisons the lithium–sodium exchange pump, leading to intracellular accumulation of lithium that takes time to abate.
  - Lithium may also be slowly eliminated from the brain after an episode of toxicity.

### Treatment

- Ensure adequate hydration.
- Induce emesis or lavage followed by ion exchange resin, if patient is alert.
- Obtain baseline EKG.
- Obtain
  - Serum lithium
    - Continue to monitor for secondary peaks after initial decline.
  - Creatinine
  - Electrolytes
  - Blood glucose
  - Urinalysis
    - Look for albuminuria.
- Hemodialysis
  - Apply if
    - Serum lithium > 2–3 mM and patient deteriorating.
    - Fluid/electrolyte imbalance unresponsive to supportive measures.
    - Declining creatinine clearance or urine output.
    - Serum lithium does not decrease by 20% in first 6 hours.
  - Goal: Reduce serum lithium level to < 1 mM within 8 hours.
  - Rebound of lithium level a few hours after hemodialysis may require repeat hemodialysis.
- For less severe intoxication
  - Restore fluid/electrolyte balance.
    - Correct sodium depletion.

- Intravenous 0.9% sodium chloride if sodium depletion suspected.
  - 1–2 liters in first 6 hours
- IV diuretics not effective.
- Increase lithium excretion with
  - Sodium bicarbonate
  - Urea
  - Mannitol
  - Acetazolamide
  - Aminophylline
- Treat seizures with benzodiazepine or short-acting barbiturate.

Lithium can be restarted after patient has recovered clinically
- 48 hours in younger patients
- 4–5 days later in geriatric patients.
- Clinical recovery is not reliably correlated with lithium levels.
  - Intracellular lithium levels may still be toxic.
- Lithium should be restarted very slowly or the lithium extrusion pump may be reinjured.

The outcome of lithium poisoning is variable.
- 70–80% recover fully.
- 10% have persistent toxicity with
  - Cognitive impairment
  - Ataxia
  - Polyuria
  - Dysarthria
  - Spasticity
  - Tremor
- 10% mortality
- In geriatric patients, signs of neurotoxicity may persist for 3–10 weeks before recovery.


## PRECAUTIONS

Between 33% and 45% of patients stop lithium during the first year of treatment.
- It is important to monitor closely for nonadherence, especially during the first year.
- Common causes of lithium discontinuation include
  - Dislike of laboratory tests.

- Side effects
  - Weight gain
  - Cognitive impairment
  - Hair loss
  - GI side effects
  - Tremor
  - Affective blunting
- Missing "highs"
- Treatment-emergent depression

Lithium should not be used in the presence of
- Immediate risk of overdose
- Vomiting, diarrhea, or dehydration
- Sick sinus syndrome

Significant precautions include:
- Renal insufficiency
  - Lithium is eliminated almost entirely by the kidneys.
  - Lower and less frequent dosing and more careful monitoring of levels are necessary in the presence of renal insufficiency.
- Pregnancy
  - Risk of Ebstein's anomaly, neonatal effects, and the need to monitor levels closely preterm.
  - Risk of lithium is probably less than that of anticonvulsants but more than risks of verapamil, antipsychotics, and ECT.
  - Need to balance potential risks of medication and potential risks of illness.
- Brain damage
  - Lithium is useful for agitation and mood disorders in brain-damaged patients.
  - Lithium has neuroprotective properties.
  - Risks in these patients
    - Inability to remember dosing and monitoring
    - Cognitive side effects
    - Neurotoxic interactions with other centrally acting medications
- Low-salt diet or diuretic therapy
  - Lithium is conserved along with sodium, resulting in higher lithium levels.
  - Adjust lithium dose carefully and monitor closely if diet or diuretic is changed.
  - Use sodium-potassium-sparing diuretic, if possible.

- Vigorous exercisers
  - Excessive sweating leads to sodium loss, which results in increased lithium retention as kidneys attempt to conserve sodium.
  - Advise patient to drink plenty of electrolyte-containing fluids during exercise.

## ADVICE FOR CARETAKERS

Patients should be advised not to go on a diet without notifying clinicians. Warn patients about risks of

- Salt restriction
- Diuretics
- Vomiting
- New exercise program, especially in hot weather or at high altitutde

High rate of nonadherence warrants regular questioning about how patient feels about the medication.

Ensure that patient understands that lithium level should be drawn 12 hours after last dose and before morning dose, if such dosing is employed.

## NOTES FOR PATIENT AND FAMILY

Tell physicians treating other conditions about use of lithium, and be sure to tell clinician prescribing lithium about other medications that are prescribed.

A Medic Alert card or bracelet indicating lithium use is a good idea.

Side effects of lithium are not necessarily signs of toxicity.

- If the dose is increased more slowly, tolerance to side effects is more likely to develop.
- GI side effects are reduced by taking lithium with meals or a snack.
- Possible signs of toxicity include
  - Confusion
  - Muscle twitching
  - Diarrhea that was not present previously
  - Coarse tremor

If a dose is forgotten

- It can be taken within 8 hours.
- Otherwise, wait for the next scheduled dose.

# CHAPTER SIX

# *Anticonvulsants, Calcium Channel-Blockers, Antipsychotics in Bipolar Disorder, and Antiaggression Agents*

Carbamazepine was first studied as a possible antimanic agent in the early 1960s (Okuma, 1983). Subsequently, a theory emerged that the antikindling action of anticonvulsants like carbamazepine could prevent bipolar recurrences, which are thought to be promoted partly by kindling and behavioral sensitization. However, the pathophysiology of the progression of bipolar disorder undoubtedly is multifactorial, and carbamazepine has a variety of actions in addition to reduction of kindling. Furthermore, some anticonvulsants are not mood stabilizers, some anticonvulsants may make bipolar illness worse, and some mood stabilizers do not have any antiepileptic properties.

Although the use of carbamazepine, valproate, and lamotrigine (to some extent) has greatly expanded the armamentarium for treating bipolar illness, many patients cannot tolerate, or do not respond to, these treatments. A number of additional antimanic drugs/mood stabilizers have been developed. Extensive experience has accumulated with the benzodiazepines, especially clonazepam and lorazepam, in the treatment of mania. Calcium channel-blocking agents (CCBs) have been studied in placebo-controlled studies. Atypical antipsychotic drugs are all effective for mania. Even though they are in widespread use in maintenance treatment, their efficacy for this indication remains to be clarified fully.

In addition to their uses in mood disorders, lithium, anticonvulsants, benzodiazepines, and antipsychotic drugs have been used to treat nonspecific aggressive and impulsive behavior associated with personality and neurological disorders. Beta-blockers and several other treatments also are used for this purpose.

This chapter reviews the use of anticonvulsants, CCBs, atypical antipsychotics, benzodiazepines, and beta-blockers in

- Bipolar disorder
- Atypical psychosis

295

- Flashbacks in chronic hallucinogen use
- Aggression and impulsive behavior
- Posttraumatic stress disorder
- Pathological gambling

Conditions treated with anticonvulsants discussed elsewhere include:
- CNS depressant withdrawal (Chapter 8)
- Unipolar depression (Chapter 3)
- Schizophrenia (Chapter 1)
- Anxiety disorders (Chapter 17)
- Binge eating disorder (pp. 131–132)

Table 6.1 provides a basic overview of the drugs discussed in this chapter.

**Table 6.1  Names, Dose Forms, Colors**

| GENERIC NAMES | BRAND NAMES | DOSE FORMS (MG)* | COLORS |
|---|---|---|---|
| carbamazepine | Tegretol | t: 100/200<br>su: 100 mg/5 ml | t: red-speckled/pink<br>su: yellow-orange |
| clonazepam | Klonopin | t: 0.5/1/2 | t: orange/blue/white |
| divalproex | Depakote ER<br>Depakote | t: 500<br>t: 125/250/500 | t: gray<br>t: salmon-pink/<br>peach/lavender |
| divalproex<br>  sodium-coated<br>  particles | Depakote Sprinkle | c: 125 | c: white-blue |
| gabapentin | Neurontin | c: 100/300/400 | c: white/yellow/<br>orange |
| lamotrigine | Lamictal** | t: 25/100/150/200 | t: white/peach/<br>cream/blue |
| levetiracetam | Keppra | t: 250/500/750<br>su: 100 mg/mL | t: blue/yellow/<br>orange |
| oxcarbazepine | Trileptal | t: 150/300/600<br>su: 60 mg/mL | t: all yellow |
| topiramate | Topamax | t: 25/100/200 | t: white/yellow/<br>salmon |
| valproic acid | Depakene | c: 250<br>s: 250 mg/5 ml | c: orange<br>s: red |

* c = capsules; s = syrup; su = suspension/concentrate; t = tablets.
** Beware of potential dispensing error confusing Lamictal vs. Lamisil.

## PHARMACOLOGY

In addition to their antiseizure effect, anticonvulsants have a variety of cellular actions. The metabolism of these medications differs from agent to agent.

Carbamazepine
- Multiple cellular actions
  - Antikindling
  - Reduction of polysynaptic responses and inhibition of posttetanic potentiation
  - Blockade of voltage-sensitive sodium channels
  - Calcium channel blockade
- Half-life
  - Initial dose 25–65 hours
  - Repeated doses 12–17 hours
- Protein binding: 76%
- Induces its own metabolism (autoinduction).
  - Results in decrease in level with continued treatment.
  - Repeated dosage increases often necessary before consistent blood level is obtained.
  - Also induces metabolism of many other CYP450 3A4 and 2C19 substrates, including estrogen.
- Metabolized by oxidation.
  - Major metabolite is a 10, 11-epoxide.
    - Half-life is 5–8 hours.
    - Responsible for autoinduction and many side effects.

Valproic acid/divalproex
- Valproic acid and divalproex have similar actions, but divalproex has fewer GI side effects (15% vs. 29%).
- Cellular actions
  - Increases brain levels of GABA.
  - Inhibits an enzyme responsible for GABA catabolism.
  - May potentiate postsynaptic GABA responses.
  - Sodium channel-blocker causing decrease in glutamate release.
  - May affect potassium channels or have a direct membrane-stabilizing effect.
- Absorbed rapidly.
  - Peak level in 3–8 hours.
  - Absorption most rapid with syrup.
    - Peak level in ½–2 hours

- Half-life: 6–16 hours.
  - Usually needs bid dosing.
  - Half-life shorter when combined with enzyme inducers (e.g., carbamazepine).
- Depakote ER (extended-release divalproex) reaches peak level in 7–14 hours.
  - Same elimination half-life as immediate release
  - Fewer GI side effects
  - Once daily dosing
- Excreted as glucuronide
- Protein binding: > 90%

Lamotrigine
- Cellular actions
  - Inhibits voltage-sensitive sodium channels and stabilizes neuronal membranes.
  - May modulate presynaptic release of excitatory amino acids.
  - Has neuroprotective effect that protects against excitotoxic injury (Wang, Sihra, & Gean, 2001).
  - Blockade of presynaptic calcium influx through N- and P-type calcium channels.
  - Inhibits amygdala and cortical-kindled seizures.
- Rapidly and completely absorbed.
- High bioavailability
- Half-life: 23–37 hours
  - Shorter half-life when combined with enzyme inducers such as carbamazepine
  - Longer half-life when combined with valproate
- Protein binding: 55%
- Extensively metabolized.
  - Autoinduction of metabolism
  - Primarily excreted in urine as inactive 2-N-glucuronide conjugate.

Oxcarbazepine
- Keto derivative of carbamazepine
- Cellular actions
  - Blockade of voltage-sensitive sodium channels
  - Enhancement of potassium efflux
  - Stabilization of neuronal membranes
  - Inhibition of repetitive neuronal firing

- Diminution of propagation of synaptic impulses
- No known action on neurotransmitters or receptors
- Metabolized by reduction (carbamazepine metabolized by oxidation).
  - Major metabolite is a 10-monohydroxy derivative (MHD) rather than 10,11-epoxide.
    - Fewer adverse effects
    - Weak inducer of CYP3A4
    - Less autoinduction of metabolism
- Should be taken bid.

Gabapentin
- Cellular actions
  - Structural analogue of GABA.
  - Does not interact with GABA receptors.
  - Not converted to GABA.
  - Not an inhibitor of GABA uptake or degradation.
  - Increases brain GABA levels in a dose-dependent fashion.
    - Increases GABA synthesis and release.
  - Binds to voltage-activated calcium channels.
  - Inhibits voltage-gated sodium channels.
  - Appears to have neuroprotective properties by inhibiting glutamate either by
    - Activating the glutamate metabolizing enzyme glutamate dehydrogenase, or by
    - Competitive inhibition of glutamaic aminotransferase
  - Reduces release of dopamine, norepinephrine, and serotonin.
- Not protein bound
- Not metabolized
  - Excreted largely unchanged by kidneys.
  - Hepatic impairment does not affect levels.
  - Renal insufficiency leads to drug accumulation.
- Half-life: 5–7 hours
  - Requires tid dosing.
- Saturable transport across blood–brain barrier.
  - Higher doses not always more effective.

Topiramate
- Derivative of fructose
- Cellular actions
  - Sodium channel blockade

- Potentiation of GABA
- Blockade of kainate/AMPA (EAA) receptors
- Inhibits isoenzymes of carbonic anhydrase (CA-II and CA-IV).
  - Related to paresthesias.
  - Renal calculi in 1.5%.
- Half-life: 21 hours
- Protein binding: 13–17%
- Not extensively metabolized
- Renal excretion


### Laboratory Investigations

There is no evidence that routine monitoring predicts serious adverse reactions to anticonvulsants (Morihisa, Rosse, & Cross, 1994; Preskhorn, Burke, & Fast, 1993).

- In studies of laboratory abnormalities in epileptic patients taking various anticonvulsants, the incidence of increased aspartate aminotransferase, alanine aminotransferase, alkaline phosphatase, or gamma glutamyl transpeptidase has ranged from 25–75% (Anderson et al., 1996; Jacobsen, Mosekilde, Myhre-Jensen, & Wildenhoff, 1967; Verma & Haidukewych, 1993; Wall, Baird-Lambert, Buchanan, & Farrell, 1992).
  - These abnormalities are probably related to enzyme induction and have not been associated with clinical or biopsy evidence of hepatocellular damage (Callaghan, Majeed, O'Connell, & Oliveira, 1994; Wall et al., 1992).
  - No evidence that routine liver function tests can identify rare cases of hepatotoxicity with either medication (see side effects, pp. 341–342).
- It may be reasonable to obtain baseline studies to identify risk factors such as preexisting neutropenia, thrombocytopenia, or abnormal liver function.
  - Additional routine laboratory monitoring is unnecessary in the absence of signs and symptoms of drug toxicity or conditions that increase the risk of adverse reactions (Pellock & Willmore, 1991), such as
    - Baseline abnormalities
    - Neurodegenerative disease
    - History of significant adverse drug reactions
  - Obtain appropriate laboratory tests for patients who develop signs or symptoms of bone marrow or liver toxicity, such as bruising,

bleeding, rash, abdominal pain, vomiting, jaundice, or lethargy (Schoeneberger, Tanasijevic, Jha, & Bates, 1995).

- Risk of agranulocytosis with carbamazepine is about 2/525,000.
  - Baseline CBC does not identify patients at risk.
  - Routine CBCs are not effective in early detection of agranulocytosis
    - An idiosyncratic and unpredictable condition
  - More effective to obtain CBC if patient develops clinical evidence of bone marrow suppression.

## DOSES

Table 6.2 summarizes the dosing parameters of anticonvulsant drugs used in the treatment of mania.

Four valproate formulations are available.

- Divalproex sodium (Depakote)
  - Enteric coated
  - Equal amounts valproic acid and sodium valproate
  - Lower risk (50%) of GI side effects than Depakene
  - Twice daily dosing
  - Loading doses of 20 mg/kg of divalproex have been used successfully in acutely manic inpatients.
    - Rapid control of agitation and hyperactivity
    - Decreased length of stay

**Table 6.2  Anticonvulsant Doses for Treating Mania/Hypomania**

| GENERIC NAMES | STARTING DOSES (MG/DAY)* | DAYS TO REACH STEADY STATE LEVEL | USUAL THERAPEUTIC DOSES (MG/DAY) | HIGH/LOW DOSAGE RANGE (MG/DAY) |
|---|---|---|---|---|
| carbamazepine | 50–100 | 4–6 | 600–1800 | 200–3000 |
| clonazepam | 0.5–1 | 5–8 | 2–8 | 0.5–16 |
| gabapentin** | 300 | 1–3 | 600–1800 | 900–3600 |
| lamotrigine | 25 | 4–7 | 100–200*** | 50–500 |
| levetiracetam[†] | 500 | 2 | 1000–2000 | 500–3000 |
| oxcarbazepine | 150–300 | 2–3 | 1200–2400 | 600–3000 |
| topiramate | 50 | 3–5 | 300–400 | 25–1000 |
| valproic acid | 500–1500 | 3–6 | 1000–1500 | 750–5000 |

\* Inpatient starting doses are higher and dosage increase can be faster
\*\* No more effective than placebo in two studies
\*\*\* Lower doses may be needed with divalproex due to VPA increasing lamotrigine levels and higher doses may be needed with carbamazepine because of induction of lamotrigine metabolism.
[†] Doses are for epilepsy; insufficient data on possible doses for mania

- When drug accumulates after discharge, side effects may increase rapidly, and some patients discontinue medication.
- More gradual increase in dose of any mood stabilizer is often better tolerated with more long-term treatment adherence (see p. 258).
- Depakote Sprinkle
  - Capsule can be opened to sprinkle over food.
  - Easier to adjust dose in small increments.
  - Fewer GI side effects.
- Depakote ER
  - Consists of equal amounts free and bound valproic acid and sodium valproate.
  - Once daily dosing
  - May have less weight gain than Depakote.
    - Possibly because of lower blood level peak after each dose, causing GI discomfort that is relieved by eating.
  - Serum levels may be 8–20% lower with Depakote ER than with Depakote.
    - Dose should be about 20% higher than immediate-release Depakote.
  - Little controlled research in mood disorders
- Valproic acid (Depakene capsules)
- Sodium valproate (Depakene capsules and syrup)
- Topiramate
  - Starting dose: 25 mg
  - Increase dose by 25 mg/week to 50–400 mg/day.
  - In open label trials, topiramate has been started at 25–50 mg and titrated in 25–50 mg increments to 150–1300 mg/day (mean daily dose 100–300 mg/day).
    - Slower dosage titration is better tolerated.
    - Doses > 500 mg may not be necessary.

Optimal frequency of dosing
- Carbamazepine: tid
- Valproate: bid (once daily for ER form)
- Lamotrigine: once daily
- Oxcarbazepine: bid
- Topiramate: bid

Children need more frequent dosing and, at times, higher mg/kg doses (not necessarily higher absolute doses) to achieve therapeutic levels.

Managing small-dosage increments or a formulation for patients who cannot swallow pills or when it is difficult to divide pills into small enough doses:

- Mix contents of a capsule or crushed tablet into a tablespoon or more of applesauce, cottage cheese, or oatmeal.
  - Take whatever portion of the food corresponds to the desired dose (e.g., one teaspoon of a one-tablespoon mixture = half the dose of the pill).
- Push a capsule into a piece of banana and blend at slow speed with orange juice concentrate and water.
  - Banana keeps the capsule from breaking.
- Discard the unused portion.

### Plasma level monitoring

- A retrospective analysis of results of a multicenter trial suggested a better response of acute mania at valproate serum levels around 100 mg/dL (Bowden, Brugger, & Swan, 1994). More recent work suggests a higher response rate as the level increases.
  - However, it has not been shown that therapeutic drug monitoring improves the response rate with any anticonvulsant (Preskhorn et al., 1993).
- Usual suggested therapeutic level of carbamazepine in bipolar disorder is 4–12 ng/mL.
  - Many patients have a thymoleptic response at higher or lower levels (Preskhorn et al., 1993).
  - Although neurotoxicity is more likely at carbamazepine levels greater than 25 ng/mL, less severe adverse effects are not correlated with serum level and may appear after months at a stable dose (Preskhorn et al., 1993).
  - Decrease in carbamazepine levels and clinical response is a common manifestation of carbamazepine inducing its own metabolism.
    - Repeated dosage increases may be necessary over months before metabolizing enzymes are saturated.
  - It might be appropriate to measure carbamazepine levels if an initial response fades and autoinduction of metabolism or noncompliance is suspected (Janicak, 1993).
- In a random sample of 330 epileptic inpatients who had 855 AED-level determinations (Schoeneberger et al., 1995), only 27% of levels were obtained for standard indications (apparent toxicity, seizure recurrence, change in dose), and only 51% of these tests were sampled correctly (i.e., steady state trough or 12-hour level). The majority of the AED levels that were drawn without clinical justification were deter-

mined daily, although daily changes in level would not be expected in this setting. Just four of the AED levels were markedly elevated; all of these were drawn too soon after administration of the drug to be valid. Eliminating tests that did not have a clinical indication would have saved $300,000.

- Most appropriate use of anticonvulsant levels:
  - Increase dose gradually until patient has full response.
  - Measure 12-hour level when patient is well.
    - Therapeutic level for that patient
  - If patient deteriorates, compare new level with patient's previously demonstrated therapeutic level.

## CLINICAL INDICATIONS AND USE

### General Information

#### CARBAMAZEPINE

- Effective for
  - Acute nondysphoric mania
  - Rapid cycling
  - Mixed bipolar depression
  - Impulsive and aggressive behavior in brain-damaged patients
  - Psychosis secondary to partial complex seizures
  - Some aspects of benzodiazepine withdrawal
- Possibly effective for
  - Mixed mania
  - Prevention of manic recurrence
  - Prevention of recurrence of depression
- Onset of action 2–3 weeks.
- Patients (N = 94) with at least two bipolar episodes who were currently in remission were randomly assigned to carbamazepine (mean level 6.8 mg/L) or lithium (mean level 0.75 mM) for prophylaxis and were followed for 2 years (Hartong, Moleman, Hoogduin, Broekman, & Nolen, 2003).
  - Carbamazepine was associated with a constant risk of recurrence of about 40%/year.
  - Lithium produced significantly fewer episodes when it was started in a stable patient.
  - When lithium was instituted while patients were in remission, there were almost no recurrences.

- When lithium was started during an acute episode after other mood stabilizers were stopped, it was not as effective in preventing relapse during the first 3 weeks of treatment.

DIVALPROEX

- Effective for
  - Typical mania
  - Mixed mania
  - Prevention of manic recurrence
  - Bipolar disorder with prominent anxiety
  - Panic disorder
  - Agitation in brain-damaged patients

  In the prevention of manic recurrence:

- A 52-week randomized double-blind placebo-controlled study discontinued whatever medications produced remission and then randomized 372 patients, who recovered from an acute episode of mania within 3 months to divalproex, lithium, or placebo (Bowden et al., 2000).
  - There was no difference between divalproex and placebo in the primary outcome measure (i.e., time to recurrence of any mood episode).
  - However, divalproex was superior to placebo in lower rate of discontinuation for depression or mania and superior to lithium in reducing deterioration of depression scores.
  - The lack of effect of divalproex on the primary outcome measure reduces confidence in divalproex as a maintenance treatment.
- In a study supported by the manufacturer, 40 adolescents with a manic, hypomanic, or mixed episode were assigned to open-label divalproex to obtain 12-hour levels of 45–125 μg/mL (mean level 83), for an average of 40 days open-label phase, followed by an 8-week double-blind placebo-controlled phase (Wagner et al., 2002).
  - 10% had lithium added.
  - 53% used other concomitant medications.
  - 23 subjects discontinued the open-label phase and 17 continued to the double-blind phase (mean duration 36 days).
    - 82% discontinued the double-blind phase prematurely, mostly because of loss of efficacy.
  - During the open-label phase, 61% had at least a 50% improvement in mania ratings.
- Possibly effective for
  - Prevention of depressive recurrence
  - Rapid cycling

- In an open 16-week trial in nine patients with active comorbid substance abuse (polysubstances: alcohol and cocaine) and bipolar disorder who had never received valproate, divalproex produced significant reductions in mania and depression rating scale scores and significant decreases in days and amount of substance use (Brady, Sonne, Anton, & Ballenger, 1995).
- Not helpful for acute depression.
- Onset of action is 3–5 days.

### LAMOTRIGINE

- Approved in 2003 for prevention of recurrence of bipolar depression.
- Effective acutely for bipolar depression.
- Not effective for prevention of manic recurrence.
- May be helpful as adjunct in rapid cycling with prominent depression.
- Can be administered in one bedtime dose.
- Doses of 400 mg probably not more effective than 200 mg.
- A 2001 review of three double-blind studies, three open-label studies, and two case series involving 401 bipolar patients treated with lamotrigine found (Zerjav-Lacombe & Tabarsi, 2001):
    - Most patients were nonresponders or partial responders to mood stabilizers.
    - Overall, 50–83% responded to 50–400 mg/day of lamotrigine.
    - Switching to mania was rare in these studies.
- An open trial of lamotrigine or lithium for 1 year in 14 patients with rapid cycling bipolar disorder (Walden, Schaerer, Schloesser, & Grunze, 2000) found that three of seven patients (43%) on lithium had < four episodes and the rest (57%) had four or more episodes; six of seven (86%) of lamotrigine patients had < four episodes, and three of the seven (43%) had no episodes over the year of follow-up.
    - This study is limited by small N, lack of statistical significance, absence of placebo, and possibility that patients with worse illnesses were assigned to lithium.
- A complicated study began with the open-label addition of lamotrigine to ongoing treatment and titrated to response in 324 patients with rapid cycling bipolar disorder (Calabrese et al., 2000).
    - Stabilized patients were tapered off other medications and randomly assigned to lamotrigine or placebo monotherapy for 6 months.
    - Of the 324 patients who received open-label lamotrigine, 182 entered the double-blind phase (i.e., only 56% responded acutely to open treatment).

- There was no difference between lamotrigine and placebo in the primary outcome measure (i.e., time to additional pharmacotherapy).
- However, the secondary efficacy measure (i.e., time to premature discontinuation) was 41% of lamotrigine vs. 26% of placebo patients remaining in the study over the 6 months without relapse.
    - The finding that the primary measure did not show a difference makes this outcome less impressive.
- Adults with a DSM-IV current or recent manic or hypomanic episode who had a past history of at least one manic/hypomanic and one depressive episode were either started on or switched from other medications to lamotrigine, with a 6-week titration to a target dose of 200 mg/day (Bowden et al., 2003).
    - Patients who responded to 8–16 weeks of open-label treatment with lamotrigine were randomized to double-blind treatment with lamotrigine (this time with a dose of 100–400 mg), lithium titrated to a serum level of 0.8–1.1 mM, or placebo and were followed for up to 18 months.
    - Of 349 patients who began open-label treatment, 175 were sufficiently stable to be randomized (i.e., about half the patients deteriorated or dropped out during acute open treatment with lamotrigine).
    - Lamotrigine and lithium were equivalently better in terms of statistical significance than placebo in lengthening the time until treatment had to be changed to manage an affective recurrence.
        - Lamotrigine but not lithium was significantly better than placebo in prolonging the time to recurrence of depression, whereas lithium but not lamotrigine was significantly better than placebo in prolonging the time to a manic, hypomanic, or mixed episode.
        - 400 mg lamotrigine was no better than 200 mg.
    - Findings suggest that lamotrigine is better for bipolar depression than for mania or hypomania.
    - Lamotrigine usually should be combined with lithium or another established mood stabilizer that has antimanic properties.

## OXCARBAZEPINE

- No placebo-controlled studies in bipolar disorder
- Review of charts of 13 outpatients treated with oxcarbazepine for refractory bipolar disorder found mild improvement in six patients (46%) and moderate improvement in two patients (16%; Ghaemi, Ko, & Katzow, 2002).
- In an open study, 12 manic patients received oxcarbazepine for 14 days; it was then withdrawn for 7 days, then reinstituted for 2 weeks (Hummel et al., 2002).

- The final dose of oxcarbazepine was 900–2100 mg/day.
- Mean YMRS scores were lower in the on- than in the off-oxcarbazepine periods, and one-third of patients had at least a 50% reduction in YMRS scores.
    - But 50% of patients were withdrawn early from the study.
- Two older open 2-week studies found oxcarbazepine to be equivalent to haloperidol and lithium in treating acute mania.
- Many clinicians feel that oxcarbazepine is equivalent to carbamazepine in bipolar disorder, but no formal comparisons have been conducted.
- Usual dose in bipolar disorder is probably around 1800–3000 mg/day.

GABAPENTIN

- Effective for anxiety and depression.
- Probably useful
    - In chronic pain
    - Augmenting antidepressant in unipolar depression
- In an open trial, 43 patients with bipolar disorder with depression, mixed states, or mania who were resistant to standard mood stabilizers (persistent symptoms for at least 6 months, causing clinically significant distress or impairment) received adjunctive gabapentin (mean dose 1272 mg, range 600–2400) for 8 weeks (Perugi et al., 2002).
    - 18 patients (42%) were responders (CGI score of 2, or moderate improvement).
    - Mean HRSD scores improved significantly, whereas mean YMRS scales did not show significant reduction.
    - Of the 18 patients who improved, 17 maintained improvement of depression for 4–18 months.
    - The presence of panic disorder and alcohol abuse were significant predictors of response to addition of gabapentin.
- In a 12-week open trial of gabapentin (mean dose 1725 mg/day) added to mood stabilizers or atypical antipsychotics in 22 bipolar patients with a depressive episode that had lasted an average of 18 weeks, HRSD scores decreased 53%, with 55% having moderate or marked improvement (HRSD decreased 78%; Wang et al., 2002).
- However, a double-blind controlled study found gabapentin < placebo for mania, and gabapentin = placebo for bipolar depression (Pande, Crockatt, Janney, Werth, & Tsaroucha, 2000).
- Similarly, a double-blind 6-week study in refractory bipolar disorder found lamotrigine > gabapentin = placebo (Frye et al., 2000).
- Double-blind randomized assignment to lamotrigine, gabapentin, or placebo monotherapy with crossover to the other agents involved

35 patients with refractory bipolar disorder and 10 with refractory unipolar depression (Obrocea et al., 2002).

- Response, defined as much or very much improved on CGI, was 51% for lamotrigine, 28% for gabapentin, and 21% for placebo.
- Lamotrigine was most likely to produce response in male patients with fewer medication trials, but the N was small and the patients heterogeneous.

## TOPIRAMATE

- Open-label trials suggest efficacy of topiramate as adjunctive treatment for mania, bipolar depression, and rapid cycling (Suppes, 2002).
  - Most of these studies show a trend only.
- No positive controlled studies in the treatment of bipolar disorder.
  - Helpful for some patients, whereas others experience mania induction.
  - In four open-label trials, 46% of 92 patients had significant improvement of CGI or YMRS on topiramate (Suppes, 2002).
  - Topiramate 25–200 mg/day was added openly for 10 days to mood stabilizers in 11 moderately manic patients (Grunze et al., 2001).
    - After 1 week, seven patients had > 50% decrease in YMRS.
    - Symptoms worsened when topiramate was withdrawn and improved again when it was reinstituted.
  - Open-label topiramate monotherapy was given to 10 hospitalized manic patients for up to 28 days (Calabrese, Keck, McElroy, & Shelton, 2001).
    - Mean YMRS score decreased from 32 to 22.
    - Three patients had at least 50% reduction.
    - Results were interpreted as suggesting an antimanic effect, but only a minority of patients responded and, on average, patients were still manic.
  - Absence of placebo limits interpretation of results.
- Topriamate seems most useful when combined with other mood stabilizers.
- A prospective double-blind placebo-controlled 21-day study of bipolar I inpatients compared 512 mg/day of topiramate, 256 mg/day, and placebo (Suppes, 2002). A high placebo response resulted in no difference between groups in intent-to-treat analysis.
- An open study randomly assigned 36 outpatients with bipolar depression (bipolar I or II) to topiramate (mean dose 176 mg/day) or bupropion SR (mean dose 250 mg/day) for 8 weeks (McIntyre et al., 2002).
  - Thirteen patients discontinued the study, most for adverse effects.

- The percentage demonstrating a 50% or greater reduction in HDRS scores were equivalent (56% and 59%, respectively).
    - There were no affective switches over the short study.
  - These results support an antidepressant action of topiramate, which could be complicated during long-term treatment of bipolar disorder.
- Topiramate 100–400 mg/day was added as adjunct for 6 months to lithium, carbamazepine, or valproate taken by 34 patients, 11 with depression, 17 with mania, 3 with hypomania, and 3 with mixed symptoms (Vieta, Torrent, Garcia-Ribas, & Gilabert, 2002).
  - 59% of the manic patients had 50% improvement of YMRS scores.
  - 55% of depressed patients had 50% improvement in HRSD scores.
  - 15 patients relapsed during treatment.
  - 9 patients did not complete the study.
- A randomized controlled trial of two doses of topiramate (256 and 512 mg/day) in 97 patients found no significant difference between either dose or placebo in YMRS scales.
  - GAS scores did improve significantly more with 512 mg topiramate than with 256 mg or placebo (Yatham et al., 2002).
- May be more effective for PTSD and anxiety.
- Effective as migraine prophylaxis.
- Effective for bulimia (see pp. 131–132).
- Often used to treat weight gain caused by mood stabilizers.
  - Topiramate (mean dose 135 mg/day) given to patients who had gained a mean of 13 kg on SSRIs resulted in an average loss of 4.2 kg (Van Ameringen, Mancini, Pipe, Campbell, & Oakman, 2002).
  - Similar weight loss over 1 year in bipolar patients who had gained weight on antimanic drugs.
- High rate of drug discontinuation because of adverse effects.
  - Cognitive dysfunction (most common side effect)
  - Sedation
  - Paresthesias
  - Kidney stones

## ZONISAMIDE

- Open-label trial in bipolar disorder positive, but controlled study was negative.
- An open-label study of 24 patients with mania or excited schizophrenia (N = 3) found moderate–marked improvement after 4–5 weeks with 100–600 mg of zonisamide (Kanba, Yagi, & Kamijima, 1994).
- A controlled study in bipolar disorder was negative.

- Promotes weight loss in bipolar patients without exacerbating symptoms.
- In a 16-week randomized double-blind placebo-controlled trial of zonisamide (mean dose 427 mg) in 51 of 60 moderately obese nonpsychiatric patients followed by 16-week single-blind extension (Gadde et al., 2003):
    - All received dietary counseling.
    - In the double-blind phase, the zonisamide group lost 5.9 kg, vs. 0.9 kg for the placebo group ($p < 0.001$).
    - Considering just the patients who completed this phase, zonisamide patients lost 6.4 kg and placebo patients lost 1.1 kg ($p < 0.001$).
    - 10/19 zonisamide patients and none of 17 placebo patients had lost at least 10% of their body weight by week 32 ($p < 0.001$).
- Most common side effect: cognitive dysfunction.

## LEVETIRACETAM

- S-enantiomer derivative of pyrrolidine acetamide
    - R-enantiomer inactive
- Anticonvulsant that blocks N-type calcium channels
- No P450 effects
- Usual antiepileptic dose 2000–4000 mg/day
- In 10 acutely manic inpatients receiving levetiracetam added to haloperidol (5–10 mg/day; Grunze, Langosch, Born, Schaub, & Walden, 2003):
    - Levetiracetam started at 500 mg bid.
    - Increased to mean dose 3125 mg/day, given bid.
    - After 2 weeks on levetiracetam, anticonvulsant was abruptly withdrawn.
    - Patients were off levetiracetam from days 14–21.
    - Levetiracetam reintroduced from days 21–28.
    - Mean YMRS scores had decreased from 29.6 to 17.2 by day 14.
    - Mean YMRS increased to 20.9 during "off" days (14–21).
    - Mean YMRS decreased to 14.7 by end of second "on" phase.
- No controlled studies

## TIAGABINE

- Approved for partial epilepsy
- In an open trial, 17 patients with refractory bipolar disorder in the Stanley Foundation Bipolar Network were given open-label addition of tiagabine to ongoing antimanic drugs (Suppes et al., 2002).
    - Four patients dropped out after the first visit.
    - The remaining 13 took an average of 8.7 mg/day of tiagabine for a mean of 38 days.

- No patient was able to continue the medication for > 9 months.
- On the CGI Scale for Bipolar Disorder, 3 patients were much or very much improved and 10 (77%) were unchanged or worse.
  - The medication was of no real benefit.
- Three patients had seizures as a tiagabine side effect.

### Bipolar Disorder in Children

- A 6–8-week study in 42 outpatient children and adolescents (mean age 11) with manic or mixed episodes randomly assigned patients to open treatment with lithium, divalproex, or carbamazepine (Kowatch et al., 2000).
  - Response rates (at least 50% improvement of YMRS and CGI improvement scores) were
    - 53% with divalproex
    - 38% with lithium
    - 38% for carbamazepine (nonsignificant differences)
    - Effect sizes were 1.63, 1.06, and 1.00, respectively, all of which indicate major effects.
    - Of the original sample of 42, 35 continued in an open trial for another 16–18 weeks; 30 of these patients (85%) were responders at the end of the continuation phase, and 37% were on just one mood stabilizer and no other medications.

### Refractory Bipolar Disorder

Anticonvulsants may be more effective than lithium for
- Mixed and psychotic mania
- Rapid and ultradian cycling
- Head injury
- Nonspecific EEG abnormalities
- Bipolar disorder with comorbid substance dependence

Patients who do not respond to lithium can have an anticonvulsant added. If patient responds, an attempt can be made to withdraw lithium very slowly. Reinstitute previous lithium dose if symptoms worsen
- Because the illness is physiologically more complex, many patients with refractory bipolar disorder require combinations of medications, including
  - Lithium
  - One or more anticonvulsant
  - Antipsychotic medication, especially clozapine

- Lithium and carbamazepine may have additive neurotoxicity.
  - Worsened by concomitant use of antipsychotics.
- Valproate has fewer interactions with both carbamazepine and lithium.
  - Carbamazepine lowers valproate levels.
  - Valproate increases carbamazepine levels.

## Initiating and Discontinuing Therapy

Slow initiation of treatment with anticonvulsants is better tolerated and less likely to result in more rapid control of mixed mania/hypomania than depression, resulting in treatment-emergent lethargy or depression.

- Whenever possible, anticonvulsants should be withdrawn slowly.
  - Withdrawal seizures may occur in nonepileptic patients when chronic anticonvulsant therapy is discontinued rapidly.

### VALPROIC ACID

- Divalproex is preferred preparation because of fewer GI side effects.
- Improvement usually begins within 4–14 days.
- Faster improvement of mania occurs with rapid oral loading.
  - Start at 20 mg/kg in divided dose.
  - Manic patients can be discharged sooner.
  - Eventual drug accumulation may result in side effects after patient is discharged.
    - Causes outpatient noncompliance.
- Slower rate of increase in inpatients may lead to better long-term treatment adherence.
  - Start with 250 mg tid or 10–15 mg/kg.
  - Increase by 250 mg every 3–4 days.
  - Give tid until patient stable, then switch to bid dosing.
  - Obtain serum level 3–4 days after dosage adjustment.
    - Aim for 12-hour level around 100 μg/mL.
  - Treat agitation, hyperactivity or severe insomnia with adjunctive antipsychotic or benzodiazepine.
- In outpatients
  - Start with 62.5–125 mg hs.
  - Increase bedtime dose to 250–500 mg.
  - Then add small daytime dose.
  - Increase total dose slowly to reduce risk of limiting side effects and adverse effects on mood (see p. 258).

- When patient stable, it may be possible to switch to ER formulation and cautiously increase dose.
  - Since smallest ER dose is 250 mg, slow titration with small dosage increments is not possible.
- Early side effects are less bothersome with slower dosage increase.
  - GI (nausea, diarrhea)
  - Sedation
  - Tremor
  - Increased appetite

### CARBAMAZEPINE

- Improvement somewhat slower than with divalproex, probably because sedation is less marked.
- Carbamazepine is generally given bid and hs to reduce side effects and maintain therapeutic level when autoinduction of metabolism occurs.
- For inpatients with severe mania
  - Start with 200 mg bid or tid.
  - Increase dose by 100–200 mg/day q 3–4 days to 800–1000 mg/day.
  - Then increase dose more slowly until patient stable.
- For outpatients
  - Begin with 50–100 mg hs.
    - Elixir and chewable tablet permit slow dosage titration.
  - Increase dose by 50–100 mg q 1–2 weeks to 200 mg hs, then start adding daytime doses.
  - Initial improvement followed by decreased benefit suggests auto-induction of metabolism.
    - If no adverse effects, continue to increase dose.
- Carbamazepine also can be used to
  - Augment antidepressants in unipolar depression.
  - Treat PTSD.
- Common early side effects are more likely to occur with rapid dosage increase:
  - Ataxia
  - Diplopia
  - Dizziness
  - Blurred vision
  - Drowsiness
  - Confusion
- Obtain baseline CBC and reconsider administering carbamazepine to patients with significantly low white or red cell count.

- Subsequent routine CBCs will not reliably identify rare cases of bone marrow suppression.
- Routine LFTs not useful in preventing hepatotoxicity.
- If small mild rash occurs (10%), stopping medication and restarting a few weeks later or simply continuing medication results in resolution of rash in about 50%.
  - Discontinue carbamazepine for more extensive or severe rash.
- Do not combine with clozapine.

## GABAPENTIN

- In absence of controlled data demonstrating efficacy in bipolar disorder, gabapentin is not a first-line treatment.
- Most appropriately used for major depression, anxiety, neuropathic pain.
- Antidepressant effect may be helpful or troublesome in bipolar disorder.
- Usually prescribed for outpatients.
- Begin with 50–100 mg hs.
- Increase dose by 50–100 mg q 3–7 days.
- Give tid.
- Target dose probably 900–3600 mg/day.
  - Higher doses are not transported as efficiently into brain.

## LAMOTRIGINE

- Since lamotrigine is more effective for depression than mania, it is usually combined with other mood stabilizers for patients with persistent bipolar depression.
- Not recommended for bipolar disorder in patients < 16.
  - An epilepsy study in children found lamotrigine to be well tolerated.
  - No bipolar data.
- Risk of serious rash (Stevens–Johnson syndrome or toxic epidermal necrolysis) about 0.1%.
  - Risk appears to be much lower with slow dosage titration.
  - Manufacturer recommends increasing dose by no more than 25 mg/week.
  - Rate of dosage increase of 50 mg/week in 350 patients was not associated with increased risk of rash, but N may have been too small to detect increased risk (Bowden et al., 2003).
- Need for slow dosage increase makes lamotrigine most appropriate for outpatients.
- Usual dose is 25–200 mg/day.
  - Dose of 400 mg was no more effective than 200 mg in trial mentioned above.

- Lamotrigine can be given in one daily dose.
  - Sedative side effect better tolerated in hs dose.
- Start with 12.5–25 mg hs.
- Increase dose by 12.5–25 mg q 1–2 weeks.
  - Slower, if patient becomes activated or develops adverse physical effects.
- More aggressive dosing recommended when lamotrigine combined with enzyme-inducing antiepileptic drugs such as carbamazepine.
  - Increase once a week by 50 mg for 4 weeks.
  - Then increase by 100 mg.
  - Give bid.
  - However, rapid dosage increase not always well tolerated, and once daily dosing is often possible.
- More cautious dosing recommended when lamotrigine is combined with divalproex.
  - Start with 12.5 mg/day for 2 weeks.
  - Then increase by 25 mg/week.

OXCARBAZEPINE

- Only two small 2-week trials in mania
  - Equivalent to lithium and to haloperidol
  - No placebo-controlled trials
- Although a derivative of carbamazepine, the two medications do not always have the same spectra of action.
- Inform patients of limited scientific data before starting medication.
- Oxcarbazepine should be given bid.
- Inpatient dosing:
  - Start with 150 mg bid.
  - Increase dose by 150–300 mg q 3–5 days.
- Outpatient dosing:
  - Start with 75–150 mg hs.
  - Increase dose by 75 mg/week.
- Target dose probably is 1800–3000 mg/day.
- If patient develops nervousness, twitching, or confusion, obtain serum sodium determination.
  - Hyponatremia occurs in 2.5%.
  - Mild hyponatremia may be corrected in compliant patient with water restriction.
  - Lithium may counteract SIADH caused by oxcarbazepine or carbamazepine.

TOPIRAMATE

- Start with 25 mg.
- Increase dose by 25–50 mg/week.
- Give bid.
- Monitor for cognitive impairment.
- Consider nephrolithiasis if patient develops dysuria or abdominal pain.

## Benzodiazepines in Bipolar Disorder

Most benzodiazepines can be useful in the treatment of mania.
- Lorazepam and clonazepam are used most frequently.
- Antidepressant effect and short duration of action of alprazolam make it a poor choice.
- Useful for agitation, hyperactivity, and insomnia.
- No specific mood-stabilizing effect separate from improving sleep.
- Usually used adjunctively
  - Combined with antimanic and/or antipsychotic drug.
  - Occasionally used as initial monotherapy to reduce hyperactivity sufficiently for patient to comply with more specific treatments.
- Doses vary with severity of symptoms.
  - Acute mania
    - 1–6 mg/day lorazepam
    - 1–3 mg clonazepam
  - Hypomania or anxiety associated with mood instability
    - 0.5–4 mg/day lorazepam
    - 0.25–2 mg/day clonazepam
- Clonazepam and lorazepam are frequently used as adjuncts or substitutes for antipsychotic drugs in the treatment of mania.
  - Reduction of insomnia can improve the mood disorder.
- In a typical double-blind crossover design of 10 days of each drug in acutely manic patients admitted from the emergency room, clonazepam was significantly more effective than lithium in rapidly reducing mania (Chouinard, Young, & Annable, 1983).
  - More rapid onset of improvement in agitation and related symptoms
- A case series of 20 patients who received addition of clonazepam to lithium demonstrated that clonazepam could replace antipsychotics (Sachs, Rosenbaum, & Jones, 1990).
- Chronic use of benzodiazepines in bipolar disorder may aggravate depression.

### Calcium Channel-Blocking Agents (CCBs)

Mania and bipolar depression are both associated with increased free intracellular calcium ion concentration in peripheral cells such as platelets and lymphocytes.

- Lithium, valproate, and carbamazepine have been found to reduce hyperactive intracellular calcium signaling in bipolar patients but not controls (Dubovsky, Lee, & Christiano, 1991).
- Verapamil was superior to placebo in about 30 small controlled studies and case series and negative in three (Dubovsky & Buzan, 1997).
  - Negative trials lasted less than 2 weeks and/or used inadequate dosing schedules of verapamil.
- Nimodipine was superior to placebo and similar to lithium in an 18-month on/off study (Manna, 1991) and was effective in open and controlled trials alone and as an adjunct in refractory ultradian cycling (Pazzaglia, Post, Ketter, George, & Marangell, 1993).
- Verapamil (phenylalkylamine) and nimodipine (1,2-dihydropyridine) bind to different calcium antagonist binding sites in the brain and may have different spectra of action.
- Consider verapamil for
  - Typical mania
  - Lithium-responsive bipolar disorder in patients who cannot tolerate lithium
  - Bipolar disorder associated with dementia or head injury
    - Verapamil less likely to cause cognitive impairment than other mood stabilizers.
  - Bipolar disorder in patient with medical condition that may be improved by verapamil.
    - Hypertension
    - Supraventricular tachycardia
    - Migraine headache
    - Tardive dyskinesia
    - Achalasia
    - Raynaud's disease
  - Bipolar illness during pregnancy
    - Verapamil used to treat premature labor and fetal and maternal arrhythmias (Byerly, Hartmann, Foster, & Tannenbaum, 1991).
    - Verapamil was effective for bipolar disorder in 32 pregnant patients and was not associated with any fetal anomalies (Wisner et al., 2002).

- Consider nimodipine for
  - Inability to tolerate other mood stabilizers
  - Problematic medication interactions
  - Refractory ultradian cycling (as an add-on treatment)
  - Bipolar disorder in demented patients
  - Partial response to existing mood stabilizers
  - Not a practical treatment for mania that requires urgent intervention because of dosing schedule and slow onset of action.
- Use of verapamil
  - Onset of action in mania similar to lithium (2–4 weeks).
  - Lack of sedation may require addition of benzodiazepine or antipsychotic drug initially.
  - Extensive first-pass metabolism requires high doses.
  - Elimination half-life of 5 hours requires qid dosing.
    - In chronic therapy, half-life increases to 8 hours, and tid dosing may be effective.
  - Sustained-release preparations used to treat hypertension are not as reliably effective in mood disorders as immediate-release verapamil.
  - Dosing in mania:
    - Start with 40 mg qid.
    - Increase by 40–160 mg q 2–4 days.
    - Target dose is 120 mg qid.
  - Outpatient dosing:
    - Start with 40 mg.
    - Add additional 40 mg doses q 4–7 days.
    - Target dose is 240–480 mg/day.
    - May be possible to switch from qid to tid schedule after several months.
- Use of nimodipine
  - Very short half-life (~3 hours) requires very frequent dosing.
  - Usual dose is 180–720 mg/day (360 mg is maximum labeled dose).
  - Multiple pills are necessary because only 30 mg tablets are available.
  - Start with 30 mg.
  - Add 30 mg doses q 2–7 days to 180 mg/day total dose.
  - If necessary, increase dose further by 30 mg/week.

### Antipsychotic Drugs

NEUROLEPTICS

Neuroleptics are rapidly effective for reducing hyperactivity, insomnia, agitation, and psychosis.

- Have questionable efficacy as mood stabilizers.
- Haloperidol is reference antimanic drug in many clinical trials.
  - Doses > 10 mg/day are not more effective than lower doses but have more side effects.
  - May be augmented with benzodiazepine to reduce neuroleptic dose.
- At least two-thirds of manic patients continue neuroleptics a year after discharge (Sernyak, Godleski, Griffin, Mazure, & Woods, 1997).
  - In many cases, doses have been increased over time.
    - Suggests incomplete response to mood stabilizers.
- 37 patients with psychotic or nonpsychotic manic episode treated openly with perphenazine 4–64 mg + mood stabilizer (Zarate & Tohen, 2004):
  - Patients in remission after 10 weeks were randomly assigned to mood stabilizer + placebo (N = 19) or mood stabilizer + continued neuroleptic at same dose (N = 18).
  - Patients continuing neuroleptic had significantly
    - Shorter time to discontinuation of medication
    - Shorter time to depressive relapse
    - More dysphoria and parkinsonism
    - More depressive symptoms
- Although some patients with very unstable mood disorders benefit from chronic neuroleptic therapy, the efficacy of these medications as maintenance treatments has not been demonstrated scientifically.

ATYPICAL ANTIPSYCHOTICS

All atypicals are effective for mania. For example:

- Olanzapine manufacturer-sponsored monotherapy trials
  - 139 patients with pure or mixed mania were randomized to placebo or olanzapine starting at 10 mg and increased to 20 mg for 3 weeks (Tohen et al., 1999).
    - Olanzapine produced significantly greater reduction in Young Mania Rating Scale (YMRS) scores, with a difference in response rates of 25%.
    - In the 3-week trial, olanzapine reduced YMRS scores > placebo (14 vs. 4 points) in a subset of manic patients with a past history of rapid cycling (Sanger et al., 2003).
  - In a random assignment of 110 patients with pure or mixed mania for 4 weeks to placebo or olanzapine starting with 15 mg and increased to 20 mg (Tohen et al., 2000)
    - Significantly greater YMRS reductions occurred with olanzapine (22% > placebo).

- Olanzapine comparisons with divalproex
  - In a 3-week randomized trial in 248 manic patients, olanzapine produced a greater decrease in YMRS scores than divalproex, with 47% achieving remission on olanzapine vs. 34% with divalproex (Tohen et al., 2002a).
  - A randomized 12-week double-blind comparison of olanzapine and divalproex in 120 acutely manic patients followed patients in the hospital for 3 weeks and then as outpatients (Zajecka et al., 2002).
    - Mean Mania Rating Scale (MRS) scores decreased by 15 points with divalproex and 17 with olanzapine ($p = $ NS).
    - More patients treated with olanzapine experienced somnolence, weight gain (mean body weight increased 4 kg with olanzapine), edema, rhinitis, and slurred speech; no adverse events were more frequent with divalproex. Both drugs therefore were equally effective but divalproex was better tolerated.
- Olanzapine combination trials
  - A multicenter double-blind trial of 344 patients with a manic or mixed episode with or without psychosis who had had an inadequate response to monotherapy for 2 weeks with either lithium (serum level 0.6–1.2 mM) or valproate (serum level 50–125 μg/mL) maintained patients on therapeutic levels of lithium or valproate and randomized patients to 6 weeks of either olanzapine (5–20 mg/day) or placebo added to the antimanic drug (Tohen et al., 2002c).
    - Olanzapine addition group had decrease of YMRS scores of 13.1 points (59%) vs. 9.1 points (40.1%) with placebo addition (i.e., continued monotherapy).
    - Items that showed significantly better improvement with olanzapine than placebo included irritability, speech, thought disorder, and disruptive/aggressive behavior (but not necessarily elevated mood or increased energy).
    - Difference in remission rates (defined as YMRS ≤ 12) was significant (79% for olanzapine vs. 66% for placebo).
    - Olanzapine was significantly better than placebo in patients without psychosis but not for those with psychotic features.
    - Significantly more weight gain occurred with olanzapine addition than placebo (3.1 pounds).
- Olanzapine continuation trials
  - 114 patients who completed an acute mania trial on olanzapine were continued openly on olanzapine for 49 weeks (Sanger et al., 2001).
    - Only 41% were treated with olanzapine alone; the rest received lithium, which was added on the first open-label visit in 44%.
    - One-third of patients also received fluoxetine at some point.

- Only 40% of patients completed the study.
- YMRS scores improved from 25 to 7, and HDRS scores decreased from 12 to 5.

- In an industry-sponsored multicenter study of 543 patients with bipolar I manic or mixed episode (Tohen, 2003):
  - Open-label olanzapine + lithium for 6 weeks
  - 431 patients had YMRS ≤ 12 and HRSD ≤ 8.
  - "Remitted" patients were randomized to olanzapine 5–20 mg/day or lithium 0.6–1.2 mM for 52 weeks.
  - Olanzapine patients significantly better than lithium for (1) completing trial (47% vs. 33%) and (2) manic relapse (14% vs. 28%).
  - Equal rates of relapse to affective episode (30% and 39%) and relapse into depressive episode (16% and 15%).
  - Significantly more weight gain occurred with olanzapine (1.8 kg vs. −1.4 kg).
  - Low rate of relapse in both groups suggests that a good prognosis group was studied.

- Risperidone monotherapy trials
  - Manic patients (N = 15 per arm) were randomized for 4 weeks to 10 mg of haloperidol, 6 mg of risperidone, or 900–1200 mg of lithium (Segal, Berk, & Brook, 1998).
    - All groups had similar rates of improvement, but the total N was too small to detect a difference, and there was no placebo group.
  - In a randomized multisite double-blind 6-week trial of risperidone up to 10 mg/day vs. haloperidol up to 20 mg day in 29 patients with schizoaffective disorder—depressed and 33 with schizoaffective disorder—bipolar type, both drugs worked equally well for psychotic and manic symptoms (Janicak et al., 2001).
    - Risperidone also produced at least a 50% mean reduction of depressive symptoms in 75% of 16 patients with more severe depressive symptoms, vs. 38% of 21 patients with more severe depressive symptoms receiving haloperidol.

- Risperidone combination trials
  - Risperidone or placebo was added for 3 weeks to lithium, divalproex, or carbamazepine, which had been taken for at least 2 weeks by 151 patients with a manic or mixed episode (Yatham, Grossman, Augustyns, Vieta, & Ravindran, 2003).
    - There was at least a 50% reduction in YMRS scores in 59% of risperidone patients versus 41% of placebo patients (p < 0.05)
  - A total of 541 additional bipolar or schizoaffective patients have been studied in open-label add-on studies of risperidone for up to 6 months (Vieta, Goikolea, & Corbella, 2001).

- Risperidone was associated with improvement in manic and depressive symptoms
- Quetiapine
  - Quetiapine had antimanic effects in two placebo-controlled trials involving > 500 patients (mean dose about 550 mg).
  - In a prospective open-label investigation of addition of quetiapine to ongoing mood stabilizers for 112 days in 14 patients with rapid cycling bipolar disorder (Vieta et al., 2002)
    - Quetiapine dose gradually reduced from 443 to 268 mg/day.
    - Quetiapine addition resulted in significant reduction in severity of illness and mania scores.
    - Depressive symptoms did not change significantly.
  - In two 12-week randomized double-blind controlled studies in 604 manic patients, quetiapine (mean dose 576/day) was significantly better than placebo (Jones, 2003) for
    - Completion of study: 61% vs. 39%
    - Reduction in YMRS: 14 vs. 8 points
    - Response (≥ 50% YMRS reduction): 48% vs. 31%
  - Quetiapine was studied as an adjunct to valproate in 30 bipolar I adolescents (ages 12–18) with a manic or mixed episode (DelBello, Schwiers, Rosenberg, & Strakowski, 2002).
    - All patients received valproate 20 mg/kg.
    - On the same day that valproate was started, patients were randomly assigned for 6 weeks to addition of placebo or quetiapine 450 mg/day.
    - All patients had a decrease in YMRS scores, but the decrease was significantly (if not dramatically) greater in the valproate + quetiapine group (from 31–15 in placebo group; from 34–11 in quetiapine group).
    - Response rate was significantly greater with addition of quetiapine vs. placebo (87% vs. 53%).
- Ziprasidone
  - A 3-week controlled trial in 197 manic patients found that ziprasidone produced significantly greater improvement than placebo beginning on the second day (Keck & Ice, 2000).
  - In another multicenter 3-week placebo-controlled trial in 210 inpatients with a manic or mixed episode, 75/140 patients assigned to ziprasidone and 31/70 assigned to placebo completed the trial (Keck et al., 2003).
    - Mean ziprasidone dose was 130–139 mg/day.
    - Statistically significant difference between ziprasidone and placebo emerged at day 2 and continued throughout the trial.

- Average decrease in MRS score was 7.8 for placebo and 12.4 for ziprasidone ($p < 0.001$).
- Significantly more patients had response ($\geq$ 50% decrease in MRS score) to ziprasidone than placebo (50% vs. 35%).
  - However, ziprasidone can be too activating for some bipolar patients.
    - Induced mania in four bipolar patients (Baldassano et al., 2003).
- Aripiprazole
  - In a 12-week randomized double-blind study of 347 patients with mania or mixed episode, aripiprazole 15 mg/day was compared to haloperidol 10 mg/day (Bourin, 2003).
    - Aripiprazole significantly better than haloperidol for response rates (50% vs. 28%) and continuing medication (51% vs. 29%).
    - More EPS seen with haloperidol (36% vs. 9%).
    - Neither medication caused weight gain.
    - No placebo
- Clozapine most effective as adjunct in severely refractory bipolar disorder.
  - Clozapine vs. no clozapine added to usual treatment in refractory bipolar or schizomanic disorder (Suppes et al., 1999)
    - Patients already taking mean of four drugs.
    - 82% vs. 57% had 30% improvement at 6 months
    - More potent for mania and cycling than depression
    - Mean dose 355 mg/day

Use of antipsychotic drugs in bipolar disorder

- Acutely manic hospitalized patients can be treated initially with any antipsychotic, with or without a benzodiazepine.
  - Atypical antipsychotic is first choice
- Mood stabilizer can be started as agitation decreases.
- Use of atypical antipsychotics as primary mood stabilizers is not established.
  - May be effective as adjunctive treatment for refractory mood cycling and depression.
  - Antidepressant effects of atypicals other than clozapine sometimes destabilize mood.
    - In post-hoc analysis of two 3-week double-blind trials of olanzapine vs. placebo in mania (Baker, Milton, Stauffer, Gelenberg, & Tohen, 2003), (1) worsening of mania scores in 22% on olanzapine, 38% on placebo; (2) trial not designed to identify exacerbation of mania; (3) mood cycling and hypomania not identified; and (4) trials were too brief to be reassuring.

- All atypicals except clozapine have been found occasionally to induce mania with long-term use.

## ECT

- Most effective treatment for mania
  - May induce remission with a small number of treatments.
- Conventional wisdom that bilateral is more effective than unilateral ECT in mania may reflect poor electrode placement.
  - In studies of bilateral ECT, shunting of current through scalp.
- Lower stimulus intensity may be necessary for bipolar than for unipolar mood disorders.
- May be effective for refractory mood cycling.
  - 20 or more treatments may be necessary.
- Consider as early treatment for
  - Mania or other severe bipolar symptoms during pregnancy
  - Life-threatening bipolar disorder
  - Catatonia
  - Inability to tolerate medications
- Most medications should be withheld during ECT.
  - Increased risk of lithium neurotoxicity because of increased entry of lithium into brain with disruption of blood–brain barrier by ECT.
  - Anticonvulsants can inhibit response to ECT by raising seizure threshold.
  - Antipsychotics do not have important interactions with ECT.

Figure 6.1 illustrates a standard treatment protocol for various mania syndromes.

### Combining Anticonvulsants with Each Other and with Other Mood Stabilizers

Like many forms of cancer, bipolar disorder is a progressive illness that becomes more complex with time if it is not well controlled initially. Whereas mania and uncomplicated bipolar depression often can be treated or prevented with a simple regimen, rapid and ultradian cycling and chronic mixed states have complex physiology that rarely responds to a single mood stabilizer. If a combination of two medications is not effective, a third one may have to be added.

- Lithium + valproate
  - May be superior to either alone in preventing relapse of mania.
  - No pharmacokinetic interactions reported.
  - May cause additive weight gain, tremor, and cognitive dysfunction.

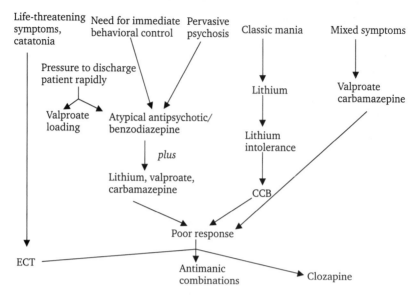

**Figure 6.1  Treatment of Mania Syndromes**

- Lithium + carbamazepine
  - Useful for rapid cycling.
  - Acute antidepressant effects reported.
  - Lithium can reverse early neutropenia associated with carba-
    mazepine treatment but will not prevent agranulocytosis.
  - No pharmacokinetic interactions reported.
  - May have neurotoxic interactions.
- Lithium + verapamil
  - May be helpful for patients refractory to one of these agents.
  - Verapamil may increase renal lithium excretion.
  - Neurotoxic interactions may occur.
  - Both agents have similar actions on SA and AV node.
    - May cause additive cardiac slowing.
- Lithium + gabapentin
  - Lithium may reduce mania risk with gabapentin.
  - Both are excreted by kidney, but have no pharmacokinetic
    interactions.
- Lithium + lamotrigine
  - Appropriate choice for bipolar depression.
  - Lamotrigine will not prevent mania (although it may be less likely
    than other antidepressants to induce mania acutely), whereas

lithium is not as effective for depression as it is for mania prophylaxis (see pp. 306–307).

- Valproate + lamotrigine
  - Valproate increases lamotrigine levels by inhibiting glucuronidation.
    - May be increased risk of rash and other adverse effects.
    - Use lower starting doses and slower dosage escalation when combining lamotrigine with valproate.
- Carbamazepine + lamotrigine
  - Carbamazepine increases lamotrigine metabolism.
  - Lamotrigine may increase levels of 10,11-epoxide metabolite of carbamazepine, with increased neurotoxicity.
- Carbamazepine + verapamil
  - Verapamil increases carbamazepine levels and may have neurotoxic interactions with it at moderate carbamazepine levels.
- Lithium + neuroleptics
  - Neuroleptic addition provides more rapid control of mania.
  - Neurotoxic interactions may cause severe adverse effects.
    - EPS
    - Delirium
    - Adverse effects more likely in hot weather or hot seclusion room (increased lithium levels with dehydration).
    - Neurological impairment sometimes irreversible.
- Lithium + atypical antipsychotic
  - Fewer interactions with lithium than with neuroleptics.
    - Delirium and mild NMS have been reported.
  - Initiate treatment of mania with atypical antipsychotic.
    - Add lithium and gradually increase dose as behavior is better controlled.
  - Combination may be more effective than either one alone.
- Valproate + neuroleptic
  - Faster control of mania
  - Increased confusion may occur.
- Valproate + atypical antipsychotic
  - In a multicenter double-blind trial of 344 patients with a manic or mixed episode, with or without psychosis, who had had an inadequate response to monotherapy for 2 weeks with either lithium (serum level 0.6–1.2 mM) or valproate (serum level 50–125 μg/mL; Tohen et al., 2002b):
    - Patients were maintained on therapeutic levels of lithium or valproate and randomized to 6 weeks of either olanzapine (5–20 mg/day) or placebo added to the antimanic drug.

- Olanzapine addition group had decrease of YMRS scores of 13.1 points (59%) vs. 9.1 points (40.1%) with placebo addition (i.e., continued monotherapy).
- Items that showed significantly better improvement with olanzapine than placebo included irritability, speech, thought disorder, and disruptive/aggressive behavior.
- Difference in remission rates (defined as YMRS ≤ 12) was statistically significant (79% for olanzapine vs. 66% for placebo).
- Olanzapine was significantly better than placebo in patients *without* psychosis but not for those *with* psychotic features.
- Olanzapine was significantly better than placebo in patients with a mixed episode but not for patients with pure mania.
- Significantly more weight gain occurred with olanzapine addition than placebo (3.1 pounds).
- Carbamazepine + antipsychotic medications
  - Carbamazepine increases neuroleptic and atypical antipsychotic metabolism and may reduce efficacy.
  - The only reports of agranulocytosis in psychiatric patients taking carbamazepine have been in patients also taking clozapine.
  - NMS rarely reported when carbamazepine combined with clozapine.
- Lithium + benzodiazepine
  - Adjunctive benzodiazepine often used initially with lithium for more rapid control of mania.
  - Combination may have neurotoxic interactions, especially with clonazepam.

### Maintenance Therapy

Lithium has best data for prevention of recurrence. Laboratory monitoring is discussed on pages 255–256 and blood level monitoring on pages 255–259. Other issues concerning maintenance therapy are discussed in the following material.

Lithium
- Probably most effective for prophylaxis at levels ≥ 0.8 mM.
- Withdrawing lithium after chronic good response may result in rebound of mood disorder and refractoriness to lithium when it is restarted.
  - More likely with rapid lithium withdrawal
- Refractoriness to lithium is not uncommon with long-term treatment.
  - Not clear whether refractoriness is an inherent characteristic of bipolar disorder or lithium maintenance, or whether it reflects con-

comitant use of antidepressants or development of medical complications that interfere with therapeutic action of lithium, such as hypothyroidism or hyperparathyroidism.

### DIVALPROEX

- Although a few studies suggest optimal valproate level is around
  100 mg/dL (Bowden et al., 1994), the most effective way to assess the
  therapeutic level for an individual patient is to measure a 12-hour level
  when the patient has had a maximal response and then regain this level
  if relapse occurs.
  - Divalproex is not supposed to induce its own metabolism; however,
    levels and clinical response often fluctuate substantially and unpre-
    dictably.
    - Decreases are more common than increases but either may occur.
- Women receiving long-term treatment with valproate should be informed about the risk of polycystic ovaries.
  - In a case-controlled study, 80% of women who started taking dival-
    proex for epilepsy before age 20 had multiple ovarian cysts and/or
    elevated testosterone vs. 27% of women taking other antiepileptic
    drugs (Isojarvi, Laatikainen, Pakarinen, Juntunen, Myllyla, 1993).
    - The risk was increased further by taking multiple anticonvulsants.
    - Of women starting anticonvulsants after age 20, 56% of those
      taking valproate had polycystic ovaries or hyperandrogenism vs.
      20% of those not taking valproate.
    - Clinical implications were not clear.
    - Only a few women had polycystic ovary (Stein–Leventhal) syn-
      drome (PCOS).
  - The risk of PCOS should be considered in women taking valproate
    long term. PCOS is characterized by
    - Menstrual irregularities
    - Infertility
    - Hirsutism, obesity, acne
    - Elevated androgens and LH/FSH ratio
    - Chronic anovulation
    - Insulin resistance
  - PCOS is associated with an increased risk of
    - Carbohydrate intolerance
    - Elevated LDL and reduced HDL
    - Endometrial cancer
    - Ischemic heart disease
    - Infertility

- A comparison of 17 patients taking valproate and 15 not taking valproate in a clinical practice found current and lifetime prevalence respectively of menstrual abnormalities in 47% and 77%, of those taking valproate (O'Donovan, Kusumaker, Graves, & Bird, 2002).
  - 7 of the 8 women taking valproate who had current menstrual abnormalities also had PCOS, with an overall prevalence of PCOS of 41% vs. 2–22% in the general population (O'Donovan et al., 2002).
- Abdominal ultrasound prior to starting valproate and 6–12 months later is prudent but is not required.

## Carbamazepine

- Carbamazepine regularly induces its own metabolism.
  - Loss of benefit after initial improvement suggests autoinduction of metabolism.
  - It may be necessary to raise the dose several times before metabolizing enzymes are saturated.
  - The primary role for serum level determinations (i.e., therapeutic drug monitoring) is to ascertain the level that is optimal for an individual patient and reestablish that level if it decreases.
- Monitoring CBC and platelet count does not prevent clinically important bone marrow suppression.
  - About 20% of patients have a mild reduction of neutrophil count during initial months of treatment.
    - Not clinically meaningful
  - Agranulocytosis and related disorders can appear without warning.
    - Obtain CBC and/or platelet count if patient develops warning signs of bone-marrow suppression (e.g., persistent fever or infection, bruising, bleeding or wound that does not heal normally).
- The only meaningful indication for LFTs is clinical evidence of hepatotoxicity.
  - Mild elevations of transaminases occur with many medications that induce their own metabolism and are not clinically meaningful.
- Hyponatremia reported in 6–31% of patients taking carbamazepine chronically.
  - Measure electrolytes if patient develops evidence of hyponatremia, such as tremor, myoclonus, confusion, or a seizure.

## Calcium Channel-Blockers

- No routine monitoring is necessary with this class of medication.
- No correlation is known between blood level and clinical response.

- Concerns that short-acting CCBs such as verapamil can increase the risk of myocardial infarction are contradicted by controlled studies in which the risk of recurrent infarction is reduced by maintenance CCBs (Rengo et al., 1996; Vaage-Nilsen, Hansen, Hagerup, Sigurd, & Steinmetz, 1995).

## Oxcarbazepine

- No laboratory monitoring is recommended for this drug.
- Incidence of hyponatremia is about 2.5%.
  - Caused by SIADH.
  - Measure electrolytes if signs or symptoms of hyponatremia occur.

## Lamotrigine

- More effective than placebo in preventing recurrence of bipolar depression but not mania.
- Although it is sometimes effective as monotherapy for maintenance therapy, lamotrigine is more predictably useful when it is combined with a primary mood stabilizer.
- Lamotrigine can induce hypomania.
- Like other medications used in bipolar disorder, lamotrigine should be gradually withdrawn during maintenance therapy to avoid causing rebound depression, hypomania, or mood cycling.

Despite lack of empirical support for the usefulness of routine laboratory monitoring, most experts recommend monitoring

- LFTs with valproate and carbamazepine
- CBCs with carbamazepine every 2–6 months.

However, no study has demonstrated that this approach reduces the risk of serious adverse events.

### Bipolar Depression

A protocol for treating bipolar depression is suggested on pages 264–268. Issues to consider when using anticonvulsants for bipolar depression include:

- Carbamazepine and possibly oxcarbazepine may be useful acutely for bipolar depression.
  - Combination of lithium + carbamazepine is acutely effective for depression in some patients.
- Valproate and verapamil are not particularly effective for depression.
- Lamotrigine is clearly effective for bipolar depression.
  - 349 recently depressed bipolar I patients switched to lamotrigine over 8–16-week open-label phase (Bowden et al., 2003).

- 175 patients who stabilized were randomized for 18 months to lamotrigine (50, 200, or 400 mg/day), lithium (0.8–1.1 mM), or placebo.
- Lamotrigine = lithium > placebo for lengthening time to affective recurrence.
- Lamotrigine significantly > placebo for lengthening time to recurrence of depressive symptoms; no increase in mania.
- Lithium significantly > placebo for increasing time to manic recurrence; no increase in depression.
- Conclusions: (1) Half of the original sample could not tolerate or responded poorly to lamotrigine; (2) lamotrigine is more effective for bipolar depression than for mania; (3) 400 mg no more effective than 200 mg; (4) Lamotrigine probably should be combined with a primary mood stabilizer most of the time.
  - Lamotrigine can be used to augment antidepressants in unipolar depression.
- Antidepressant effects of gabapentin can be useful acutely but can induce hypomania and mood cycling.
  - Especially if not combined with an established mood stabilizer.

## Panic Disorder

All benzodiazepines are effective for panic disorder in doses equivalent to 3–6 mg/day of alprazolam.
- Clonazepam
  - Twice as potent as alprazolam
  - Effective for panic disorder
- Valproate
  - Useful for panic disorder
  - Initial medication of choice for bipolar disorder associated with panic disorder/panic attacks.
- Carbamazepine is not effective for panic attacks.
- Zonisamide might be useful for anxiety, but little research has accumulated.

## Aggression

Aggressive behavior is a nonspecific event that may be associated with personality disorders, mood disorders, schizophrenia, impulse control disorders, intermittent explosive disorder, epilepsy, developmental disabilities, delirium, or dementia. Premeditated and criminal violence are not psychiatric syndromes and cannot be ameliorated by medications.

Aggression directed toward the self (e.g., self-mutilation in patients with borderline personality disorder, or biting oneself in patients with Lesch–Nyan syndrome) may respond to the same treatments used for outwardly directed impulsive aggression.

### Acute Outwardly Directed Aggression

- Neuroleptics are useful only for aggression caused by psychosis.
  - Offer patient po neuroleptic first.
    - For example, haloperidol 2–15 mg
  - Provide adequate show of force to permit patient to deescalate without losing face.
  - If patient refuses oral medication, consider 2.5–7.5 mg haloperidol IM.
  - Intravenous haloperidol or IV or IM droperidol rapidly effective for life-threatening acute agitation (see Chapter 2).
- Atypical antipsychotics have an antiagitation and antiaggression effect separate from their antipsychotic action.
  - First choice for psychotic or nonpsychotic aggression because of favorable side-effect profile and nonspecific action on aggression and agitation.
  - Start with risperidone 1–2 mg or olanzapine 5–10 mg po.
  - Consider IM ziprasiodone if patient refuses oral medication.
- Benzodiazepines can be helpful for acute aggression, especially if associated with anxiety.
  - Start with po short- or intermediate-acting benzodiazepine.
    - Lorazepam 1–2 mg
    - Oxazepam 15–30 mg
  - IM lorazepam is reliably absorbed.
    - 1–2 mg q 1–2 hours until calm
  - IV lorazepam can be administered alone or in the same syringe as haloperidol (see Chapter 2).
    - Do not administer more than 2 mg at a time.
    - Can repeat in 30 minutes if necessary.
  - IV midazolam is rapidly effective.
  - Benzodiazepines may be disinhibiting in brain-damaged and hypervigilant patients.

### Chronic Unpredictable Outwardly Directed Aggression

Treatment of agitation and aggression associated with dementia and other neurological conditions is discussed on pages 90–104. No medication is effective for chronic premeditated violence, which is usually associated with other forms of antisocial behavior.

Buspirone, propranolol, SSRIs, and trazodone can reduce chronic unpredictable aggression in non-neurological as well as neurological patients. A therapeutic effect may take 1–2 months for these and the following additional treatments.

- Anticonvulsants
  - Most effective for aggression associated with bipolar disorder.
  - Indicated for aggression associated with partial complex seizures.
  - Also useful in personality disorders and intermittent explosive disorder.
  - Valproate
    - Low doses (15–25 mg/kg/day) can decrease chronic impulsive violent behavior.
    - If lower doses not effective, increase to usual therapeutic level.
    - In a 7-week trial, 71 adolescents with DSM-IV conduct disorder were randomized to high or low-dose valproate (Steiner, Petersen, Saxena, Ford, & Matthews, 2003). High-dose valproate was significantly better in improving impulse control.
  - Carbamazepine
    - Useful for intermittent explosive disorder and aggression in patients with borderline personality disorder and PTSD.
    - Usual dose is 1200–2000 mg/day.
- Lithium
  - Especially useful for aggression in patients with bipolar disorder.
  - Reduces impulsive aggression in personality disorders and developmental disability.
  - Adjust to usual therapeutic level.
- Benzodiazepines
  - More likely to disinhibit than to reduce chronic aggressive behavior.
  - May be useful for intermittent angry outbursts in anxious patients.
  - Use longer-acting benzodiazepine for chronic aggression
    - Clonazepam
    - Clorazepate
- Antipsychotic drugs
  - All antipsychotic drugs reduce aggression caused by psychosis.
  - Atypical antipsychotics have additional antiaggressive effect in nonpsychotic patients.

CHRONIC SELF-DESTRUCTIVE BEHAVIOR

- Lithium has clearly been shown to decrease suicidality, even in the absence of significant impact on a mood disorder.
- Naltrexone decreases chronic self-injurious behavior such as cutting and biting in patients with personality disorders and developmental disabilities.
  - Usual dose is 50–100 mg/day.
- SSRIs can reduce many nonspecific forms of repetitive, impulsive aggression directed toward the self or others in patients with brain damage or personality disorders
  - Effective even if patient not depressed
  - Usual doses
    - Fluoxetine 20–60 mg/day
    - Sertraline 200 mg/day
    - Paroxetine 20–40 mg/day
- Atypical antipsychotics
  - Especially useful for chronic self-destructive behavior caused by psychosis.

## Flashbacks from Chronic Hallucinogen Use

LSD is a $5HT_2$ receptor agonist. Sensitization of this receptor may result in autonomous signaling, causing recurrence of hallucinations. SSRIs sometimes precipitate flashbacks in patients who have used LSD in the past by increasing activation of supersensitive $5HT_2$ receptors.

- Treatment involves blocking $5HT_2$ receptors.
- Short-term treatment usually sufficient.
- Cyproheptadine 4–8 mg tid
- Atypical antipsychotic drug
  - Risperidone 0.5–2 mg
  - Olanzapine 2.5–10 mg
- Carbamazepine and valproate sometimes helpful.

## Atypical Psychosis Associated with Seizure Disorders

Intermittent psychosis may be associated with seizure disorders.

- Interictal psychosis with generalized seizures
  - May resemble schizophrenia.
- Partial complex seizure spectrum disorders
  - Generalized seizures do not occur.
  - Seizure focus may or may not be in the temporal lobe.

- Intermittent signs and symptoms include
  - Episodic psychosis with complete resolution between episodes
  - Nonauditory hallucinations
  - Objects appear bigger or smaller
  - Altered state of consciousness during psychotic episodes
  - Memory for episode may be incomplete
  - Repetitive, purposeless behaviors
  - Abrupt, intense changes of mood (e.g., rage, tearfulness, sexual feelings, mystical/religious experiences)
  - EEG abnormal only 50% of time.
- May be confused with cycloid psychosis
  - Highly recurrent non-affective psychosis responsive to lithium
- Treatment is with an anticonvulsant.
  - Carbamazepine is preferable.
  - Valproate is not as predictably effective.
  - Usual anticonvulsant doses necessary.
  - Adjunctive antipsychotic medication may be necessary to treat hallucinations.

### Posttraumatic Stress Disorder (PTSD)

Antikindling effects of some anticonvulsants could make them useful in PTSD.

- A few open trials report reduction of PTSD symptoms with carbamazepine (Iancu, Rosen, & Moshe, 2002).
- A large 5-year retrospective study of carbamazepine in doses up to 800 mg suggested efficacy in veterans with PTSD (Viola, Ditzler, & Butzer, 1997).
- In an open-label trial of valproate (mean dose 365 mg) in 16 patients with PTSD (Clark, Canive, & Calais, 1999), there were
  - Decreases in intrusive recall and hyperarousal
  - Decreases in depression and anxiety
  - No change in avoidance or numbing
- A small double-blind study of lamotrigine (up to 500 mg/day) vs. placebo in 14 patients with PTSD found that 50% of 10 lamotrigine-treated patients but only one of four (25%) of placebo-treated patients had improvement of reexperiencing and avoidance/numbing (Clark et al., 1999)
- An open trial of topiramate in doses up to 100 mg/day in 35 civilians with PTSD found that topiramate decreased nightmares in 79% of patients and flashbacks in 86%, with complete suppression of nightmares in 50% and flashbacks in 50% (Berlant & van Kammen, 2002).

- There were significant reductions in mean PTSD symptom scores over 4 weeks of treatment, including reductions of reexperiencing, avoidance, and hyperarousal.

### Pathological Gambling

In a 14-week single-blind trial, both lithium (N = 15) and valproate (N = 16) produced significant and equivalent improvement of compulsive gambling in nonbipolar patients.

## SIDE EFFECTS

In general, side effects can be minimized by increasing the dose very slowly and dividing the dose more frequently. Most common adverse effects of anticonvulsants follow.

- Carbamazepine
  - Ataxia, incoordination
  - Dizziness, lightheadedness
  - Fatigue
  - Rash
- Valproate
  - GI side effects
    - Nausea, dyspepsia, diarrhea, abdominal pain
  - Sedation
  - Tremor
  - Cognitive impairment
  - Weight gain
- Lamotrigine
  - Sedation
  - Dizziness, ataxia
  - Nausea, vomiting
  - Benign rash
    - Severe rash (Stevens–Johnson or toxic epidermal necrolysis) in 1/5,000
- Gabapentin
  - Sedation
  - Agitation, jitteriness
  - Dizziness, ataxia
  - Nausea
  - Decreased libido

- Topiramate
  - Sedation, psychomotor slowing
  - Dizziness
  - Cognitive impairment
  - Kidney stones
- Tiagabine
  - GI distress
  - Dizziness
  - Asthenia
  - Sedation
  - Tremor

## Cardiovascular Side Effects

### AV CONDUCTION TIMES

These may be increased. A quinidine-like effect rarely occurs with carbamazepine.

- AV conduction delay and bradycardia with carbamazepine
  - More common in older women
- Use caution with carbamazepine in patients with heart block or those at high risk for cardiac conduction abnormalities (e.g., myotonic dystrophy).

### ORTHOSTATIC HYPOTENSION

- Common with topiramate
  - Often accompanied by ataxia

## Central Nervous System Side Effects

### COGNITIVE IMPAIRMENT

- Can occur with any anticonvulsant.
  - Most common with topiramate and valproate
  - Tolerance may not develop.
- May respond to standard doses of cholinesterase inhibitors (Chapter 2).
  - These medications may have adjunctive mood-stabilizing properties.
- A 12-day comparison of placebo, 50 mg of lamotrigine, and 900 mg of valproate in 30 normal subjects investigated adverse cognitive effects (Aldenkamp et al., 2002).
  - Lamotrigine-treated subjects had fewer drug-related cognitive complaints than valproate-treated subjects.

- Cognition seemed somewhat improved in the lamotrigine group compared to the others.

## CONFUSION

- Especially with carbamazepine and topiramate
- More likely with
  - Combination with lithium or neuroleptics
  - Older age
  - CNS disease
- May be caused by hyponatremia.

## DROWSINESS, SEDATION, DIZZINESS

- Dose related
- Occurs with all anticonvulsants.
- Fatigue common with topiramate.
- Management:
  - Increase dose slowly.
    - Start carbamazepine at 50 mg hs.
    - Increase weekly.
  - Give tid.
  - Administer larger dose hs.
  - Add modafanil (see p. 475).
    - Stimulants can destabilize bipolar mood disorders.

## IRRITABILITY

- Carbamazepine occasionally makes children and adolescents more irritable or disorganized.

## OVERSTIMULATION, IRRITABILITY

- Primarily occurs with gabapentin and topiramate.

## PARESTHESIAS

- May be caused by topiramate.

## TREMOR

- Most common with valproate, gabapentin
- Management:
  - Reduce/divide dose.
  - Add beta-blocker.

### Word-finding Difficulties

- Seen with valproate, carbamazepine, topiramate.

## Endocrine and Sexual Side Effects

### Hyperandrogenism and Polycystic Ovaries

- Occurs with valproate.
- Opinions vary about the risk of polycystic ovaries and PCOS, and whether this is a problem in women starting valproate in adulthood.
- In a group of 43 epileptic women treated for at least 2 years with valproate or other antiepileptic drugs, valproate use was associated with higher androgen levels and higher postprandial insulin levels (Luef et al., 2002).
  - Possibly due to the effect of valproate on islet cells.
- Significant differences found between 18 women with bipolar disorder taking valproate and 20 taking lithium (MacIntyre, Mancini, McCann, Srinivasan, & Kennedy, 2003).
  - 50% of valproate-treated women and 15% of those taking lithium had menstrual abnormalities.
  - 50% of women with BMI ≥ 25 and history of menstrual abnormalities also had laboratory evidence of hyperandrogenism.
- In a prospective cohort analysis of 93 women with focal epilepsy
  - Incidence of PCOS was similar in patients treated with valproate, carbamazepine, or no anticonvulsant (Bauer, Jarre, Klingmuller, & Elger, 2000).
- All studies that suggest androgenization, polycystic ovaries, and related problems with valproate are cross-sectional or retrospective.
  - In the absence of good prospective studies, there is no reason not to consider valproate a first-line treatment.

### Syndrome of Inappropriate Antidiuretic Hormone Secretion (SIADH)

- Occurs with carbamazepine and oxcarbazepine.
  - 5% with carbamazepine and 2.5% with oxcarbazepine.
- Water intoxication occurs if patient drinks too much water.
  - With normal renal and endocrine function, it is necessary to drink 1 liter/hour to produce hyponatremia.
- Management:
  - Restrict fluids.
  - Lithium increases renal water excretion.
  - Administer demeclocycline 300–600 mg bid.

### Eyes, Ears, Nose, and Throat Side Effects

BLURRED VISION OR DECREASED VISUAL ACUITY

- With topiramate
  - Eye pain may also occur.
- Topiramate can cause myopia, increase intraocular pressure, and precipitate narrow angle glaucoma (Thambi et al., 2001).
  - Multiple case reports of glaucoma precipitated by topiramate.
  - Eye problems remit when drug is withdrawn.

NASAL CONGESTION

- Occurs occasionally.

### Gastrointestinal Side Effects

CONSTIPATION

- May respond to cholinesterase inhibitor.

DRY MOUTH

- Use sugar-free candy/gum or cholinesterase inhibitor.

HEPATOTOXICITY

- Liver function tests (mainly transaminases) show increases during first 3 months of treatment with many anticonvulsants.
  - 15–30% of those taking valproate
  - Also common with carbamazepine
  - Not a sign of hepatotoxicity, but of induction of metabolism.
  - Elevated bilirubin may be an indication of hepatic damage.
  - Elevated ammonia with valproate not clearly correlated with adverse CNS effects.
    - Elevation primarily important in hepatic coma, when patient is clearly ill anyway.
    - Monitoring serum ammonia is not useful and sometimes leads to unnecessary discontinuation of valproate.
- Severe generalized rash and fever with carbamazepine may predict allergic hepatitis.
- Serious hepatotoxicity with valproate:
  - Mainly in children < 2 years old with severe neurological or metabolic disease, taking other anticonvulsants
  - With polytherapy and neurological disease, fatal hepatoxocity in
    - 1:500 < 2
    - 1:17,000 ages 2–21

- 1:37,000 ages 21–40
- 1:38,000 > 40 years old
- Caution usually advised with valproate in patients with liver disease.
  - However, a review of records of 564 VA patients with a new valproate prescription and at least one ALT level prior to, and after starting, valproate found that marked elevations of ALT with valproate were rare (Felker, Sloan, Dominitz, & Barnes, 2003).
  - ALT levels were significantly more likely to be elevated in patients with hepatitis C, but the same risk of elevated ALT was found in hepatitis patients taking antidepressants, lithium, or gabapentin as in those taking valproate.
  - Elevations of liver function tests in these patients may reflect fluctuations in the hepatitis, unreported alcohol use, or other factors rather than use of valproate. Based on these findings valproate appears safe in patients with hepatitis C, although these patients should be followed closely.

Nausea, Vomiting, Anorexia, Indigestion

- More likely if
  - Medication taken on empty stomach
  - Any dose too high
  - Dose increased too rapidly
- More frequent with valproate, lamotrigine, topiramate
  - GI side effects 15–20% with Depakene (valproic acid) vs. < 10% with Depakote (divalproex sodium).
- Management:
  - Use Depakote rather than Depakene.
  - Consider Depakote-ER if immediate-release causes intolerable GI side effects.
    - Doses of the two preparations are not equivalent.
    - Little research with Depakote-ER in mood disorders.
  - Depakote Sprinkle has fewer GI side effects and permits smaller dosage increments.
  - Administer medication with food.
  - Histamine H2 antagonist may help.
  - Ginger root capsules or broth may help nausea (see Chapter 2).

Weight Gain

- In a 1-year double-blind study, 25% of valproate patients experienced significantly more weight gain than patients on placebo (Bowden et al., 2000).

- Gabapentin can cause weight gain.
- Weight gain may occur with lamotrigine but is uncommon.
- Zonesamide and topiramate cause weight loss.

### Hematologic Side Effects

APLASTIC ANEMIA, AGRANULOCYTOSIS

- Risk of severe bone marrow suppression with carbamazepine is extremely rare; routine CBCs do not identify risk (see p. 301).

ANEMIA

- Occurs in $< 5\%$ of patients taking carbamazepine.
- Not clinically important

LEUKOPENIA

- About 20% of patients taking carbamazepine have decrease in white blood count of 25–30% .
  - Does not predict agranulocytosis.
- Leukopenia may be persistent in 2% on carbamazepine.
  - Moderate decrease in WBC ($3000–4000/mm^3$) in 76% of these patients.
  - WBC $< 3000$ in 24%.
  - Not correlated with susceptibility to infection.
  - White count returns to normal with discontinuation of carbamazepine.

THROMBOCYTOPENIA

- Platelet count $< 100,000/mm^3$
- Occurs occasionally with divalproex.
- More likely to occur at higher doses.
- Not clinically important unless patient develops bleeding, bruising, or anemia.

MUSCULOSKELETAL

- 40 epileptic adults on long-term valproate monotherapy were compared with 40 age- and sex-matched epileptic patients taking phenytoin and 40 controls (Sato et al., 2001).
  - Patients on valproate and phenytoin had similar average reductions of bone mineral density compared with controls.
    - Of the valproate patients, 23% had osteoporosis and 37% had osteopenia.
  - Serum calcium concentrations were significantly higher in valproate than phenytoin patients or controls.

- Seemed to be caused by increased bone resorption.
- However, phenytoin-treated patients also had increased bone re-sorption and reduced bone mineral density.

### Renal Side Effects

- Carbamazepine occasionally causes urinary frequency or urinary retention.
- Kidney stones develop in 1.5% of patients taking topiramate.

### Skin, Allergies, and Temperature Side Effects

#### DECREASED SWEATING

Oligohidrosis and hyperthermia, sometimes with dangerous fevers, occasionally occur with topiramate

#### FEVER, CHILLS, SWEATING, LYMPHADENOPATHY, JOINT PAIN

- Can occur with carbamazepine.

#### HAIR LOSS

- Most common with valproate
- Zinc and/or selenium supplement may help.
- Topical minoxidil can be useful but may aggravate depression.

#### HYPERSENSITIVITY WITH PULMONARY SYMPTOMS

- Occasionally caused by carbamazepine
- Hay fever symptoms
- Shortness of breath
- Pneumonia may develop.

#### RASH

- Varieties of drug rash
  - Benign morbilliform rash
    - Mildly pruritic, confluent maculopapular rash
    - Starts on trunk; may spread to face and extremities.
    - Begins 7–10 days after starting medication.
  - Erythema multiforme
    - Target-shaped lesions
    - On limbs, face, mucous membranes
    - Fever, malaise
    - Burning and pruritis in affected areas

- Joint and muscle pain
- Begins within 3 days of starting drug.
- Dangerous rashes
  - Occur with lamotrigine, carbamazepine, divalproex, phenobarbital, phenytoin.
  - Toxic epidermal necrolysis
  - Stevens–Johnson syndrome
- Approach to drug rashes:
  - Do not start a new medication within 2 weeks of a rash or viral infection.
  - Add antihistamine.
  - Avoid sunlight.
  - Do not change soaps, cosmetics, deodorants, or detergents during first few months of taking a medication that can cause a rash.
- Carbamazepine
  - Rash occurs in 3–15% of patients.
  - Milder rashes resolve spontaneously in 50%.
  - Rash does not reappear in 50% if medication withdrawn and restarted 2 weeks later.
  - Management:
    - Continue medication or stop and restart if mild, localized rash.
    - Patient may be allergic to excipients in pill, not to the active medication.
    - Try liquid or chewable form.
    - Discontinue medication if rash is extensive or associated with fever or elevated LFTs.
- Lamotrigine
  - Retrospective analysis of 12 multicenter studies of unipolar depression or bipolar disorder involving 1,955 patients treated with lamotrigine (Calabrese et al., 2002) found that
    - 8.3% of lamotrigine-treated patients and 6.4% of those receiving placebo had a benign rash.
    - Overall rate of rash for lamotrigine in open-label and controlled studies was 13.1%; two patients (0.1%) had serious rashes and one patient had Stevens–Johnson syndrome.
  - Risk of serious rash has decreased from 120:100,000 in 1993 to 1:5,000 in 2000 with introduction of slower titration guidelines.
  - Valproate increases lamotrigine levels and can increase risk of serious rash.
    - Raise lamotrigine dose more slowly if combined with valproate.
  - Any rash is cause for discontinuation of lamotrigine.

- Valproate and carbamazepine have been found to produce psoriasiform skin rashes (Brenner, Wolf, Landau, & Politi, 1994).

## PREGNANCY AND LACTATION

### Teratogenicity

- Anticonvulsants can cause major and minor anomalies.
- Major malformations
  - Occur in 2–3% of general population
  - Rate 2–4% of nonepileptic women
  - Rate 4–8% of women with epilepsy taking AEDs
  - Risk increased with higher anticonvulsant dose and with anticonvulsant polytherapy.
  - Examples:
    - Midline facial (all anticonvulsants)
    - Cardiac (all anticonvulsants)
    - Urogenital (all anticonvulsants)
    - Neural tube (1–2% with valproate, 0.5–1% with carbamazepine)
- Minor anomalies
  - Rate 4–10% of nonepileptic women
  - Rate up to 15% of women with epilepsy
- A review of studies of major malformations in infants exposed to anticonvulsants considered cleft lip/palate, congenital heart defects, hypospadias and other genitourinary anomalies, distal limb hypoplasia, clubfoot, and neural tube defects (Stoler, 2001). The reviewer noted that
  - Polytherapy increased the risk of anomalies.
  - A prospective Italian study found an overall malformation rate in epileptic women taking anticonvulsants of 9.7%, whereas epileptic women not taking anticonvulsants did not have abnormal babies.
  - Infants exposed to antiepileptic drugs had a higher frequency of malformations, microcephaly, growth retardation, and hypoplasia of the face and fingers.
    - There were no abnormalities in children of epileptic women not taking AEDs.
  - Valproate may have a higher risk of spina bifida than other AEDs; effects seem to be dose related.
  - There is a small decrease in birth weight and head circumference in infants exposed to AEDs during pregnancy.
    - Especially with carbamazepine and oxcarbazepine

- Adjusting for other relevant factors, risk of microcephaly is
  - 3.6% for any AED
  - 2.1% for infants of women with epilepsy not taking AEDs
  - 3.6% for carbamazepine monotherapy
  - 4.8% for phenobarbital monotherapy

Specific risks estimated from retrospective reviews and a few small prospective studies (Gagliardi & Krishnan, 2003).

- Valproate overall risk of fetal malformation: 11.1%
  - Neural tube defects: 1–2%
  - Fetal valproate syndrome
    - Brachycephaly
    - High forehead
    - Hypertelorism
    - Small nose and mouth
    - Low-set ears with posterior rotation
    - Long fingers and toes
    - Hyperconvex fingernails
    - Shallow philtrum
    - Small mouth
  - Lumbosacral spina bifida
  - Cardiac anomalies
  - Bleeding resulting from reduced vitamin K-dependent clotting factors
  - Liver failure
  - Developmental delays
  - Behavioral problems
- Carbamazepine overall risk of fetal malformation: 5.7%
  - Neural tube defects: 1%
  - Cranial facial defects
  - Fingernail hypoplasia
  - Short nose
  - Tetralogy of Fallot
  - Ventricular septal defects
  - Esophageal atresia
  - Vertebral anomalies
  - Limb defects
  - Esophageal atresia
  - Cavernous hemangiomas
  - Impaired vitamin K-dependent clotting

- Transient neonatal hepatic dysfunction
- Developmental delays
- Possible causes of teratogenicity
  - Toxic intermediates
  - Folic acid deficiency
  - Valproate may alter the expression of HOX genes, which are necessary for normal fetal development.
- Teratogenicity risk mostly during first trimester.

Approach to minimizing risk

- Do not start an anticonvulsant if patient is, or may become, pregnant, unless absolutely necessary.
- If anticonvulsants are unavoidable, try
  - Anticonvulsant monotherapy
  - Lowest possible anticonvulsant dose
  - Folic acid supplementation of 0.8–4 mg/day
  - Prenatal diagnostic testing at 16–18 weeks
  - Maternal serum alpha feto-protein
  - Ultrasound
- Women should not rely on oral contraceptives if they are taking
  - Carbamazepine
  - Oxcarbazepine
  - Phenobarbital
  - Phenytoin
  - Topiramate
  - Felbamate
- Anticonvulsants that do not interact with oral contraceptives include
  - Gabapentin
  - Lamotrigine
  - Levetiracetam
  - Zonisamide
  - Tiagabine
  - Valproate
- Lithium is probably safer during pregnancy than anticonvulsants.
- Verapamil has low risk of teratogenicity.
  - Verapamil was effective without apparent teratogenicity in a consecutive series of pregnant bipolar patients (Wisner et al., 2002).
  - Nimodipine was effective and well tolerated by a pregnant woman with bipolar disorder intolerant of other antimanic drugs (Yingling, Utter, Vengalil, & Mason, 2002).
- ECT is safe during pregnancy.

### Direct Effect on Newborn (3rd Trimester)

- Valproate can cause hepatotoxicity in newborn, especially if serum level > 60 μg/mL.

### Lactation

- All anticonvulsants are excreted in breast milk.
- Toxicity has been reported in infants nursing from mothers taking valproate.

## DRUG–DRUG INTERACTIONS

Table 6.3 summarizes interactions between anticonvulsants and other drugs.

## WITHDRAWAL

Anticonvulsants do not produce psychological dependence, tolerance, or addiction.
- Abrupt discontinuation can cause seizures in nonepileptic patients.
- Rapid discontinuation can result in rebound of affective symptoms.
- If possible, withdraw anticonvulsants by 10%, or one dose every few days to every few weeks.

## TOXICITY AND OVERDOSE

### Carbamazepine

- Overdose can cause
  - Nausea, vomiting, glossitis, abdominal pain
  - Agitation, restlessness
  - Irregular breathing
  - Vertigo
  - Mydriasis, nystagmus, blurred vision, diplopia
  - Anuria, oliguria, urinary retention
  - Hypotension, hypertension, tachycardia
  - Tremor, involuntary movements, athetosis, ataxia
  - Visual hallucinations
  - Abnormal reflexes
  - Seizures (especially in children)

**Table 6.3 Drug–Drug Interactions**

| DRUGS (X) INTERACT WITH: | CARBAMAZEPINE (C) | COMMENTS |
|---|---|---|
| acetazolamide | C↑ | Increases levels/toxicity. |
| alprazolam (*see* benzodiazepines) | | |
| antipsychotics | X↓ C↓ | Carbamazepine induces metabolism of many antipsychotic drugs. |
| azithromycin (*see* macrolide antibiotics) | | |
| barbiturates | C↓ | Phenobarbital increases metabolism of carbamazepine to epoxide; can lower serum level in 5 days, but without causing major clinical effects. Other barbiturates probably act similarly. |
| benzodiazepines | X↓ | Diminishes alprozolam and clonazepam plasma levels (20–50%). Other benzodiazepines potentially affected. |
| birth control pills | X↓ | Diminished oral contraceptives levels, loss of effect, pregnancy. Valproate, lamotrigine, tiagabine, and gabapentin do not induce estrogen metabolism. |
| cimetidine | C↑ | Increases acutely administered carbamazepine by 30% to produce toxicity in 2 days; chronically taking both drugs poses no particular risk. When cimetidine stopped, carbamazepine toxicity dissipates in about 1 week. Ranitidine can be substituted for cimetidine. |
| clarithromycin (*see* macrolide antibiotics) | | |
| clobazam | X↓ | Reduces plasma levels. |
| clonazepam | X↓ | Diminishes clonazepam level. |
| clozapine | X↑ C↑ | Possible synergistic bone-marrow suppression. |
| corticosteroids: dexamethasone methylprednisone prednisolone prednisone | X↓ | Carbamazepine may chronically reduce actions and levels of most corticosteroids; may need to increase steroid dose. False positive DST in patients taking carbamazepine |
| cyclosporine | X↓ | Lowers blood level. |
| danazol | C↑ | Danazol greatly raises carbamazepine levels, at times to toxicity. Other androgen derivatives (e.g., methyltestosterone) may act similarly. If used together, closely monitor carbamazepine level and adjust dose of one or both drugs. |

(*continues*)

## Table 6.3 Continued

| DRUGS (X) INTERACT WITH: | CARBAMAZEPINE (C) | COMMENTS |
|---|---|---|
| dexamethasone (*see* corticosteroids) | | |
| dextropropoxyphene | C↑ | Increases levels/toxicity. |
| digitalis, digoxin | X↑ | May worsen or cause bradycardia. |
| diltiazem | C↑ | Calcium channel blockers such as diltiazem and verapamil inhibit CYP3A4, increasing carbamazepine levels to toxic levels. Nifedipine, which does not affect carbamazepine clearance, is a safer calcium channel-blocker. Nimodipine may also be safer. |
| diuretics | X↓ | Symptomatic hyponatremia; may need periodic electrolytes. |
| doxycycline | X↓ | Carbamazepine may reduce levels of doxycycline as well as other tetracyclines. |
| erythromycin (*see* macrolide antibiotics) | | |
| ethosuximide | X↓ | Diminishes ethosuximide. |
| fentanyl | X↓ | Reduces plasma level and analgesia. |
| fluoxetine (*see* SSRIs) | | |
| fluphenazine (*see* haloperidol) | | |
| flurithromycin (*see* macrolide antibiotics) | | |
| fluvoxamine (*see* SSRIs) | | |
| gemfibrozil (*see* lipid-lowering agents) | | |
| haloperidol | X↓ | Carbamazepine reduces haloperidol levels by 50–60%, which may or may not induce symptoms in 24 h (in rapid-cyclers) to 3 weeks. Serum levels of both drugs may be normal or low. |
| isoniazid (INH) | C↑ | Carbamazepine may increase levels to toxicity usually in 1–2 days of INH; frequently happens at INH doses > 200 mg/day. Symptoms stop 2 days after INH is discontinued. INH often reduces level of carbamazepine; when INH is reduced or stopped, serum carbamazepine increases. |
| josamycin (*see* macrolide antibiotics) | | |

(*continues*)

**Table 6.3 Continued**

| DRUGS (X) INTERACT WITH: | CARBAMAZEPINE (C) | COMMENTS |
|---|---|---|
| lipid-lowering agents: gemfibrozil isonicotinic acid niacinamide nicotinamide | C↑ | Increase carbamazepine levels and high-density lipoprotein (HDL). |
| lithium | X↑ C↑ | Lithium and carbamazepine may increase each other's neurotoxicity and therapeutic effects. Additive effect to decrease thyroid function. Lower levels of each may still be therapeutic. Lithium leucocytosis may counteract carbamazepine leucopenia. |
| liquid medicinal agents or diluents | X↓ C↓ | Carbamazepine suspension can result in a rubbery orange mass when given with other liquid suspensions. May result in decreased bioavailability and absorption. |
| macrolide antibiotics: azithromycin clarithromycin erythromycin flurithromycin josamycin ponsinomycin troleandomycin | C↑ | Significantly (1–2 times) increases carbamazepine levels/toxicity; may subside in 2–3 days after antibiotics stopped. Spiramycin probably safe alternative. |
| mebendazole | X↓ | Carbamazepine may impair mebendazole's therapeutic effect at high doses; no special precautions needed. Valproic acid may be safer than carbamazepine. |
| methadone | X↓ | Carbamazepine may lower serum methadone and increase withdrawal symptoms; patients may need more methadone or should be switched to valproic acid. |
| methylprednisone (see corticosteroids) | | |
| nefazodone | C↑ | Potentially increases carbamazepine levels by inhibition of 3A4 isoenzyme. |
| neuromuscular blocking agents (see pancuronium, vecuronium) | X↓ | Shortens duration of action. |
| niacinamide (see lipid-lowering agents) | | |
| oral contraceptives (see birth control pills) | | |
| pancuronium | X↓ | Shortened neuromuscular blockade. |

(continues)

**Table 6.3  Continued**

| DRUGS (X) INTERACT WITH: | CARBAMAZEPINE (C) | COMMENTS |
|---|---|---|
| paroxetine (*see* SSRIs) | | |
| phenytoin | X↓ C↓ | Each can induce the other's metabolism. |
| phenobarbital | X↓ C↓ | Monitor both serum levels. |
| ponsinomycin (*see* macrolide antibiotics) | | |
| prednisolone (*see* corticosteroids) | | |
| prednisone (*see* corticosteroids) | | |
| primidone | X↓ | Speeds conversion of primidone to phenobarbital. |
| propoxyphene | C↑ | Consistently raises carbamazepine, at times to toxicity. |
| sertraline (*see* SSRIs) | | |
| SSRIs | X↓ C↑ | Some SSRIs (especially fluvoxamine and fluoxetine) inhibit 3A4 and increase carbamazepine levels. |
| tetracycline (*see* doxycycline) | | |
| theophylline | X↓ | Decreased theophylline half-life and levels. |
| thyroid hormones | X↓ | Accelerates elimination of thyroid hormones and may induce hypothyroidism; add thyroid. |
| TCAs | X↓↑ C↑ | Carbamazepine can accelerate metabolism of HCAs. Additive side effects (e.g., ortho-static hypotension, sedation) may occur. |
| troleandomycin (*see* macrolide antibiotics) | | |
| valproic acid | X↓ C↑ | Diminished valproic acid levels; can increase carbamazepine levels. |
| vecuronium | X↓ | Reduced level. |
| verapamil | C↑ | Verapamil inhibits CYP3A4 and raises carbamazepine levels. Discontinuing can lead to seizures because carbama-zepine abruptly declines; nifedipine may be safer. |
| viloxazine | C↑ | Increases levels/toxicity. |
| warfarin | X↓ | Impaired hypoprothrombinemic response in several days to a week; adjust anticoagu-lants when carbamazepine changed. |

(*continues*)

**Table 6.3  Continued**

| DRUGS (X) INTERACT WITH: | VALPROIC ACID (V) | COMMENTS |
|---|---|---|
| amitriptyline (*see* TCAs) | | |
| antacids | V↑ | Increase valproic acid absorption; give 1 h apart. |
| aspirin (*see* salicylates) | | |
| benzodiazepines | X↑ | Valproic acid may elevate diazepam; with clonazepam, may cause absence seizures in epileptic patients. |
| carbamazepine | X↑ V↓ | Decreases valproic acid; increases carbamazepine and epoxide metabolite. |
| cimetidine | V↑ | Increases valproic acid levels; monitor levels or switch to ranitidine. |
| chlorpromazine | V↑ | Monitor valproic acid levels or switch to alternative neuroleptic (e.g., haloperidol). |
| ethosuximide | X↑ | Decrease ethosuximide or use alternative. |
| erythromycin | V↑ | Increases level/toxicity; may occur with other macrolide antibiotics. |
| felbamate | V↑ | Increases level/toxicity; monitor levels; start and withdraw felbamate slowly. |
| lithium | X↑ V↑ | Additive neurotoxicity may occur. |
| macrolide antibiotics (*see* erythromycin) | | |
| nortriptyline (see TCAs) | | |
| phenobarbital | X↑ | Increases serum phenobarbital; may prompt toxicity. Cut phenobarbital dose by 30–75% and monitor for decreased valproate. |
| phenothiazines | V↑ | May increase valproate levels. |
| phenytoin | X↑↓ V↓ | Valproate initially lowers serum phenytoin by 30%, but in several weeks, phenytoin may exceed pre-valproate levels, with accompanying ataxia, nystagmus, mental impairment, involuntary muscular movements, and seizures. Can also increase phenytoin toxicity by displacement from binding protein. Do not increase phenytoin unless seizures occur. Phenytoin may decrease serum valproate with reduced thymoleptic effect. |
| primidone | X↑ | Valproic acid elevates serum phenobarbital, which is a metabolite of primidone. Valproic acid also inhibits phenobarbital metabolism, increasing risk of phenobarbital intoxication. |

(*continues*)

**Table 6.3  Continued**

| DRUGS (X) INTERACT WITH: | VALPROIC ACID (v) | COMMENTS |
|---|---|---|
| propoxyphene | C↑ | Increases levels/toxicity. |
| salicylates | X↑ V↑ | Salicylates may increase unbound serum valproic acid concentrations to cause valproic acid toxicity. Symptoms resolve when salicylate stopped. Bleeding time may be prolonged; decreased thrombocytes plus salicylates may yield bleeding, bruising, and petechiae. |
| TCAs | X↑ | Increases levels of nortriptyline and amitriptyline and possibly other TCAs. |
| thiopentone | X↑ | Lower anesthesia dose of thiopentone. |
| warfarin | X↑ | Increases unbound warfarin. |

↑ Increases; ↓ Decreases; ↑↓ Increases or decreases.

**Table 6.4  Effects on Laboratory Tests**

| GENERIC NAMES | BLOOD/SERUM TESTS* | URINE TESTS |
|---|---|---|
| carbamazepine | Calcium ↓<br>BUN ↑<br>Thyroid function ↓<br>**LFT ↑<br>WBC, platelets ↓<br>RBC ↓<br>Sodium ↓<br>*** TCA ↑ | Albumin ↑<br>Glucose ↑ |
| clonazepam | **LFT ↑ | |
| valproic acid | **LFT (mainly AST [SGOT], ALT [SGPT], LDH) ↑<br>WBC, platelets ↓<br>Thyroid function ↓<br>Lymphocytes ↑<br>Ammonia ↑ | Ketones ↑ |

* ↑ Increases; ↓ Decreases.
** LFT tests are AST/SGOT, ALT/SGPT, alkaline phosphatase, LDH, and bilirubin. Increases in transaminases (SGOT, SGPT, and LDH) are usually benign; increases in bilirubin and other tests suggest hepatotoxicity.
*** False positive for TCA when Abbot TCA immunoassay used.

- Management:
  - Use diuresis to speed elimination.
  - Use dialysis.
  - Treat seizures with diazepam.
    - May increase respiratory depression.

Valproate
- Overdose can cause
  - Anorexia and vomiting
  - Somnolence, ataxia, tremor
  - Rash, alopecia, increased appetite
  - Heart block
  - Coma
- Management:
  - Gastric lavage of no help because valproate is rapidly absorbed.
    - Gastric lavage or emesis may help with extended-release valproate.
  - Try hemodialysis, hemoperfusion.
  - Naloxone may reduce coma but also can precipitate a seizure by antagonizing anticonvulsant effect.

Gabapentin
- Because L-amino acid transporter that carries gabapentin into brain is saturated at higher doses, overdoses do not usually produce significant toxicity.

Lamotrigine
- Overdose can cause
  - Somnolence
  - Ataxia, dizziness
  - Headache
  - Nystagmus
  - Vomiting
  - Coma

## PRECAUTIONS

Because carbamazepine regularly induces its own metabolism, frequent dosage increases may be necessary. Valproate is not supposed to induce its own metabolism, but similar interventions are often necessary.

- Determine the patient's particular therapeutic 12-hour level once response has been optimal.
- Recheck level if response fades or patient develops side effects.

Carbamazepine and valproate should be used with caution in these settings:

- Heart block may be aggravated by carbamazepine.
  - Not a risk with valproate.
- Preexisting hematologic or liver disease warrants closer monitoring.
- Mild anticholinergic properties of carbamazepine can be problematic for patients with increased intraocular pressure, urinary retention, or dementia.
- Manufacturer's warning not to combine carbamazepine and MAOIs is based on tricyclic structure of carbamazepine and not on any actual interaction.
  - Because carbamazepine is not serotonergic, it can be combined safely with MAOIs.

## ADVICE FOR CARETAKERS

Patients should be informed about early problems with anticonvulsants:

- GI distress with valproate
- Bleeding, bruising, persistent sore throat, or failure of wounds to heal may be manifestations of bone marrow suppression.
- Physician should be informed about any rash.
- A rash with carbamazepine that is not clearly localized or that is associated with constitutional symptoms is indication to discontinue medication.
- Lamotrigine should be discontinued for any rash.
- Confusion or memory problems may indicate early neurotoxicity with carbamazepine.
  - Can occur at usual levels.
- Cognitive impairment can occur with any anticonvulsant.
  - Especially valproate and carbamazepine

## NOTES FOR PATIENT AND FAMILY

Common and important side effects of anticonvulsants include:

- Carbamazepine
  - Unsteadiness, incoordination, dizziness
  - Lightheadedness
  - Blurred vision
  - Weakness
  - Fatigue
  - Rash
  - Bruising

- Valproate
  - Nausea, abdominal pain, diarrhea
  - Increased appetite, weight gain
  - Cognitive impairment
- Lamotrigine
  - Fatigue, sedation
  - Rash
  - Increased appetite

Additional precautions

- Anticonvulsants should not be taken unless absolutely necessary if there is a possibility of patient becoming pregnant.
  - If pregnancy is suspected, do not immediately stop the medication.
    - Start taking folic acid.
    - Consult with physician immediately.
- Take valproate with food.
  - Food delays absorption without altering bioavailability.
  - If a dose is forgotten, it can be taken within 4 hours.
  - Otherwise, wait for next scheduled dose.
    - Do not take a double dose.
- Do not abruptly stop anticonvulsants without discussing with physician.
  - Withdrawal may cause a seizure.

# CHAPTER SEVEN

# Antianxiety Agents

Medications that reduce anxiety have diverse actions. Some of these actions produce sedation, and others do not. Use of most benzodiazepines as anxiolytics or hypnotics is largely based on marketing decisions; Other drugs used to treat anxiety are not necessarily sedating and are not used as sleeping pills. Primary antianxiety agents are discussed in this chapter; medications used primarily as sleeping pills are addressed in the next chapter.

This chapter covers

- Benzodiazepines
- Azapirones (e.g., buspirone)
- Adrenergic agents
- Antihistamines
- Propanediols (e.g., meprobamate)

Disorders discussed include:

- Adjustment disorder with anxious mood (p. 376)
- Agoraphobia (p. 382)
- Catatonia (pp. 392–393)
- Generalized anxiety disorder (pp. 376–379)
- Obsessive–compulsive disorder (pp. 384–389)
- Obsessive–compulsive spectrum disorders (pp. 389–390)
  - Body dysmorphic disorder
  - Eating disorders
  - Paraphilias
  - Pathological gambling
  - Pathological jealousy

- Sexual "addiction"
- Trichotillomania
- Panic disorder (pp. 379–382)
- Phobias (pp. 382–385)
- Posttraumatic stress disorder (pp. 390–392)
- Elective mutism (p. 384)
- Social phobia (pp. 382–383)

Conditions treated with antianxiety agents discussed in other chapters include:

- Aggression (Chapter 6)
- Akathisia (Chapter 1)
- CNS depressant withdrawal (Chapter 7)
- Delirium (Chapter 1)
- Dementia (Chapter 2)
- Mania (Chapter 5)
- Restless legs syndrome (Chapter 8)
- Schizophrenia (Antipsychotics, Chapter 1)

Table 7.1 provides a basic overview of the drugs discussed in this chapter.

## PHARMACOLOGY

Benzodiazepines have no central effect themselves, but they enhance the action of GABA (gamma-aminobutyric acid), the major inhibitory neurotransmitter in the CNS.

- The benzodiazepine–GABA receptor complex (Figure 7.1A) consists of allosterically linked receptors organized around a chloride ion channel (see Figure 7.1).
- When the $GABA_A$ receptor interacts with GABA, a change in the conformation of the complex occurs.
  - Chloride channels open and allow more negative charges into the neuron, thereby hyperpolarizing it (Figure 7.1B).
- Activation of the benzodiazepine receptor increases the affinity of the $GABA_A$ receptor for GABA, resulting in more chloride ion channel opening for every molecule of available GABA (Figure 7.1C).
- Benzodiazepine receptors located on noradrenergic arousal centers (e.g., the locus coeruleus) decrease arousal and activation of the sympathetic nervous system.
- Benzodiazepine receptors located in the cerebral cortex slow activity of

### Table 7.1  Names, Classes, Dose Forms, Colors

| GENERIC NAMES | BRAND NAMES | DOSE FORMS (MG)* | COLORS |
|---|---|---|---|
| **BENZODIAZEPINES** | | | |
| alprazolam | Xanax | t: 0.25/0.5/1/1 | t: white (oval)/peach/ blue/white (oblong) |
| alprazolam extended release | Xanax XR | t: 0.5/1/2/3 | t: white/yellow/blue/green |
| chlordiazepoxide | Librium | c: 5/10/25 p: 20 mg/ml | c: green-yellow/green- black/green-white |
| clonazepam | Klonopin | t: 0.5/1/2 | t: orange/blue/blue |
| clorazepate | Tranxene Tranxene-SD | t: 3.75/7.5/15 t: 11.25/22.5 | t: blue/peach/lavender t: blue/tan |
| diazepam | Valium | t: 2/5/10 p: 5 mg/ml | t: white/yellow/blue |
| halazepam | Paxipam | t: 20/40 | t: orange/white |
| lorazepam | Ativan | t: 0.5/1/2 p: 2/4 mg/ml | t: all white |
| oxazepam | Serax | t: 15 c: 10/15/30 | t: yellow c: white-pink/white-red/ white-maroon |
| *Azaspirodecanedione* buspirone | BuSpar | t: 5/7.5/10 d: 15/30 | t/d: all white |
| *Beta-Blocker* propranolol | Inderal | t: 10/20/40/60/80 | t: orange/blue green/pink/yellow |
| *α2-adrenergic agonist* clonidine | Catapres | t: 0.1/0.2/0.3 | t: tan/orange/peach |
| hydroxyzine | Atarax | t: 10/25/50/100 s: 10 mg/5 ml | t: orange/green/yellow/ red |
| | Vistaril | c: 25/50/100 su: 25 mg/ml | c: green/green-white/ green-gray |

\* c = capsules; p = parenteral; s = syrup; su = suspension; t = tablets; d = divided dose tablets.

those neurons, causing sedation and psychomotor impairment.

- Benzodiazepine receptors in pyramidal neurons have an anticonvulsant effect and cause muscle relaxation.
- Peripheral and mitochondrial benzodiazepine receptors are thought to mediate withdrawal and dependence.

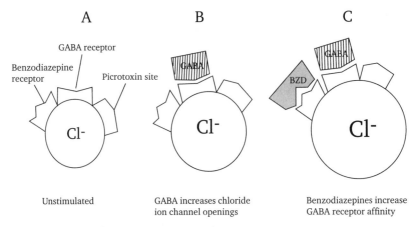

Figure 7.1 **Benzodiazepine Receptor Actions**

- At least three major benzodiazepine receptor subtypes have been identified:
  - Type 1 (omega-1): located in arousal centers
  - Type 2 (omega-2): located on pyramidal and cortical neurons
  - Type 3 (omega-3): located on peripheral sites
- An endogenous benzodiazepine receptor agonist exists in plants, but mammals cannot produce it.
- Mammals do have an endogenous inverse agonist (diazepam-binding inhibitor) of the GABA receptor, which
  - Decreases GABA receptor affinity for GABA.
  - Reduces chloride ion channel openings.
  - Depolarizes rather than hyperpolarizes neurons of arousal.
  - Primary function is probably to set the tone of arousal centers to an adaptive level.

There are four benzodiazepine classes:
- 2-keto
  - Diazepam, chlordiazepoxide, halazepam, clorazepate
  - Metabolized by oxidation.
  - Some (clorazepate, halazepam) are prodrugs.
    - They have no action themselves but are metabolized to desmethyldiazepam, which is biologically active.
  - Active drug (e.g., diazepam) or active metabolite has long-elimination half-life.
    - Half-life of desmethyldiazepam is 30–200 hours.

- 3-hydroxy
  - Lorazepam, oxazepam, temazepam
  - All are active.
  - Shorter elimination half-lives
  - Metabolized by glucuronidation to inactive compounds.
- Triazolo
  - Alprazolam, triazolam, estazolam, midazolam
  - All are active, without active metabolites.
  - Short elimination half-lives
  - Metabolized by oxidation.
- 7-nitro
  - Clonazepam
  - Active compound
  - No active metabolites
  - Metabolized by nitroreduction and oxidation.
- Medications and illnesses that interfere with hepatic oxidation (e.g., cimetidine) can antagonize oxidative metabolism of 2-keto and triazolo compounds.

Figure 7.2 summarizes benzodiazepine metabolism.

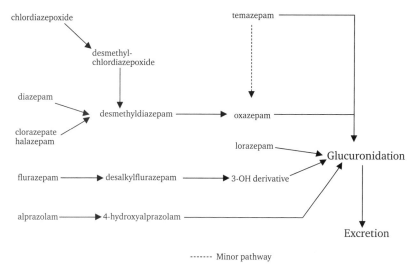

------- Minor pathway

**Figure 7.2  Simplified Benzodiazepine Metabolism**

### Features of Benzodiazepines

Regardless of chemical class, benzodiazepines can be categorized according to three dimensions:

- Lipid solubility
  - Benzodiazepines that are more lipid soluble (e.g., diazepam, alprazolam) are absorbed more rapidly orally and enter the brain rapidly along a concentration gradient.
    - Results in rapid onset of action.
    - As soon as the concentration gradient reverses itself, highly lipid-soluble benzodiazepines leave the brain rapidly, resulting in a more rapid offset of action.
  - Highly lipid-soluble benzodiazepines are distributed more widely in adipose tissue.
  - Less lipid-soluble benzodiazepines (e.g., lorazepam) enter and leave the brain slowly, resulting in slower onset of action but more sustained effect.
- Elimination half-life
  - Long half-life benzodiazepines (e.g., diazepam) are more likely to accumulate with multiple doses.
    - Drug accumulation more likely when a medication is given more frequently than its half-life.
  - Discontinuation syndromes with long half-life benzodiazepines are
    - Slower to appear
    - More prolonged
    - More attenuated
  - Benzodiazepines with shorter half-lives and simpler metabolism (e.g., oxazepam, lorazepam) are safer in patients with impaired hepatic metabolism (e.g., geriatric patients, those with liver disease).
- Potency
  - Higher-potency medications, which have more affinity for receptors, require lower doses to produce the same effect.
    - Examples of high-potency benzodiazepines are midazolam, triazolam, alprazolam, estazolam.
  - High-potency benzodiazepines are associated with more intense discontinuation syndromes.

The interaction of all three dimensions predicts the clinical features of a benzodiazepine.

- The combination of high potency, high lipid solubility, and short half-life (e.g., alprazolam, midazolam) is associated with
  - Rapid onset of action

- Brief duration of action
- Interdose withdrawal
- More severe and abrupt discontinuation syndromes
- Low potency, low lipid solubility, and long half-life (e.g., clonazepam) predict
  - Slow onset of action
  - Accumulation with continued dosing
  - Slower onset of discontinuation syndromes
  - More prolonged discontinuation syndromes

Effects with acute dosing are not the same as with chronic dosing of longer half-life benzodiazepines.

- With single doses, lipid solubility and distribution half-life are more important.
  - Lorazepam is low in lipid solubility, resulting in a slow onset of action.
    - Slow departure from the brain and slow distribution results in a longer duration of action after a single dose, even though it has a fairly short elimination half-life.
  - Diazepam, which is higher in lipid solubility, enters and leaves the brain more rapidly and distributes more widely.
    - This results in more rapid but shorter duration of action after a single dose, even though diazepam has a longer elimination half-life.
- With chronic dosing, elimination half-life plays a more important role.
  - Once the drug has entered a steady state, transfer of medication from the bloodstream to the brain occurs at a constant level.
  - Medications with shorter half-lives must be given more frequently to maintain a steady-state concentration.
  - Long half-life benzodiazepines that are higher in potency and lipid solubility (e.g., diazepam) often have to be taken more frequently than would be predicted by their rate of elimination from the body, because single additional doses result in blood and brain level peaks that return rapidly to baseline.
- Short half-life benzodiazepines that have high potency and high lipid solubility must be taken frequently in chronic as well as acute treatment.
  - Alprazolam often must be given every 2–3 hours to prevent interdose withdrawal.

## CLINICAL INDICATIONS AND USE

### General Information

PROPANEDIOLS

The only currently available propanediol is meprobamate. This drug is generally a poor choice for the treatment of anxiety, as are the barbiturates, because it

- Has dangerous side effects
- Is fatal in overdose
- Causes dangerous withdrawal syndromes
- Induces metabolizing enzymes, requiring dosage escalation

BENZODIAZEPINES

Benzodiazepines are best used to treat time-limited anxiety that arises in response to identifiable stressors. Some patients, however, take these medications chronically. Predictors of a good response to benzodiazepines include

- Acute symptoms
- Precipitating stress
- High levels of anxiety
- Low levels of depression
- Previous good response
- Awareness that problem is mental
- Desire to be treated with a medication
    - Many anxious patients prefer not to receive medications

Treatment of anxiety with benzodiazepines results in

- Marked improvement in 25–35%
- Moderate improvement in 40%
- Minimal improvement in 25%

Benzodiazepines are among the most effective and safest antianxiety agents. However, their use, especially chronically, can also pose problems. Among these are:

- Side effects such as sedation and psychomotor impairment.
- Drug dependence
- Discontinuation syndromes
- Interdose withdrawal with short-acting benzodiazepines
    - Especially alprazolam

- Interactions with other CNS depressants
  - Especially alcohol
- Benzodiazepines can reinforce passive approach to illness and desire for immediate relief from a pill.
  Physical dependence consists of tolerance and withdrawal.
- Tolerance develops to sedative effects of benzodiazepines but not to anxiolytic effect.
  - Tolerance to psychomotor impairment may occur.
- Discontinuation syndromes can occur with
  - three to four times the usual daily dose for a few weeks
  - Usual therapeutic doses for 8 months or more

Three kinds of syndromes may occur when benzodiazepines are discontinued.

- Relapse
  - Return of original anxiety
  - Gradual over weeks to months
- Rebound
  - Intensification of original anxiety
  - Rapid over days to weeks
  - Abates over weeks
- Withdrawal (discussed in Chapter 8, pp. 441–449)
  - New physiological signs and symptoms, such as
    - Autonomic signs (e.g., hypertension, tachycardia)
    - Diaphoresis
    - Muscle twitching
    - Confusion
    - Delirium
    - Seizures
  - Appears within hours to weeks, usually lasts days to weeks.
  - Subtle withdrawal symptoms have been reported for a year after discontinuation of long-acting benzodiazepines taken for extended periods of time at therapeutic doses.
  - Withdrawal appears later and lasts longer, but is more attenuated, with long half-life, low-potency benzodiazepines.
  - Gradual benzodiazepine discontinuation after chronic use often prevents severe withdrawal symptoms.
  - Withdrawal is more difficult with alprazolam.
    - As dose is reduced below 1 mg, benzodiazepine receptors paradoxically down-regulate, resulting in fewer receptors available to declining molecules of the benzodiazepine.

- Switching to a longer-acting benzodiazepine and withdrawing that medication may be better tolerated.

Escalating the dose to prevent withdrawal is more likely with

- Use of high-potency, short half-life, very lipid-soluble benzodiazepines (e.g., alprazolam).
- Waiting until anxiety is intolerable before taking the medication prn.
- Taking medications regularly at an interval significantly longer than the duration of action.
  - Taking higher doses increases this problem because a greater concentration gradient develops after each dose, resulting in more intense withdrawal after initial relief.
- Benzodiazepine misuse is rare in medical practice when benzodiazepines are prescribed for anxiety. Risk factors include
  - History of misuse of drugs or alcohol
  - Losing prescriptions
  - Taking high doses at some times and no medication at others
- Benzodiazepines with a higher risk of misuse include
  - Alprazolam
  - Diazepam
  - Lorazepam
- The risk of misuse is lower with long half-life low-lipid soluble benzodiazepines such as
  - Chlordiazepoxide
  - Clonazepam
- Benzodiazepines sometimes aggravate depression, but more frequently they do not aggravate or improve it.
  - Alprazolam is the only benzodiazepine that has been found to have antidepressant properties.

ANTIDEPRESSANTS

Most antidepressants are effective for anxiety disorders.

- Bupropion may be least reliable for severe primary anxiety disorders, but it is sometimes useful in primary care settings.
- Controlled studies for TCAs, especially imipramine and clomipramine, in panic disorder:
  - Therapeutic doses of TCAs may be lower in panic disorder.
- A number of TCAs, especially desipramine and doxepin, have been effective in controlled studies of GAD.
  - A randomized placebo-controlled comparison of imipramine (mean dose 143 mg), trazodone (mean dose 255 mg), and diazepam (mean dose 26 mg) in 230 patients with GAD found moderate–marked

improvement in 73% on imipramine, 69% with trazodone, 66% with diazepam, and 47% on placebo (Rickels, Downing, Sweizer, & Hassman, 1993).

- TCAs also useful for separation anxiety in children.
- Controlled studies support use of citalopram, escitalopram, paroxetine, and venlafaxine for GAD.
  - An 8-week randomized placebo-controlled trial of paroxetine 20 or 40 mg/day in GAD found a 62% response rate with 20 mg paroxetine, 68% response rate with 40 mg paroxetine, and 46% response rate with placebo (Rickels et al., 2003).
    - Remission (HAM-A total score ≤ 7) was achieved in 30%, 36%, and 20% of groups, respectively.
  - All SSRIs are probably equally effective.
  - Venlafaxine effective in GAD in controlled trials.
    - A survival analysis of two placebo-controlled randomized 6-month studies of once daily venlafaxine XR 75–225 mg/day (flexible dose) or 37.5–150 mg (fixed dose) in GAD found that placebo-treated patients discontinued treatment due to lack of efficacy significantly more frequently than venlafaxine-treated patients (Montgomery, Mahe, Haudiquet, & Hackett, 2002).
    - Appears effective for other anxiety disorders.
- All antidepressants other than bupropion are effective for panic disorder.
  - For example, a 10-week double-blind comparison of escitalopram, citalopram, and placebo in 366 patients with panic disorder found both SSRIs to be significantly > placebo in reducing panic attack frequency (Stahl, Gergel, & Li, 2003).
  - An open 3-month trial of 30 mg mirtazepine in 45 patients with panic disorder, with or without agoraphobia (11 with comorbid major depression), found it to be effective in reducing anticipatory anxiety and the number and severity of panic attacks (Sarchiapone et al., 2003).
    - Presence of depression did not influence the results.
- MAO inhibitors are the most effective medications for panic disorder and social phobia.
- A 12-week industry-sponsored double-blind controlled study of generalized social anxiety disorder found that sertraline (mean dose 159 mg) produced significantly greater reductions than placebo in Liebowitz Social Anxiety Scale scores (−31.0 vs. −21.7) and significantly more patients with CGI-I ratings of much, or very much, improved (56% vs. 29%; Liebowitz et al., 2003).
- A placebo-controlled multicenter study had single-blind acute treatment for 12 weeks and double-blind maintenance phase for 24 weeks (Stein, Versiani, et al., 2002).

- Of 435 patients who entered a single-blind 12-week study, all of whom received paroxetine titrated up to a maximum of 50 mg/day (mean dose 37 mg), 323 responded and were randomized to continue paroxetine or switch to placebo over a 3-week period. The placebo-controlled phase lasted 24 weeks.
- Mean dose of paroxetine for the 136 patients who completed the double-blind phase was also 37 mg; 161 patients were assigned to placebo.
- 84% of paroxetine patients and 75% of placebo patients completed the study.
- Relapse rates were 14% for paroxetine and 39% for placebo.
  - Estimated probability for relapse at any time was 3.29 times greater for placebo ($p < 0.001$).
- Paroxetine produced significantly greater reduction of scores on the Liebowitz Social Anxiety Scale, Social Phobia Inventory, and Sheehan Disability Scale.

- The antianxiety action of antidepressants is independent of sedation.
- All antidepressants can increase anxiety initially.
  - Anxiety is associated with hyperactive noradrenergic arousal systems.
  - Because of interactions between noradrenergic and serotonergic neurons, even SSRIs can increase norepinephrine neurotransmission.
  - Eventually, noradrenergic activity down-regulates, resulting in decreased anxiety.
  - Dropout rates are higher in patients who develop early jitteriness.
  - Benzodiazepines often used to reduce initial activation.
    - Once antidepressant has taken effect, it may be possible to withdraw the benzodiazepine.

### Beta-Adrenergic Blockers

Beta-blockers antagonize hyperactivity in central and peripheral adrenergic stress-response systems, including the sympathetic nervous system.

- Reducing peripheral signs of activation (e.g., tachycardia, tremor) may decrease cues to anxiety, especially performance anxiety.
- Most useful for patients with
  - Palpitations
  - Tachycardia
  - GI symptoms
  - Tremor
  - Sweating
- Less useful for psychic anxiety

Propranolol
- Blocks beta-1 (cardiac) and beta-2 (pulmonary) receptors.
  - Because circulating catecholamines stimulate bronchiolar relaxation, propranolol contraindicated in asthma.
  - Also reduces mobilization of glucose by catecholamines.
    - Risk of dangerous hypoglycemia in diabetes mellitus
  - Reduced ability to increase heart rate may impair exercise tolerance.
- Rapid withdrawal can cause rebound hypertension.
- Do not give propranolol to patients with
  - Significant bradycardia
  - Hypotension
  - Heart failure
  - Asthma
  - Diabetes
- In treatment of performance anxiety, a single dose of 5–20 mg is sufficient.
  - Determine the optimal dose before patient faces the performance situation.
- Doses of 40–120 mg/day can be used as adjunctive treatment for physiological symptoms of anxiety.
  - Also used to treat tremor and sweating caused by adrenergic medications.
  - Monitor pulse and blood pressure.
    - Do not allow heart rate to fall below 60.
- Central effects of propranolol can cause sedation and sexual dysfunction.
  - Propranolol has not been found to induce or exacerbate depression predictably.
- Alternative lipid-soluble beta-blockers that enter the brain and are better tolerated (have less hypotension and bradycardia than propranolol) but not as well studied include
  - Pindolol
  - Metropolol
  - Acebutolol
- Beta-blockers that are not as lipid soluble and do not cause central side effects include
  - Atenolol
  - Nadolol
- Elimination half-lives (hours)
  - Propranolol: 4
  - Nadolol: 22

- Atenolol: 7
- Propranolol LA
  - Slow-release form has longer duration of action.
- For elderly patients and patients with impaired hepatic function, choose beta-blockers that are directly excreted by the kidneys:
  - Atenolol
  - Carteolol
  - Nadolol
- Beta-blockers, especially propranolol, are useful for unpredictable aggressive behavior in demented and brain-damaged patients (see p. 101).
  - Also may be useful for intermittent explosive disorder.
  - Starting dose is 10 mg.
  - Increase to 10 mg qid.
  - Then increase each dose to 20–80 mg qid.
  - Some patients require and tolerate higher doses.
  - Onset of action takes about a month.

## CLONIDINE

Used for hyperactivity in ADHD.
- Usually not a practical treatment for anxiety.
- Start with 0.1 mg.
- Increase to 0.2–0.6 mg/day.
- Significant risk of adverse effects, including
  - Sedation
  - Depression
  - Cognitive impairment
  - Rebound hypertension if withdrawn too rapidly

## ANTIHISTAMINES

Antihistamines are sometimes used to treat anxiety, but apparent reduction in anxiety is often an artifact of sedation.
- Examples
  - Hydroxyzine
    - 25–100 mg/day
  - Diphenhydramine
    - 25–50 mg/day
- May be useful for patients who have to be sedated for an EEG.
  - Minimal effect on EEG
- Tolerance develops rapidly to sedation, making use as hypnotics unreliable.
- Anticholinergic side effects limit use in cognitively impaired patients.

## AZAPIRONES

Azapirones are partial agonists of 5HT1A receptors. These receptors are both presynaptic and postsynaptic. A partial agonist effect at both sites enhances low endogenous serotonin neurotransmission and reduces excessive serotonin neurotransmission

- Relationship of this action to the actual therapeutic effect is unclear.
- Only buspirone is currently available.
- Gepirone is currently undergoing phase-III trials.
- Used primarily for GAD in doses of 15–30 mg/day.
  - May also be helpful for social anxiety.
  - May be adjunct in treatment of PTSD.
  - Not effective in panic disorder or OCD.
- Higher doses (45–90 mg/day) have antidepressant properties and are probably more reliable in treating anxiety.
  - Can be useful in augmentation of antidepressants in depression accompanied by anxiety.
- Patients previously treated with benzodiazepines do not respond as well to buspirone.
  - Onset of action is much slower (around 1 month, as for antidepressants).
  - No acute response occurs that reassures patient that medication is working.
  - Patients switched from benzodiazepines to buspirone may experience prolonged subtle discontinuation syndromes not suppressed by buspirone because the medication classes are not cross-reactive.
- Advantages
  - No sedation, cognitive impairment, or weight gain
  - No impairment of driving
  - No risk of dependence, withdrawal, or drug seeking
- Disadvantages
  - Because onset of action is slow and continued treatment is necessary, cannot be used prn or for acute anxiety.
  - Not as effective as benzodiazepines.
- Because it has serotonergic properties, buspirone should not be combined with MAOIs.

## ANTICONVULSANTS

Antidepressants with actions on GABAergic systems have antianxiety properties.

- Valproate found effective for panic disorder.

- Divalproex was given openly in doses to produce serum levels of 45–90 µg/mL to patients with panic disorder and mood instability refractory to other drugs (Baetz & Bowen, 1998).
  - The 10 of 13 patients who completed the study all had statistically significant improvement of depression, anxiety, mood instability, panic attacks, and quality of life.
- Initial choice for bipolar disorder with comorbid anxiety.
- Gabapentin can be useful for anxiety and depression.
  - 103 patients with panic disorder were randomly assigned to 8 weeks of double-blind treatment with gabapentin or placebo (Pande et al., 2000).
    - The dose of gabapentin was increased, as needed, to 600–3600 mg/day.
    - There was no overall difference between gabapentin and placebo in scores on the Panic and Agoraphobia Scale. However, gabapentin was superior to placebo in patients with initial higher scores on this scale.
  - A study of social phobia randomly assigned 69 patients to double-blind treatment with 900–3600 mg/day of gabapentin or placebo for 14 weeks (Pande et al., 1999).
    - Gabapentin produced significantly more reduction of social phobia symptoms than placebo on both clinician- and patient-rated scales.
  - Not reliable as mood stabilizer.
  - Must be taken tid.
  - Can cause excessive sedation or activation.
- Pregabalin is an anticonvulsant GABA analogue related to gabapentin with anxiolytic and antidepressant properties.
  - Rapidly absorbed
  - Does not bind to plasma proteins
  - Plasma half-life 6 hours
  - Linear pharmacokinetics
  - Excreted unchanged by kidneys
  - Not effective for mania
  - Well tolerated
  - A 4-week double blind study of pregabalin 150 or 600 mg/day, lorazepam 6 mg/day, or placebo in 276 patients with GAD found (Pande et al., 2003):
    - Hamilton anxiety scale scores decreased significantly more in all active treatment groups compared with placebo.
    - The decrease in anxiety scores was similar for both doses of pregabalin and for lorazepam.

- Frequency of responders (≥ 50% improvement) was significantly greater for 600 mg pregabalin (46%) and lorazepam (61%) than placebo (27%).
  - Withdrawal symptoms were similar to placebo.
- Most common side effects
  - Dizziness
  - Weight gain averaged 2.2 kg with 600 mg/day in study summarized above (Pande et al., 2003).
  - Somnolence
  - Dry mouth
- Tiagabine
  - Anticonvulsant that inhibits GABA reuptake pump.
  - Does not appear to cause physical dependence, tolerance, or withdrawal.
  - Five patients whose treatment with SSRIs or TCAs was augmented with tiagabine 10–16 mg/day had improvement of refractory anxiety (Schwartz, 2002).
- Consider anticonvulsants for
  - Patients with history of drug misuse
  - Anxious patients with comorbid mood disorders

### Antipsychotic Drugs

Antipsychotic drugs are not considered first choices for nonpsychotic anxiety.
- They may be useful for anxiety associated with feelings of disorganization or loss of boundary in patients with personality disorders.
  - Use low doses if possible.
- Anxiety secondary to organic brain disease sometimes responds better to antipsychotics, with fewer cognitive side effects and less disinhibition than benzodiazepines.
- Despite lack of extensive clinical experience, atypical antipsychotics are preferable to neuroleptics.
  - Risperidone 0.5–2 mg/day
  - Olanzapine 2.5–10 mg/day
- An 8-week double-blind study of olanzapine up to 20 mg (N = 7) or placebo (N = 5) found olanzapine significantly superior to placebo for social phobia.
  - However, only four olanzapine patients and three placebo patients completed the entire study (Barnett, Kramer, Casat, Connor, & Davidson, 2002).

- Patients with insomnia may prefer a sedating antipsychotic.
  - Most useful when risk of substance abuse.
  - Sedation may be frightening to hypervigilant anxious patients.

## CLINICAL INDICATIONS AND USE

### Adjustment Disorder with Anxious Mood

Rapid onset of action makes benzodiazepines the first choice for acute situational anxiety. Such situations may include

- Psychosocial stress or crisis
- Acute medical illness or hospitalization
  - Anxiety increases catecholamine release, which can be dangerous for patients with myocardial injury (e.g., recent MI).
    - Minimization of acute anxiety can reduce the risk of arrhythmia.
- Time-limited intermittent stressor (e.g., planned airplane trip by someone who is afraid of flying)
  - Stresses involving performance anxiety are treated differently (see pp. 284–285).

Guidelines for treatment of situational anxiety

- Benzodiazepine dosing prn is useful for intermittent stress or fluctuating response to an ongoing stress.
  - Patients who need a rapid response do best with a highly lipid-soluble, relatively high-potency agent such as alprazolam or diazepam.
  - Lorazepam and oxazepam, which have shorter half-lives, have a slower onset of action after a single dose because they are less lipid soluble.
    - Patients who experience rapid onset of benzodiazepine effect as frightening or dysphoric should receive one of these benzodiazepines instead of one that is very lipid soluble.
- If stress is pervasive and ongoing, or if patient is medically ill, give benzodiazepine regularly.
  - Benzodiazepines with half lives > 24 hours are likely to accumulate with regular dosing
  - If taken prn, time dosing to coincide with reexposure to the stressor.
- If stress becomes chronic, consider transition to antidepressant or buspirone.

### Generalized Anxiety Disorder (GAD)

GAD is characterized by chronic excessive worry with both psychic and somatic symptoms. Because GAD is persistent or relapsing, indefinite treatment is usually indicated. Behavioral and cognitive techniques should always be considered; these are not only effective but enhance feelings of mastery over anxiety.

## Benzodiazepines

- Placebo response rate is high (50–60%) and spontaneous fluctuation of symptoms is common, making evaluation of medication trials < 6 months' duration difficult.
- It is often recommended that benzodiazepines not be used chronically for GAD because of concerns about drug dependence and adverse effects.
  - In the average office setting, benzodiazepine misuse is uncommon in the absence of a history of substance abuse.
  - A review of records of 2,440 Medicaid patients taking benzodiazepines (460 new and 1,980 ongoing prescriptions) showed that the median dose remained constant at about 10 mg diazepam equivalent for at least 2 years of continuous use (Soumerai et al., 2003).
    - Dosage was escalated in only 1.6%.
    - Most common when patients filled duplicate benzodiazepine prescriptions within first 7 days.
  - Tolerance develops to sedative but not anxiolytic effects.
  - Transition to an antidepressant or other alternative may be possible over many months.
    - Some patients require chronic treatment with a benzodiazepine.
  - Chronic use of very short-acting benzodiazepines such as alprazolam is usually troublesome because of interdose withdrawal and difficulty eventually withdrawing medication.
- If a benzodiazepine is used chronically for GAD, begin with a preparation with an intermediate (e.g., oxazepam, lorazepam) or long (e.g., clonazepam, chlordiazepoxide) half-life.
- If benzodiazepine is withdrawn, decrease dose very gradually over 3–6 months to reduce risk of rebound and withdrawal symptoms.
  - Relapse during the first year after withdrawing benzodiazepine around 50–70%.
- If another medication is to be substituted, maximize treatment with that medicine before beginning to withdraw the benzodiazepine.

## Buspirone

Buspirone has fewer adverse effects than benzodiazepines but is less predictably effective, especially with more severely anxious patients.

- Initial benefit may begin in 2–4 weeks.
  - Full response takes 4–6 weeks.

- Buspirone must be taken regularly.
- Buspirone is initial choice for patients with history of substance abuse or pulmonary disease and for patients who operate heavy equipment, trucks, airplanes, etc.
- Switching directly from a benzodiazepine to buspirone is often unsuccessful.
    - Buspirone is not cross-reactive with benzodiazepines and does not prevent rebound or withdrawal.
    - Patients accustomed to rapid relief after taking a benzodiazepine are disappointed when buspirone does not have the same effect.
    - Add buspirone first and maximize dose. Attempt to reduce dose of benzodiazepine very slowly once response to buspirone has been assessed.
- Dose for moderate anxiety
    - Start at 5 mg bid–tid.
    - Increase by 5 mg q 4–7 days, to 30 mg.
    - If no response after 4 weeks, increase to 45–60 mg.
- Dose for severe anxiety
    - Start with 5–10 mg tid.
    - Increase by 5 mg q 2–4 days, to 45–90 mg.
- Dose for augmentation of antidepressant in anxious depression
    - Start with 5 mg tid.
    - Increase gradually to 45–90 mg/day, given tid.

## ANTIDEPRESSANTS

- Most antidepressants other than bupropion are effective for GAD without depression.
- Doses are similar to doses for depression.
- In patients with primary anxiety, and with both depression and anxiety, all antidepressants can cause initial activation characterized by
    - Increased anxiety
    - Agitation
    - Tremor
    - Insomnia
    - Sweating
- Early jitteriness most frequent in patients with panic attacks.
- Caused by noradrenergic effect of antidepressants, which occurs with SSRIs as well as norepinephrine reuptake inhibitors, because increasing serotonin activity secondarily enhances norepinephrine release.

- Management of antidepressant-induced jitteriness:
  - Start with very low antidepressant doses (e.g., 1–2 mg fluoxetine equivalent).
  - Increase dose slowly (e.g., q 1–2 weeks).
  - Administer benzodiazepine first. When anxiety is completely suppressed, add antidepressant. Once antianxiety effect of antidepressant is manifested, start slowly withdrawing benzodiazepine.
- If insomnia is significant, use a more sedating antidepressant at bedtime or combine nonsedating antidepressant with a hypnotic (see Chapter 8).
  - It may be possible to withdraw hypnotic once anxiety has remitted.

### ANTICONVULSANTS

Several anticonvulsants have antianxiety properties that can be useful in GAD, especially when concerns exist about substance dependence and the patient cannot tolerate an antidepressant.

- Gabapentin is the most reliable.
- Divalproex is sometimes useful but may be difficult for anxious patients to tolerate.

### BETA-BLOCKERS

Beta blockers are primarily helpful when GAD is accompanied by prominent autonomic symptoms such as palpitations, sweating, or tremor.

- Beta-blockers that are less lipid soluble may reduce these symptoms with lower risk of dysphoria, sexual dysfunction and sedation than propranolol.
- Can be added prn for comorbid performance anxiety.

## Panic Disorder

Cognitive–behavior therapy (panic control therapy), with systematic desensitization for avoidance, should be a component of the treatment of panic disorder. The relapsing nature of panic disorder is an indication for indefinite treatment with effective medications.

### BENZODIAZEPINES

- Most published experience is with alprazolam.
  - Start with 0.125–0.25 mg one–four times per day.
  - Increase dose slowly to 2–6 mg/day.
    - Some patients require higher doses.

- Short elimination half-life, high lipid solubility, and high potency increase likelihood of interdose withdrawal that occurs at shorter intervals than would be predicted from half-life alone.
  - Some patients note rebound anxiety 2–3 hours after each dose.
  - Have patient take medication frequently enough to avoid rebound anxiety.
  - Attempting to wait as long as possible before the next dose in order to avoid becoming dependent on alprazolam may make the patient more preoccupied with anxiety and its relief, increasing the risk of drug misuse.
  - Withdrawal of alprazolam can be complicated by paradoxical down-regulation of benzodiazepine receptors as the dose is reduced below 1 mg.
  - Management: (1) cross over slowly to a longer-acting benzodiazepine and then very gradually withdraw that medication; (2) wait until the new medication achieves steady state before starting to withdraw alprazolam.
  - In view of high comorbidity of panic disorder and bipolar disorder, it is important to bear in mind that alprazolam is the only benzodiazepine that has been reported to induce mania.
- Equivalent doses of other benzodiazepines are effective, but sedation can be a limiting side effect at these doses.
  - For example, 40–60 mg/day of diazepam

## ANTIDEPRESSANTS

- Preferable to benzodiazepines
- Fewer concerns about adverse effects with ongoing treatment, especially with high doses of benzodiazepines
- Comorbid depression occurs in 50–90% of panic disorder patients.
  - Antidepressants are effective for panic disorder whether or not depression is also present.
  - Reduction in anxiety may be attributable to down-regulation of noradrenergic neurotransmission in locus coeruleus
    - Facilitates exposure to panicogenic situations, which may be final common pathway of effective treatments.
- Many patients need usual therapeutic doses, but some patients do well with lower doses.
- TCAs, especially imipramine, have been most widely studied in panic disorder.
  - These medications are now second-line treatments for panic disorder because they are more difficult to tolerate than newer antidepressants.

- Initial choice is SSRI or venlafaxine.
  - Controlled data for venlafaxine, paroxetine, fluvoxamine, citalopram, escitalopram
  - Less data for nefazodone and mirtazepine
- Principles of using antidepressants for panic disorder, with or without depression:
  - Start with very small dose (e.g., 2.5–5 mg escitalopram, 5 mg desipramine).
  - Increase dose by the same small amount no more frequently than once every 1–2 weeks.
  - Have patient call after each dosage increase.
    - Anxious patients, especially those with panic attacks, are hyper-vigilant for anything that feels dangerous or out of place.
    - Contact with clinician increases patient's sense of safety.
    - Encouraging patient to call only for side effects may increase patient's vigilance for adverse events.
  - For mild antidepressant-induced jitteriness
    - Add benzodiazepine and increase dose until jitteriness remits before escalating antidepressant dose.
  - For more severe jitteriness after starting an antidepressant, or history of severe reactions to other antidepressants
    - Withdraw antidepressant and maximize benzodiazepine first; then reinstitute antidepressant slowly.
  - Relaxation training, self-hypnosis, and related techniques also may reduce antidepressant-induced activation and give patient a greater feeling of control and engagement with treatment.

## MAO INHIBITORS

- MAOIs are probably more effective than other antidepressants for panic disorder and possibly for depression with prominent anxiety.
- Improvement is gradual.
- More activating MAOIs (e.g., selegeline, tranylcypromine) may be more difficult for anxious patients to tolerate than less activating MAOIs (e.g., phenelzine, isocarboxazid).
- Start with no more than one pill and increase dose slowly.
- Anxious patients need more reassurance about need for dietary restrictions.

## VALPROATE

- GABAergic action provides potential anxiolytic effect.
- Moderately effective for panic disorder

- Initial choice for patients with comorbid bipolar disorder and panic disorder

### VERAPAMIL

- May be useful as adjunct in panic disorder.
- Usual dose is 160–320 mg/day.

### TREATMENT RESISTANCE

- Complex and refractory panic disorder often requires combination therapy.
  - Antidepressant + benzodiazepine
  - Antidepressant + valproate or verapamil
  - TCA + MAOI
- Cognitive and behavioral techniques should be added whenever medications are not fully effective.
  - Panic control therapy is especially useful.

## Phobic Disorders

Specific phobias are treated with exposure and relaxation. Medications are seldom appropriate for these conditions. When medications are used for other phobic disorders, an important action may involve reducing arousal sufficiently to promote exposure, which is the primary therapeutic mechanism.

### AGORAPHOBIA

- May occur with or without panic disorder.
- Anxiety in situations in which a panic attack might occur or from which escape may be difficult or help may be unavailable
- Medication treatment is the same as for panic disorder.
  - Alprazolam 2–6 mg/day
  - Antidepressants in usual doses
    - SSRIs
    - TCAs
    - MAOIs
- If medication does not facilitate sufficient spontaneous exposure, formal exposure/systematic desensitization should be considered.

### SOCIAL PHOBIA (SOCIAL ANXIETY DISORDER)

- Occurs in various forms in 8–13% of population.
- Major depression and substance abuse (usually as self-treatment for anxiety in social settings) are frequently comorbid with social phobia.

- Antidepressants are initial treatment.
  - Response may take 6–10 weeks.
  - SSRIs are first choice.
    - Controlled data available for paroxetine, citalopram.
    - Others are probably equally effective.
  - Venlafaxine may be effective when other agents do not produce complete improvement.
  - MAOIs most effective in usual antidepressant doses.
- Alprazolam may be useful, but caution is required because of high co-morbidity with substance dependence.
  - Benefit is lost when medication discontinued.
  - Clonazepam (0.5–3 mg/day) reduces social anxiety within 1–6 weeks.
  - It may be possible to reduce dose after 6 months of treatment.
  - Other benzodiazepines useful mostly as prn agents when anxiety-provoking social situations are anticipated.
- Buspirone
  - May be somewhat helpful in doses of 45–90 mg/day.
  - Onset of action takes up to 12 weeks.
- Gabapentin
  - Better than placebo in a small study

## PERFORMANCE ANXIETY

Performance anxiety is a specific form of social anxiety that is usually treated with beta-blockers in anticipation of performance situations.

- Commonly used agents
  - Metropolol 25–50 mg
  - Atenolol 25–50 mg
  - Propranolol 5–20 mg
- Beta-blockers decrease distress in social situations by antagonizing signs and symptoms of autonomic arousal, such as
  - Tachycardia
  - Palpitations
  - Tremor
  - Sweating
  - Dry mouth
  - Butterflies in stomach
- Protocol for use of beta-blockers for performance anxiety:
  - Take test dose of 5–10 mg propranolol or equivalent to determine that it will be tolerated.

- Visualize the anxiety-provoking situation.
  - Increase the dose if the initial dose does not seem helpful.
  - Take the medication 2 hours prior to performance situation.
  - Increase dose by 10 mg propranolol or equivalent until anxiety is prevented.
  - Take medication regularly in morning when frequent repeated episodes of performance anxiety are anticipated (e.g., walking into a classroom each day)
- Benzodiazepines can reduce acute performance anxiety, but they also impair performance.
- Chronic and repeated performance anxiety is an indication for a trial of an SSRI or MAOI.

Elective Mutism

Elective mutism may be an early-onset social phobia variant.

- SSRI (e.g., fluoxetine 10–30 mg/day) can be useful.
- Benzodiazepines are occasionally helpful.

## Separation Anxiety Disorder

- TCAs such as imipramine have best data but require special precautions when used in children (pp. 126–127).
  - Start with 10–25 mg imipramine at bedtime and increase gradually.
  - When recovery occurs, it is usually within 6–8 weeks.
  - Try to withdraw medication after 3 months.
  - For school phobia
    - Start with 10 mg imipramine at bedtime in younger children, 25 mg for older children.
  - Target dose around 3.5–5 mg/kg/day.
- SSRIs may be effective, but little controlled data.

## Obsessive–Compulsive Disorder (OCD)

Although serotonergic antidepressants are most reliably helpful for OCD, the disorder is associated with increased CSF serotonin turnover, and serotonin reuptake inhibitors (SRIs) reduce serotonin turnover in OCD.

- Suggests that increased serotonergic transmission is a compensatory response to intrusive experience caused by faulty circuits between inhibitory frontal and striatal behavior-generating systems.
  - Compensatory response is further facilitated by SRI.

- A meta-analysis of 36 randomized controlled trials of clomipramine and SSRIs in OCD revealed that both classes of medication were better than placebo for OCD, obsessions, and compulsions (Piccinelli, Pini, Bellantuono, & Wilkinson, 1995).
  - Effect sizes for clomipramine were 1.31–1.47.
  - Effect sizes for SSRIs were 0.47–0.52.
- Response rates with SRIs are inferior to behavior therapy.
  - 10–15% have remission.
  - 40–50% have response.
    - Average response is about 50% reduction of symptoms.
    - 70% have some response.
  - Response is lost when medication is withdrawn.
  - Exposure + response prevention:
    - 70–80% have response after average 20 sessions.
    - Higher dropout rate than with antidepressants because treatment is more stressful.
    - Response is sustained over years after treatment discontinued.
    - Adding antidepressant does not measurably increase good response to behavior therapy, but combination of treatments is important in management of treatment resistance.

## SRIs

- Clomipramine has best reported response rate (50%) in intention to treat (LOCF) analyses.
  - This is probably a function of fewer dropouts in clomipramine trials, which were conducted when alternative medications were not available and patients were more motivated to remain in treatment.
  - Head-to-head comparisons suggest equal efficacy of SRIs in equivalent doses.
- Response to SRIs may take 3 months.
  - Higher doses than those used to treat depression are often necessary.
- Clomipramine
  - Target dose 200–250 mg/day
    - Higher doses associated with increased seizure risk.
    - Serum concentrations may rise to dangerous levels when higher clomipramine doses are combined with stimulants or with 2D6 inhibitors such as fluoxetine or paroxetine.
  - Clomipramine is a pure SSRI, but is has a desmethyl metabolite that is a norepinephrine reuptake inhibitor and can cause noradrenergic effects.

- Common adverse effects leading to discontinuation include
  - Sedation
  - Anticholinergic side effects
  - Weight gain
  - Noradrenergic side effects such as tremor, sweating
- SSRIs
  - Usually first choice because most are better tolerated than clomipramine.
  - Usual doses in OCD
    - Fluoxetine: 60–120 mg/day
    - Sertraline: 150–200 mg/day
    - Paroxetine: 40–80 mg/day
    - Fluvoxamine: 200–300 mg/day (best data in OCD; divided dose necessary)
    - Citalopram: 40–80 mg/day
    - Escitalopram: Probably 20–60 mg/day
  - Side effects such as sexual dysfunction, tremor, dizziness, and anticholinergic side effects with clomipramine may predict treatment response, probably because they are indications of higher doses.

### Venlafaxine

- Use (mean dose 232 mg) reviewed in 39 patients with DSM-IV OCD, 29 of whom had not responded to SRIs (Hollander et al., 2003).
  - 27 patients (76%) were much improved or very much improved on CGI.
  - 24% of those who had failed previous SRI trials were improved or very much improved.
  - No assessment of specific OCD symptoms included.

Published research on pharmacological treatment of OCD in children and adolescents consists of one randomized controlled trial of sertraline and three of fluoxetine; a multicenter trial of paroxetine is underway.

- A double-blind study randomly assigned 43 patients, ages 6–18, to placebo or fluoxetine in doses of 60 mg for the first 6 weeks and then up to 80 mg (Liebowitz et al., 2002).
  - Patients who responded after 8 weeks entered a maintenance phase for another 8 weeks, during which they continued the same treatment; nonresponders were offered open treatment with fluoxetine.
  - After the acute (first 8-week) phase, 57% of fluoxetine patients vs. 32% of placebo patients were improved or very much improved on CGI-I, but the difference was not statistically significant.

- During the maintenance phase, mean child Y-BOCS (Yale–Brown Obsessive–Compulsive Scale) scores continued to decrease with fluoxetine but increased on placebo.
  - Significantly more patients during this phase responded to fluoxetine (57%) than placebo (27%) by week 16.
  - It may therefore take longer to see a response to SSRIs in OCD than in depression.

Treatment resistance predicted by
- Obsessions or mental rituals without behavioral compulsions or rituals
- Overvalued or delusional obsessions
- Severe comorbid depression
- Prominent hoarding
  - Associated with denial, secretiveness, projection, and limited treatment compliance

Management of treatment resistance:
- Maximize antidepressant dose.
- Combine SRIs.
  - Add clomipramine to an SSRI.
    - Consider pharmacokinetic interactions with fluoxetine and paroxetine.
    - Reduce dose of clomipramine to 50–75 mg first, then increase dose cautiously after SSRI is in steady state.

Augment an SRI
- Lithium most reliably helpful, probably because it is also serotonergic.
  - Additive serotonergic side effects
  - Not always effective
- Antianxiety medications
  - Buspirone was found helpful in open but not in controlled studies
    - May be useful for comorbid anxiety
  - Gabapentin
    - Useful primarily for associated anxiety
    - May be useful in promoting exposure.
- Antipsychotic medication
  - Most likely to be useful for patients with comorbid tics, overvalued obsessions, or schizoid/schizotypal traits.
  - Early reports suggested emergence of OCD symptoms in schizophrenia patients treated with clozapine.
    - Only seen in a small percentage of patients.
    - Could be chance occurrence.

- Small controlled studies suggest that risperidone, quetiapine, pimozide, and haloperidol can augment SRIs in refractory OCD.
    - Uncontrolled data suggest similar benefit with olanzapine.
- A chart review of 18 adults with OCD who responded to addition of an antipsychotic drug to an SRI and later discontinued the antipsychotic found that 15 of the 18 relapsed, 13 of them by 8 weeks after stopping the antipsychotic drug (Maina, Albert, Ziero, & Bogetto, 2003).
- SRI–neuroleptic interactions
    - Neuroleptics increase antidepressant levels.
    - Fluoxetine, paroxetine increase antipsychotic drug levels.
    - Additive down-regulation of $5HT_2$ and $5HT_7$ receptors
    - Additive sexual dysfunction and EPS
    - Increased risk of TD
- Opiates
    - Sometimes useful as adjuncts for severe refractory OCD
    - Morphine sulfate 10 mg/day
    - Tramadol 50 mg bid
    - Euphoria and drug dependence can be significant problems.

Neurosurgery for highly refractory OCD ($\sim$1/400 patients)
- Interruption of fibers from frontal cortex to basal ganglia
- Anterior cingulotomy
- Stereotactic subcaudate tractotomy
- Anterior capsulotomy
- Response rates:
    - Almost 40% well
    - 30% much improved
    - 25% improved
    - 12% no change or worse

### OCD with Pediatric Autoimmune Disorder Associated with Streptococcal Infection (PANDAS)

- Probably caused by hyperimmune response to streptococcus acting on caudate, basal ganglia, globus pallidus.
- Diagnosis based on at least two recurrences of OCD precipitated by group-A beta-hemolytic streptococcus infection.
- May be misdiagnosed as Tourette's.
- About 25% of patients who develop rheumatic fever will develop Sydenham's chorea, with abnormal gait and diffuse choreiform movements.
    - Half of patients with Sydenham's chorea develop OCD symptoms.

- Diagnosed with positive cultures for group-A streptococcus or increasing antibody titers.
- Specific treatments
  - Intravenous immunoglobulin G three times/week for 2 weeks.
    - Reduces tics by 25% and OCD symptoms by 45%.
    - Less effective than plasmapheresis.
  - Plasmapheresis
    - Administer 5 full-volume exchanges over 2 weeks.
    - Normalizes enlargement of striatal structures.
    - Reduces tics and OCD symptoms by 50–60%.
    - Improvement continues after treatment discontinued.

## Obsessive–Compulsive Spectrum Disorders

- Obsessional preoccupations without strong impulsive component:
  - Hypochondriasis
  - Pathological jealousy
  - Body dysmorphic disorder
- Obsessional ideas with prominent impulsivity:
  - Bulimia (see pp. 131–132)
  - Trichotillomania
  - Anorexia nervosa (see pp. 131–132)
  - Pathological gambling
  - Paraphilias (see pp. 522–523)
  - Sexual addictions
  - Compulsive shopping
- Management:
  - Evaluate carefully for bipolar disorder (especially with pathological gambling, sexual preoccupations, compulsive shopping, and bulimia).
  - Exclude rare cases of transsexualism in patients who consider their bodies ugly only because they are of the wrong gender.
  - SSRIs in antiobsessional doses are at least somewhat helpful, but not always as effective as in OCD
  - Trichotillomania responds only modestly to SSRIs.
    - Habit control therapy effective in the majority of cases.
    - A 12-week randomized trial found habit reversal, a type of behavior therapy, to be much more effective than 60 mg of fluoxetine, which was less effective than a waiting list control, for trichotillomania (effect sizes 3.80, 0.42, and 1.09, respectively; van Minnen, Hoogduin, Keijsers, Hellenbrand, & Hendriks, 2003).

- Opioid antagonists (e.g., naltrexone 50–100 mg/day) may reduce hair pulling and picking at skin.

## Posttraumatic Stress Disorder (PTSD)

Pharmacological treatment of PTSD is directed at specific dimensions of the disorder rather than the overall diagnosis.

- Dimensions of PTSD include
  - Reexperiencing
  - Emotional numbing/avoidance
  - Hyperarousal, easy startling
  - Kindling and behavioral sensitization promote recurrence and chronicity.
  - Frequent comorbidity with
    - Mood disorders
    - Substance abuse
    - OCD
    - Panic disorder and phobias in women
- Response may take 8 weeks or more.

### SSRIs

- First-line treatment
- Placebo-controlled studies for sertraline, fluoxetine
- Open studies for paroxetine, fluvoxamine
- Reduce arousal and intrusive thought and behavior.

### MAO Inhibitors

- Older studies show efficacy, especially for arousal, depression, and intrusive recall.
- Potent REM suppression reduces nightmares.

### Nefazodone

- Open trials
- Useful for improving sleep

### Mirtazepine

- Open trials
- Reduced nightmares and insomnia associated with nightmares in PTSD (Lewis, 2002).

Benefit also reported with amitryptiline, imipramine, brofaramine (RIMA that is not available in the United States).

### ANTICONVULSANTS

- Carbamazepine
  - 400–200 mg/day
  - Antikindling
  - Decreases anger, impulsivity, mood swings, recurrence
  - Blood levels of no value
- Topiramate
  - Reduces flashbacks, nightmares, anxiety, and depression.
  - Mean dose 150 mg/day
    - Range 35–500 mg
  - A review of records of 35 adults with chronic civilian PTSD found that topiramate (12.5–500 mg/day) as monotherapy or adjunct decreased nightmares in 79% and flashbacks in 86% of patients (Berlant & van Kammen, 2002).
    - 91% responded at ≤ 100 mg/day.
- Lamotrigine
  - Small trials
  - Useful for reexperiencing, avoidance/numbing

### BENZODIAZEPINES

- Useful for anxiety and hyperarousal
- Can facilitate exposure, but state-dependent learning may occur.
- May be disinhibiting.
- Avoid in patients with comorbid substance abuse.

### POSTSYNAPTIC ALPHA-1 ADRENERGIC ANTAGONISTS

- Clonidine
  - Helpful for arousal and insomnia
  - Sedation difficult to tolerate.
  - May aggravate depression.
  - Difficult to withdraw.
- Prazosin
  - Helpful for nightmares
  - Hypotension a common side effect
- Yohimbine (alpha-2 antagonist) increases arousal and worsens PTSD symptoms.

### ANTIPSYCHOTIC DRUGS

- 37 combat veterans with chronic PTSD with psychotic features who were taking antidepressants completed at least 1 week of a 5-week randomized, placebo-controlled trial of addition of risperidone (Hamner et al., 2003).

- Psychotic symptoms decreased significantly more with risperidone than placebo.
- PTSD symptoms also decreased more with risperidone, but the difference was not significant.

- In a VA study, 19 patients with combat-related PTSD unresponsive to 12 weeks treatment with maximally tolerated doses of SSRIs were randomly assigned to 8 weeks of double-blind addition of placebo or adjunctive treatment with 10–20 mg/day (mean dose 15 mg) of olanzapine (Stein, Kline, & Matloff, 2002).

  - Mean reductions of PTSD scores were seven times as great with olanzapine vs. placebo.
  - Sleep also improved significantly more with olanzapine than placebo.
  - Depression scores decreased slightly but significantly more with olanzapine.
  - Patients taking olanzapine gained an average of 13 pounds

Opioid antagonists

- Naltrexone for numbing and self-mutilation

Figure 7.3 summarizes approaches to treating PTSD.

### Catatonia

Features of catatonia include

- Immobility, mutism, withdrawal, posturing, grimacing: 75%
- Staring, rigidity, negativism: 50%
- Waxy flexibility, echolalia, echopraxia, stereotypy, verbigeration: < 50%

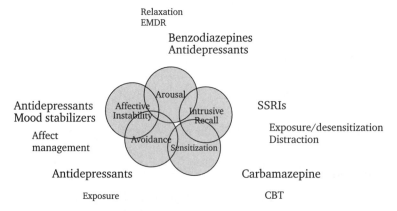

**Figure 7.3 Targeting PTSD dimensions**

Common causes of catatonia:

- Neurological illness
- Bipolar disorder (often accompanies neurological dysfunction in catatonia)
- Psychotic depression
- Neuroleptic-induced
- Schizophrenia is not commonly associated with catatonia unless this is an adverse reaction to antipsychotic medications.

Acute treatment of catatonia:

- Discontinue neuroleptics.
- Assess for NMS.
- ECT is most effective.
- Lorazepam 1–2 mg IM, repeated as needed.
  - Increases mobility and cooperativeness.
    - Facilitates accurate diagnosis.
  - Reduces risk of dehydration, starvation, pulmonary embolus.
  - Can be continued in dose of 1–2 mg po q 4–6 hours.
- Clonazepam 0.5–1 mg can be substituted for lorazepam in continuation treatment.

## SIDE EFFECTS

### Cardiovascular/Respiratory Side Effects

BRADYCARDIA

- Can be caused by all beta-adrenergic blocking agents.
- May interfere with exercise tolerance.
- Consider withdrawing medication if pulse rate is < 60.
- If bradycardia not significant at 300–500 mg/day of propranolol, it is not likely to develop at higher doses.

BRONCHOSPASM

- Nonselective beta-blockers (e.g., propranolol) antagonize bronchial muscle relaxation by catecholamines.
  - Should not be prescribed for asthmatics.
- Discontinue medication if wheezing develops.
- Cardioselective beta-blockers safer when bronchospasm is a risk.
  - Acetabutalol, atenolol, betaxolol, metropolol

### Hypotension, Dizziness, Lightheadedness

- Clonidine and beta-blockers can cause significant hypotension.
- Hypotension does not increase further as propranolol dose exceeds 500 mg/day.
- Benzodiazepines, buspirone, and newer antidepressants are much less likely to cause hypotension than TCAs and MAOIs.
- Management:
  - Obtain baseline pulse and blood pressure before starting clonidine or propranolol and then during first few days of treatment.
  - Measure lying blood pressure and then blood pressure after standing for 60 seconds.
  - For hypotension, recommend that patient
    - Sit up for 1 minute before standing from a lying position.
    - Stand up slowly.
    - Wait 30 seconds before walking.
    - See page 39 for additional management strategies.

### Raynaud's Phenomenon

- Beta-blockers may aggravate Raynaud's.

### Respiratory Depression

- Avoid benzodiazepines in patients with COPD, sleep apnea and related disorders.

## Central Nervous System Side Effects

### Amnesia

- All benzodiazepines can impair memory.
  - Memory impairment common with benzodiazepines that accumulate (e.g., clonazepam) and lipid-soluble benzodiazepines (e.g., diazepam).
- Retrograde amnesia commonly caused by withdrawal from high-potency, short half-life, highly lipid-soluble benzodiazepines.
  - 70% of patients have amnesia for surgery when midazolam used for anesthesia.

### Delirium

- Elderly, cognitively impaired, and brain-damaged patients may develop confusion, disorientation, or clouded sensorium.

- May be caused by small benzodiazepine doses.
- Propranolol also can cause confusion due to relative hypotension.
  - Not dose related

## Depression

- Not frequently caused by benzodiazepines or beta-blockers.
- Risk of benzodiazepine-induced depression is probably higher with
  - High benzodiazepine doses
  - Clonazepam
- Alprazolam has antidepressant properties

## Excitement

- Paradoxical excitement and disinhibition are more common in children, the elderly, and cognitively impaired or brain-damaged patients.

## Incoordination, Ataxia

- Usually associated with high benzodiazepine doses.

## Mania

- Alprazolam is the only benzodiazepine to be reported to induce mania.
  - Probably related to its antidepressant effect.
  - Try to avoid alprazolam in patients with bipolar disorder.

## Psychomotor Impairment

- All benzodiazepines can impair psychomotor function.
  - Especially driving and operating heavy equipment
- A single 10 mg dose of diazepam impairs driving to a degree equivalent to meeting criteria for a DUI (driving under the influence).
- Data from 225,796 patients, over 20 years old, who got a first prescription of a benzodiazepine were compared with 97,862 controls (Neutel, 1998):
  - New use of a benzodiazepine was associated with an increased risk of a traffic accident within the first 4 weeks.
  - The greatest risk was with flurazepam.
  - OR for an accident was 6.1 for those under 60 and 3.4 for those over 60.
- Alprazolam 1 mg or placebo was administered in a double-blind design; a 100 km driving test in normal traffic was performed an hour later, and psychomotor tests were performed 2.5 hours later. Subjects were crossed over to the other condition 2 weeks later (Verster, Volkerts, & Verbaten, 2002).

- Driving was significantly impaired by alprazolam compared to placebo, evidencing especially more
  - Weaving
  - Speed variability
  - Excursions out of lane
- Equivalent to impairment with BAL (blood alcohol level) of 0.15%.
- Alprazolam also produced impairment compared to placebo on cognitive testing of
  - Tracking
  - Reaction time
  - Attention
  - Memory scanning
- Tolerance develops to sedation but not psychomotor impairment.
- Driving should be assessed independently.
- Truck drivers and airline pilots should not take benzodiazepines.

## RAGE REACTIONS

- Disinhibition may cause violent outbursts.
  - More likely in patients with brain damage and in patients who cannot tolerate reduction of hypervigilance
  - More likely with highly lipid-soluble benzodiazepines that have rapid onset of action
- May respond to atypical antipsychotic medication.

## SEDATION

- Benzodiazepines, clonidine, and propranolol can cause significant sedation.
- Buspirone is not sedating.
- Longer-acting benzodiazepines are often more sedating, but some short-acting benzodiazepines can produce significant sedation for some patients.

Management:
- Increase dose very slowly.
  - If patient remains below threshold for severe sedation, tolerance often develops.
  - If patient is severely sedated at low dose, tolerance is less likely to develop.
    - Give two-thirds of clonidine dose at bedtime.

- Switch from propranolol to less sedating beta-blocker.
- If patient has had a good response and sedation is the only limiting side effect, consider treating with modafinil (will not necessarily improve psychomotor function).

STUTTERING

- Reported primarily with alprazolam.

## Endocrine and Sexual Side Effects

Propranolol and clonidine frequently cause sexual dysfunction.
- Clonidine occasionally causes gynecomastia.
- Buspirone may reduce sexual dysfunction caused by SSRIs.

## Eyes, Ears, Nose, and Throat Side Effects

BLURRED VISION

- Rare with benzodiazepines
- More common with antihistamines
- May respond to cholinesterase inhibitor.

GLAUCOMA

- Some benzodiazepines (e.g., alprazolam, clonazepam) may precipitate narrow angle glaucoma.

## Gastrointestinal Effects

DRY MOUTH

- May occur with clonidine, benzodiazepines, antihistamines.
- Nasal congestion and dry mouth can occur with trazodone.

## Renal/Urinary Side Effects

INCONTINENCE

- A study of a large Italian database of 4,583 patients (mean age 77) in home care programs found that patients taking benzodiazepines were 1.44 times more likely to be incontinent at least twice a week (Landi et al., 2002).
  - Risk was highest for benzodiazepines that are oxidized before being glucuronidated and excreted, especially if they have long elimination half-lives (odds ratio for incontinence 1.75)

Table 7.2 General Antianxiety Doses

| GENERIC NAMES | BENZODIAZEPINE DOSE EQUIVALENTS | USUAL DOSE FOR ANXIETY (MG/DAY) | HIGH/LOW DOSE RANGE FOR ANXIETY (MG/DAY) | GERIATRIC DOSE (MG/DAY) |
|---|---|---|---|---|
| alprazolam | 0.5 | 0.5–3.0 | 0.25–8 | 0.25–0.5 |
| buspirone | N/A | 30–45 | 15–900 | 15–30 |
| chlordiazepoxide | 10.0 | 25–75 | 5–200 | 5–30* |
| clonazepam | 0.25 | 0.5–1.5 | 0.25–5 | 0.25–1.0* |
| clonidine | N/A | 0.2–0.6 | 0.1–2.0 | 0.2–0.4 |
| clorazepate | 7.5 | 15–67.5 | 7.5–90 | 15–60* |
| diazepam | 5.0 | 4–30 | 2–40 | 1–10 |
| halazepam | 20.0 | 40–80 | 20–100 | 20–40 |
| hydroxyzine | 100.0** | 100–300 | 50–500 | 10–50 |
| lorazepam | 1.0 | 2–6 | 1–10 | 0.5–1.5 |
| meprobamate | 800.0 | 400–1200 | 400–1600 | 200–600 |
| oxazepam | 15.0 | 30–60 | 30–120 | 10–30 |
| propranolol | N/A | 30–80 | 30–240 | 30–60 |

* Because of long half-lives, not generally recommended for use in elderly or those with impaired hepatic function. Use lorazepam or oxazepam instead.
** Represents sedative equivalent.

## PREGNANCY AND LACTATION

Panic disorder usually does not remit during pregnancy.

- Continued symptoms associated with increased risk of preeclampsia, preterm labor, prolonged labor, stillbirth, fetal hypoxia, and lower Apgar score in newborn.
- Behavioral treatments may be as effective as antidepressants and benzodiazepines and should be considered during pregnancy, if not tried previously.

### Teratogenicity

- Concerns about risk of cleft lip/palate with low-potency benzodiazepines have not been confirmed in large studies.
- Insufficient experience with high-potency benzodiazepines to be certain that they are not teratogenic, but no evidence that they are.
- Any risk of teratogenicity is substantially less after the first trimester.
- Buspirone appears not to be teratogenic in animals, but insufficient human data.
- No evidence of behavioral teratogenicity due to benzodiazepines.
- SSRIs may be clearly safer than benzodiazepines as treatments for anxiety during first trimester.

## Direct Effects on Newborn

- Benzodiazepines can prolong labor.
- Benzodiazepines with active metabolites (e.g., diazepam, chlordiazepoxide) are eliminated slowly by the fetus and may cause hypotonia, decreased feeding, respiratory depression, and sedation in the newborn.
  - Risk of adverse effects is greater if benzodiazepine is combined with other sedating medications.
  - With clonazepam
    - Hypotonia and lethargy in the newborn persist for about 5 days.
    - Respiratory depression, for about 10 days.
- Short half-life benzodiazepines without active metabolites (e.g., lorazepam) are safer.
- Benzodiazepine withdrawal in newborn may be manifested as irritability, temors, myoclonus, hyperreflexia, abnormal sleep, bradycardia, cyanosis.
  - As in adults, withdrawal appears sooner and is more severe but does not last as long with short-acting benzodiazepines.
  - Withdrawal may last months with long-acting benzodiazepines such as clonazepem.
  - To reduce risk of withdrawal in newborn, gradually discontinue benzodiazepines prior to delivery.
- Propranolol and atenolol may cause intrauterine growth retardation, hypoglycemia, bradycardia, respiratory depression, and hyperbilirubinemia in neonate.
  - Monitor newborn closely for 1 or 2 days if mother was taking a beta-blocker preterm.
- If anxiety is severe and carries risk of obstetrical complication:
  - Consider benzodiazepines with simpler metabolism and intermediate half-life (e.g., lorazepam, oxazepam).
  - Do not use parenteral diazapem containing sodium benzoate as a preservative.
    - It can antagonize binding of bilirubin to albumin and cause kernicterus.
  - Consider SSRI or TCA.

## Lactation

- All medications used to treat anxiety are excreted in breast milk.
- Exposure to a benzodiazepine in breast milk can cause
  - Sedation

- Respiratory depression
- Weight loss
- Anorexia
- Impaired temperature regulation
- Withdrawal syndromes if breast milk levels are inconsistent
- Oxazepam appears to have lowest ratio of newborn:maternal levels ($<$ 10%).
- If benzodiazepines are to be used during lactation
  - Use shorter-acting preparation.
  - Tell mother to nurse before taking medication.
  - Assess infant plasma benzodiazepine level.
  - Monitor infant closely.

Table 7.3 summarizes interactions between benzodiazepines and other drugs.

Table 7.4 presents the effects on laboratory tests.

## WITHDRAWAL

Discontinuation syndromes and their treatment are similar for benzodiazepines, barbiturates, and other hypnotics, and are discussed in the next chapter.

### Clonidine

- Rapid discontinuation causes autonomic hyperactivity, with
  - Hypertension
    - May persist 7–10 days.
  - Tachycardia
  - Sweating
  - Nervousness
  - Headache
  - Stomachache
- Clonidine withdrawal begins about 18 hours after the last dose.
- Withdrawal of clonidine doses $>$ 0.6 mg/day may be life-threatening.
- Management of withdrawal:
  - Restart clonidine, if possible.
  - Taper gradually over 2 weeks.
  - Use IV vasodilators for severe hypotension.

## Table 7.3 Drug–Drug Interactions

| DRUGS (X) INTERACT WITH: | BENZODIAZEPINES (B) | COMMENTS |
|---|---|---|
| alcohol | X↑ B↑ | Alcohol increases risk of lethality of benzodiazepine overdose. |
| aluminum hydroxide (*see* antacids) | | |
| aminophylline (*see* bronchodilators) | | |
| amiodarone | B↑ | Increases levels of clonazepam and probably other oxidatively metabolized benzodiazepines. |
| antacids (aluminum hydroxide, magnesium hydroxide) | B↓ | Slows rate but not total amount of GI absorption. Probable clinical effect is to slow onset, perhaps peak magnitude of effect, and prolong duration of effect of single doses. In single but not repeated doses, interfered with transformation of clorazepate to desmethyldiazepam. |
| anticholinergics | B↓ | Slow time to peak absorption but not total amount absorbed. |
| antifungal imidazoles (*see* ketoconazole) | | |
| barbiturates (*see also* sedatives) | X↑ B↓↑ | Phenobarbital (and probably others) speed benzodiazepine metabolism and reduce levels. Potentiate each other's effects. |
| birth control pills | B↑↓ | Oral contraceptives may increase 2-keto and triazolo compounds while reducing 3-hydroxy agents.* |
| *bronchodilators:* aminophylline theophylline | B↓ | Rapidly antagonize diazepam, lorazepam, and probably other benzodiazepine effects; increase benzodiazepine doses. |
| caffeine | B↓ | Caffeine (250–500 mg) antagonizes benzodiazepines. |
| carbamazepine | B↓ | Decreases alprazolam and clonazepam levels 20–50%. |
| cimetidine | B↑ | May slow oxidative metabolism (*not* 3-hydroxy agents*) and increase benzodiazepine side effects. Ranitidine and famotidine appear less apt to interact with benzodiazepines than cimetidine. |
| digitalis | B↑ | Increases benzodiazepine levels. |
| digoxin | X↑ | Digoxin serum levels increased; monitor levels. |

(*continues*)

**Table 7.3** Continued

| DRUGS (X) INTERACT WITH: | BENZODIAZEPINES (B) | COMMENTS |
|---|---|---|
| disulfiram | B↑ | Increases levels of oxidatively metabolized benzodiazepine* (*not* 3-hydroxy agents) and has additive sedative properties. May need to lower benzodiazepines or switch to 3-hydroxy agents. |
| erythromycin (*see* macrolide antibiotics) | | |
| estrogen (*see* birth control pills) | | |
| fluconazole (*see* ketoconazole) | | |
| fluoxetine (and probably paroxetine and sertraline) | B↑ | Increases levels of diazepam and alprazolam and probably other oxidatively metabolized benzodiazepines except clonazepam or triazolam (and probably not lorazepam or oxazepam). |
| food | B↓ | Slows absorption; for rapid effect, take on empty stomach. |
| isoniazid (INH) | B↑ | INH increases effects of benzodiazepines that require oxidative metabolism*; lower benzodiazepine dose or switch to 3-hydroxybenzodiazepines.* |
| *ketoconazole:* fluconazole miconazole traconazole | B↑ | Increases oxidatively metabolized benzodiazepines but not hydroxy.* |
| levodopa (L-dopa) | X↓ | Benzodiazepines may reduce antiparkinson effect; seen with triazolam and temazepam. Oxazepam and flurazepam have not caused this problem. Carbidopa-levodopa agents may help. |
| magnesium hydroxide (*see* antacids) | | |
| MAOIs | B↑ | Greater intoxication with increased benzodiazepine levels. |
| *macrolide antibiotics:* azithromycin clarithromycin erythromycin | B↑ | Decreases clearance of triazolo-benzodiazepines (alprazolam, triazolam, estazolam); increases benzodiazepine levels and toxicity. Spiramycin okay. Azithromycin possibly okay. |
| metoprolol | B↑ | May slightly increase 3-keto compounds.* Minimal clinical changes noted; does not occur with atenolol. |

(*continues*)

## Table 7.3 Continued

| DRUGS (X) INTERACT WITH: | BENZODIAZEPINES (B) | COMMENTS |
|---|---|---|
| miconazole (*see* ketoconazole) | | |
| paroxetine (*see* fluoxetine) | | |
| phenytoin (*see also* sedatives) | B↑↓ | Possibly increases benzodiazepine levels, including diazepam and clonazepam; may increase oxazepam clearance with decreased levels. |
| physostigmine | B↓ | Reverses benzodiazepine effects; sometimes used after benzodiazepine OD. |
| primidone (*see* sedatives) | | |
| probenecid | B↑↓ | May increase lorazepam levels and side effects. May affect other benzodiazepines, but more likely other 3-hydroxy compounds.* |
| propoxyphene | B↑ | May increase oxidatively metabolized benzodiazepines (*not* 3-hydroxys).* |
| propranolol | B↑ | May slightly increase levels 3-keto compounds.* Minimal clinical changes noted; does not occur with atenolol. |
| rifampin | B↓ | Reduces diazepam's effects, and probably other oxidatively metabolized benzodiazepines (*not* 3-hydroxy agents).* |
| sedatives (alcohol, antihistamines, sedative-hypnotics, TCAs, low-potency antipsychotics) | X↑ B↑ | Potentiate each other's sedative effects. Disinhibition increased with alcohol and barbiturates (including primidone) |
| sertraline (*see* fluoxetine) | | |
| SSRIs (*see* fluoxetine) | | |
| theophylline (*see* bronchodilators) | | |
| tobacco smoking | B↓ | Decreases benzodiazepine levels; dosage adjustment may be necessary if patient stops smoking. |
| traconazole (*see* ketoconazole) | | |
| valproic acid | B↑ | Increases unbound diazepam levels and may inhibit its metabolism while increasing its effects. May also increase levels of other oxidatively metabolized benzodiazepines.* |

*(continues)*

**Table 7.3  Continued**

| DRUGS (X) INTERACT WITH: | ALPRAZOLAM (A) | COMMENTS |
|---|---|---|
| TCAs | X↑ | Increases TCA levels 20–30%. |

| DRUGS (X) INTERACT WITH: | ANTIHISTAMINES (A) (E.G., DIPHEN-HYDRAMINE/HYDROXYZINE) | COMMENTS |
|---|---|---|
| alcohol | X↑ A↑ | Additive CNS depression. |
| anticholinergics (see also page for list) | X↑ A↑ | Increased anticholinergic effects. |
| antipsychotics | X↓ A↑ | Hydroxyzine may block antipsychotic actions. Increased CNS depression; increased anticholinergic effects. |
| narcotics | X↑ A↑ | Additive CNS depression. |
| TCAs | X↑ A↑ | Additive CNS depression; increased anticholinergic effects. |
| sedatives (benzo-diazepines, barbiturates) | X↑ A↑ | CNS depression. |

| DRUGS (X) INTERACT WITH: | BUSPIRONE (B) | COMMENTS |
|---|---|---|
| cimetidine | B↑ | May see more minor side effects (e.g., lightheadedness). |
| food | B↓↑ | Decrease absorption speed but increases total amount in body. |
| haloperidol | X↑ | Increased haloperidol levels. |
| MAOI | X↑ | Possibility of serotonin syndrome. |

| DRUGS (X) INTERACT WITH: | CLONAZEPAM (C) | COMMENTS |
|---|---|---|
| carbamazepine | C↓ | In 5–15 days, carbamazepine may diminish clonazepam by 19–37%. Seizure effect unknown. Unclear if other benzodiazepines react to carbamazepine like clonazepam. Pure 3-hydroxy compounds (lorazepam, oxazepam, temazepam) are less apt to react similarly.* |

(continues)

## Table 7.3 Continued

| DRUGS (X) INTERACT WITH: | CLONAZEPAM (C) | COMMENTS |
|---|---|---|
| phenytoin | C↓ | Lowers plasma clonazepam with reduced clonazepam effect. |
| primidone | C↓ | May slightly decrease clonazepam level, but effect is not significant. |

| DRUGS (X) INTERACT WITH: | CLONIDINE (C) | COMMENTS |
|---|---|---|
| acebutolol | X↑ C↑ | Potentiate each other. |
| alcohol | X↑ C↑ | Enhanced sedation and decreased BP. |
| antipsychotics | X↑ C↑↓ | Isolated, severe hypotension or delirium, but usually not a problem. More common in patients with impaired cardiac function. May decrease hypotensive effect. |
| beta-blockers (*see* acebutolol) | | |
| caffeine | C↓ | Diminished clonidine effect. |
| cocaine | X↑ C↓ | BP rise. |
| diuretics | X↑ C↑ | BP drop. |
| enalapril | X↑ | May accelerate potassium loss. |
| fenfluramine | C↑ | Possible increased clonidine effect. |
| insulin | X↓ | Hyperglycemia. |
| labetalol | X↓ C↓ | Precipitous BP drop if both drugs are stopped together. |
| levodopa | X↓ | Parkinsonian symptoms may emerge. |
| lithium | X↓ | Can decrease hypotensive effect. |
| marijuana | X↑ C↑ | Weakness on standing. |
| naloxone | C↓ | May reduce clonidine's antihypertensive action; if so, change clonidine to another antihypertensive or stop the narcotic antagonist. |
| nicotinic acid (Niacin) | X↓ | Clonidine may inhibit nicotinic flushing; no special precautions. |
| nitrates | C↑ | BP drop. |
| nitroprusside | C↑ | A few cases of severe hypotensive reactions. |
| propranolol (*see also* clonidine entry under beta-blockers below.) | X↑ | |

(*continues*)

**Table 7.3 Continued**

| DRUGS (X) INTERACT WITH: | CLONIDINE (C) | COMMENTS |
|---|---|---|
| TCAs | C↑↓ | May lead to hypotension, especially imipramine and desipramine. More often may decrease clonidine's effects and may augment the hypertensive response to abrupt clonidine withdrawal. Maprotiline may interfere less with clonidine than might TCAs, although little clinical evidence. Consider alternative antihypertensive. Carefully monitor patients when clonidine is reduced; gradually tapering clonidine might lower risk. |

| DRUGS (X) INTERACT WITH: | CLORAZEPATE (C) | COMMENTS |
|---|---|---|
| primidone | X↑ | Combined use may cause depression, irritability, and aggressive behavior. |

| DRUGS (X) INTERACT WITH: | DIAZEPAM (D) | COMMENTS |
|---|---|---|
| ciprofloxacin | D↑ | Increased levels. |
| digitalis, digoxin | X↑ | Diazepam may increase digoxin and digitalis. |
| gallamine | X↑ | Prolonged neuromuscular blockade. |
| isoniazid (INH) | D↑ | INH may increase diazepam. |
| succinylcholine | X↓ | Reduces neuromuscular blockade and its side effects (i.e., fasciculations, muscle pain, increased potassium, and CPK). |

| DRUGS (X) INTERACT WITH: | LORAZEPAM (L) | COMMENTS |
|---|---|---|
| loxapine | X↑ L↑ | Isolated respiratory depression, stupor, and hypotension. |
| scopolamine | X↑ L↑ | IM lorazepam may increase sedation, hallucinations, and irrational behavior. |

| DRUGS (X) INTERACT WITH: | BETA-BLOCKERS PROPRANOLOL (P) | COMMENTS |
|---|---|---|
| acebutolol | X↑ P↑ | Increased antihypertensive effects of both drugs; adjust doses. |

(*continues*)

## Table 7.3 Continued

| DRUGS (X) INTERACT WITH: | BETA-BLOCKERS PROPRANOLOL (P) | COMMENTS |
|---|---|---|
| albuterol | X↓ P↓ | Decreased albuterol and β-adrenergic blocking effects. Avoid propranolol in bronchospastic disease; cardioselective agents safer. |
| alcohol | P↑↓ | May see variable changes in BP; no special precautions. Slows rate of propranolol absorption. |
| aluminum and magnesium hydroxides | P↓ | Decrease absorption of beta-blockers, such as propranolol (by 60%), atenolol hydroxides (by 35%), and metoprolol (by 25%). Clinical results unclear. Avoid combination; otherwise, ingest antacids and propranolol one hour apart. Calcium carbonates may be okay. |
| amiodarone | P↑ | Bradycardia, arrhythmias. |
| anesthetics | X↑ | Beta-blockers and local anesthetics, particularly those containing epinephrine, can enhance sympathomimetic side effects. Acute discontinuation of blockers prior to local anesthesia may increase anesthetic's side effects. Do not stop chronic beta-blockers before using local anesthetics. Avoid local anesthetics containing epinephrine in patients on propranolol. |
| anticholinergics | P↓ | ACAs can block beta-blockers' bradycardia. |
| antidiabetics | X↑ P↓ | Blunted recovery from both hypo- and hyperglycemia; decreased tachycardia. Cardioselective beta-blockers, such as metoprolol, acebutolol, and atenolol, are preferable in diabetics, especially if prone to hypoglycemia. |
| antihistamines | X↓ | Decreased antihistaminic effect. |
| antihypertensives | X↑ | Increased antihypertensive effect. |
| anti-inflammatory agents | X↓ | Decreased anti-inflammatory effect. |
| antipsychotics (*see also* anticholinergic) | X↑ P↑ | Increased antipsychotic levels with chlorpromazine, thioridazine, thiothixene, resulting in increase of each other's effects, such as hypotension, toxicity, and seizures. Monitor serum levels or decrease dose. Propranolol level not affected. |
| antipyrine | X↑ | Propranolol, and possibly metoprolol, may increase antipyrine. |
| barbiturates | P↓ | Barbiturates may lower propranolol. |

beta-blockers (*see* acebutolol)

(*continues*)

**Table 7.3 Continued**

| DRUGS (x) INTERACT WITH: | BETA-BLOCKERS PROPRANOLOL (p) | COMMENTS |
|---|---|---|
| benzodiazepines (*see* propranolol entry under benzodia-zepines above) | | |
| *calcium channel-blockers:* bepridil diltiazem verapamil | x↑ | Additive effects on SA and AV node cause increased bradycardia and hypotension; heart block may develop. |
| carbamazepine | p↓ | Might induce beta-blocker metabolism and decrease propranolol; combine with caution. |
| chlorpromazine | x↑ p↑ | Levels of both increase. |
| cimetidine (*see* etinidine) | | |
| clonidine | x↑ | Beta-blockers can aggravate rebound hypertension in patients withdrawn from clonidine within 24–72 h. Symptoms include tremor, insomnia, nausea, flushing, and headaches. Patients receiving propranolol with clonidine should be withdrawn from propranolol *before* the clonidine to reduce danger of rebound hypertension. Noncardioselective beta-blockers more likely to cause this reaction than cardioselective beta-blockers. Metoprolol or another cardioselective beta-blocker may be preferable to propranolol. |
| cocaine | x↑ | Irregular heartbeat. |
| dicumarol | x↑ | Propranolol may produce small increases in dicumarol; effect on prothrombin times is unknown. |
| digitalis | x↑ p↑ | Propranolol can potentiate bradycardia from digitalis; monitor heart rate. |
| disopyramide | p↑ | Negative inotropic effects. |
| epinephrine | x↑ | Noncardioselective beta-blockers (e.g., propranolol, timolol) substantially raise systolic and diastolic BPs and drop heart rate, sometimes resulting in arrhythmias and stroke. Cardioselective beta-blockers (e.g., metoprolol) are safe. Whereas beta-agonist sympathomimetics (e.g., epineph-rine) are dangerous, pure beta-agonist sympathomimetics (e.g., isoproterenol) are safer. Avoid combining noncardioselective beta-blockers and beta-agonist |

(*continues*)

## Table 7.3 Continued

| DRUGS (x) INTERACT WITH: | BETA-BLOCKERS PROPRANOLOL (P) | COMMENTS |
|---|---|---|
| | | sympathomimetics; this includes injecting epinephrine as a local anesthetic. |
| ergot alkaloids | X↑ | Propranolol may increase vasoconstriction. Using an ergotamine suppository, a patient on 30 mg/day of propranolol developed purple and painful feet. Adverse drug reactions (ADRs) more common with noncardioselective beta-blockers; use cardioselective beta-blockers. |
| etinidine | P↑ | May substantially raise concentrations of propranolol and probably other beta-blockers that undergo hepatic metabolism (e.g., metoprolol, labetalol). Ranitidine, famotidine, or nizatidine may be safer than etinitidine if an $H_2$ blocker is required. |
| furosemide | P↑ | May increase propranolol levels. |
| glucagon | X↓ | Propranolol may blunt glucagon's hyperglycemic action. |
| indomethacin | P↓ | Indomethacin, piroxicam, naproxen, and possibly other nonsteroidal anti-inflammatory drugs (NSAIDs) diminish propranolol's hypotensive effect. Sulindac and salicylates have minimal effect. NSAIDs and other beta-blockers can be unpredictable. If BP increases, may need to increase propranolol or decrease or stop indomethacin. |
| isoproterenol | P↑↓ | Noncardioselective beta-blockers (e.g., propranolol) are risky to combine with isoproterenol in asthmatic patients. Safer to use cardioselective β-blockers (e.g., labetalol or metoprolol), but *no beta-blocker is absolutely safe for asthmatic patients.* |
| lidocaine | X↑ | Lidocaine may rise with propranolol, metoprolol, or nadolol. |
| marijuana | X↓ | Propranolol delays the increase in heart rate and BP from marijuana and may prevent marijuana's impairment of learning tasks and eye-reddening effect. |
| methyldopa | X↓ | Patients taking a beta-blocker and methyldopa may develop hypertension; monitor. Hypertensive reactions may be helped by IV phentolamine. |
| MAOIs | X↓ P↓ | Depression occasionally worsens on beta- |

*(continues)*

**Table 7.3  Continued**

| DRUGS (X) INTERACT WITH: | BETA-BLOCKERS PROPRANOLOL (P) | COMMENTS |
|---|---|---|
| | | blockers. Anticholinergic MAOIs, such as phenelzine, may antagonize reduction of heart rate by beta-blockers. |
| naproxen (*see* indomethacin) | | |
| nonsteroidal anti-inflammatory drugs (NSAIDs; *see* indomethacin) | | |
| nylidrin | X↓ | Propranolol may reduce nylidrin's greater gastric acid secretion and volume; no special precautions. |
| phenylephrine | X↑ | Phenylephrine added to propranolol may trigger hypertensive episode. Phenyl-ephrine 10% eye drops have on rare occasions produced acute hypertensive episodes and cerebral hemorrhage. |
| phenytoin | P↑ | Increased propranolol effect. |
| piroxicam (*see* indomethacin) | | |
| prazosin | X↑ | Beta-blockers may increase the "first-dose" hypotensive response to prazosin. Start prazosin cautiously in patients on beta-blockers. |
| propoxyphene | P↑ | Increases highly metabolized beta-blockers (e.g., propranolol, metoprolol), but not beta-blockers excreted by kidneys (e.g., atenolol, nadolol). |
| quinidine | X↑ P↑ | Propranolol may inflate quinidine level and foster lightheadedness, hypotension, slower heart rate, and fainting. |
| rifampin | P↓ | May decrease propranolol and metoprolol levels; consider increasing dose or chang-ing to another beta-blocker when rifampin is added. |
| reserpine | X↑ | Increased reserpine effect with excessive sedation, hypotension, fainting, vertigo, and depression. |
| terbutaline | X↓↑ | Propranolol may antagonize terbutaline-induced bronchodilation, whereas cardio-selective β-adrenergic blockers have little effect on terbutaline and are safer. |
| theophylline | X↑↓ | Propranolol raises theophylline levels but |

(*continues*)

**Table 7.3 Continued**

| DRUGS (X) INTERACT WITH: | BETA-BLOCKERS PROPRANOLOL (P) | COMMENTS |
|---|---|---|
| | | antagonizes bronchodilation; cardioselective agents are safer. |
| tobacco smoking | P↓ | Decreases propranolol level and may produce arrhythmias. If smoking halted, propranolol level increases. Smoking patients need higher propranolol doses. Atenolol, and other beta-blockers not dependent on liver metabolism, are safer. |
| tocainide | X↓ | May worsen congestive heart failure. |
| TCAs | X↓ P↓ | Depression occasionally increases on beta-blockers. Highly anticholinergic TCAs can antagonize cardiac slowing by beta-blockers. Maprotiline toxicity may arise after propranolol added. |
| tubocurarine | X↑ | Propranolol may prolong neuromuscular blockade. |
| verapamil (*see* calcium channel-blockers) | | |
| warfarin | X↑ | Propranolol may produce small increases in warfarin; effect on prothrombin times is unknown. |

↑ Increases; ↓ Decreases; ↑↓ Increases and decreases.
\* *Oxidatively metabolized* includes 2-keto compounds (clorazepate, chlordiazepoxide, diazepam, flurazepam, halazepam, prazepam) and triazolo-compounds (alprazolam, estazolam, triazolam). *Not oxidatively metabolized* are 3-hydroxy compounds (lorazepam, oxazepam, temazepam, and, partially, clonazepam).

- Avoid beta-blockers.
    - May increase rebound hypertension.
    - If clonidine has been administered along with propranolol, discontinue propranolol before withdrawing clonidine.

### Propranolol

Abrupt discontinuation of propranolol may increase hypertension or coronary artery spasm in patients with preexisting cardiac disease.

### Buspirone

Buspirone has not been associated with discontinuation syndromes, other than relapse of the underlying anxiety disorder.

**Table 7.4 Effects on Laboratory Tests**

| GENERIC NAMES | BLOOD/SERUM TESTS | URINE TESTS |
|---|---|---|
| benzodiazepines | WBC ↓, RBC ↓, LFT ↑ | None |
| buspirone | LFT ↑ | None |
| clonazepam | LFT ↑ | None |
| clonidine | glucose (transient) ↑<br>plasma renin activity ↓ | aldosterone ↑<br>catecholamines ↑ |
| hydroxyzine | None | 17-Hydroxycorticosteroids ↑ |
| propranolol and atenolol | LFT ↑<br>$T_4$ ↑, $rT_3$ ↑, $T_3$ ↓<br>BUN (with severe heart disease) ↑<br>antinuclear antibodies (ANA) ↑ | None |

\* ↑ Increases; ↓ Decreases; f = falsely; r = rarely; LFT = SGOT, SGPT, LDH, bilirubin, and alkaline phosphatase.

- However, buspirone will not prevent or treat withdrawal from CNS depressants.

## TOXICITY AND OVERDOSE

### Benzodiazepines

Benzodiazepines occasionally are fatal in overdose, but most fatalities have occurred when they are combined with other CNS depressants such as alcohol. Tolerance to sedative effects may result in overdose not being associated with severe sedation.

Benzodiazepine overdose/intoxication can be manifested by

- Drowsiness
- Ataxia
- Dysarthria
- Vertigo
- Psychomotor impairment
- Confusion
- Lethargy
- Hypotension
- Lethargy

- Coma
- Cardiac/respiratory arrest (very rare)

Management of benzodiazepine overdose:

- Flumazenil
  - Benzodiazepine receptor antagonist
  - Usual dose 1–3 mg IV
  - Response occurs in 6–10 minutes.
  - Intoxication may recur 20–30 minutes later.
  - Flumazenil may precipitate benzodiazepine withdrawal, resulting in
    - Agitation, anxiety
    - Seizures in 1.1% (more common if previous benzodiazepine dependence)
  - Risk of benzodiazepine withdrawal with flumazenil may be reduced with infusion of 0.1 mg/minute.
- Noradrenergic agent for hypotension
  - Norepinephrine infusion 4–8 mg in 1000 mL D5W or D5S
  - Metaraminol
    - 10–20 mg sc or IM
    - 0.5–5 mg IV
    - Infusion of 25–100 mg in 500 mL D5W
- Increase renal excretion of benzodiazepine.
  - Forced diuresis
  - Somotic diuretic
  - IV fluids
  - Hemodialysis is not effective.

### Buspirone

Dysphoria at higher doses discourages gradual intoxication. In overdose:

- No human fatalities reported.
- Animal $LD_{50}$ appears to be 160–550 times therapeutic dose.
- Overdose can cause
  - Nausea, vomiting
  - Dizziness
  - Drowsiness
  - Miosis
- Hemodialysis unnecessary.

### Clonidine

Overdose of clonidine can cause

- Hypotension
- Bradycardia
- Lethargy, somnolence
- Irritability
- Weakness
- Hyporeflexia
- Miosis
- Vomiting
- Respiratory depression
- Cardiac conduction defects, arrhythmias
- Seizures
- Transient hypertension

Management of clonidine overdose:

- Treat hypotension with
  - IV norepinephrine or metaraminol, as above
  - IV fluids
    - Add dopamine, if necessary.
- IV atropine 0.3–1.2 mg for bradycardia.
- IV furosemide 20–40 mg over 1–2 minutes for hypertension
  - IV tolazoline 10 mg every 30 minutes, if necessary
- Hemodialysis is not effective.

### Hydroxyzine

Overdose of this and other antihistamines causes exaggerated sedation and anticholinergic side effects.

- Signs and symptoms include
  - Drowsiness
  - Confusion
  - Delirium
  - Constipation
  - Urinary retention
  - Hypotension
- Management is the same as for other anticholinergic compounds (see Chapter 2).
- Hemodialysis is not helpful.

### Meprobamate

Like the barbiturates, meprobamate is very dangerous in overdose.

- $LD_{50}$ in humans is a 7–10 day supply.
- Combining overdose of meprobamate with alcohol increases lethality of overdose.
- Signs and symptoms of overdose include
  - Drowiness, lethargy, stupor
  - Ataxia
  - Coma
  - Hypotension
  - Shock
  - Respiratory failure
  - Death
- Osmotic diuretics (e.g., mannitol), peritoneal dialysis, or hemodialysis can eliminate meprobamate.

### Propranolol

Treatment of specific signs of propranolol overdose:

- Bradycardia
  - IV atropine 0.3–1.2 mg
  - If no response, isopreteronol 1–2 mg in 500 mg D5S or D5W
- Cardiac failure
  - Digitalis/diuretics
- Hypotension
  - IV epinephrine 0.5 mL of 1:1000 epinephrine in 10 mL saline
  - Levarterenol 4–8 mg in 1000 mg D5S or D5W
- Bronchospasm
  - Isoproterenol, as above
  - Aminophylline 500 mg IV slowly

## PRECAUTIONS

### Benzodiazepines

Relative contraindications to benzodiazepines include

- Hypersensitivity to this class of medication
- Chronic obstructive pulmonary disease
- Sleep apnea

- Job as airline pilot
- Job as truck driver or other operator of heavy equipment
- History of CNS depressant addiction

Benzodiazepines should be used cautiously in

- Elderly or debilitated patients
  - Avoid long-acting benzodiazepines with active metabolites (e.g., diazepam, chlordiazepoxide).
- Patients with a history of abuse of other substances

### Buspirone

Because it does not act on the GABA–benzodiazepine receptor complex, buspirone does not prevent or treat CNS depressant withdrawal.

### Clonidine

Clonidine should not be co-administered with stimulants, because it will counteract their actions. Care is necessary when prescribing clonidine to patients with

- Coronary insufficiency
- Recent myocardial infarction
- Hypotension
- Chronic renal failure
- Generalized rash

### Propranolol

Contraindications to propranolol include

- Cardiogenic shock
- Sinus bradycardia
- Congestive heart failure
- Significant hypotension
- Bronchial asthma
  - Metoprolol, atenolol, and labetalol are less likely to cause bronchospasm.

Propranolol should be used cautiously in the presence of

- Persistent angina
- Impaired myocardial function
- Glaucoma
  - Propranolol may increase intraocular pressure.

- Diabetes mellitus
- Chronic obstructive pulmonary disease
- Hepatic failure
  - Atenolol and nadolol are not metabolized by the liver.
- Depression
  - Risk of depression with propranolol is lower than originally thought, but sexual dysfunction and fatigue are common.

## ADVICE FOR CARETAKERS

Benzodiazepines have a rapid onset of action, making it possible to estimate therapeutic and adverse effects quickly. Problems to be aware of include

- Impaired driving
  - Inform patients that they may not be aware of driving in an impaired manner.
  - Common errors include slowed reflexes, going around corners too quickly.
  - Impairment is increased with any concomitant use of alcohol or other CNS depressants.
  - Have someone independently check the patient's driving.
- Tolerance and withdrawal
  - Inform patients about warning signs of intoxication and withdrawal (pp. 441–449).
    - Ensure that patient understands risk of seizures.
- Caffeine and other anxiogenic substances can counteract antianxiety effect of benzodiazepines but not psychomotor impairment.

Whereas some patients who have been taking benzodiazepines chronically for anxiety may be able to switch gradually to an antidepressant, others respond best to benzodiazepines without significant adverse effects. If the dose has not been escalated, the patient is not impaired, and the medication is effective, then there may be nothing wrong with continuing the medication—assuming that the patient is monitored regularly.

Parenteral administration of medications involves

- IM
  - Inject slowly into upper-outer quadrant of gluteus.
  - Rotate injection sites.
  - Ensure that preparation is designed for IM and not IV use.
  - Absorption of all benzodiazepines other than lorazepam is *slower* after IM than oral administration.

- IV
  - IV lorazepam 0.5–1 mg, with or without haloperidol, is used for delirium or agitation.
  - IV diazepam 2.5–10 mg q 1–4 hours may be used for agitation or seizures but usually not for anxiety.
    - Do not exceed 30 mg in 8 hours.
- Parenteral benzodiazepine preparations should be protected from light.

## NOTES FOR PATIENT AND FAMILY

Despite concerns about patients becoming addicted to benzodiazepines, it is more common for patients to try to hold off as long as they can before taking a dose of a benzodiazepine for episodic or chronic anxiety.

- This approach *increases* the risk of addiction.
  - It focuses the patient's attention on anxiety and its relief.
  - The patient spends increasing amounts of time thinking about the medication.
  - When anxiety has to build to intolerable levels before taking another benzodiazepine dose seems justified, more medication is required to suppress symptoms. Interdose withdrawal may be more likely to occur following higher single doses, leading to more symptoms with which the patient becomes preoccupied.
  - Taking the medication regularly, in a manner consistent with its onset and offset of action, produces better results. For example:
    - Alprazolam may have to be taken every 2–3 hours because its high-potency, high-lipid solubility and fairly short half-life result in rapid onset and offset of action.
    - Longer-acting benzodiazepines (e.g., diazepam) are often taken twice a day, even though their half-life predicts the need for less frequent dosing.
    - High-lipid solubility results in the drug leaving the brain faster than it is eliminated from the body.
  - If patient forgets a dose, it can be taken within a few hours.
    - Otherwise, patient should wait for the next dose.
  - If patient not sure whether or not he or she took a short-acting medication (e.g., alprazolam), it is safer to take another dose than to wait for the next scheduled dose.

Important side effects of benzodiazepines include

- Sedation
  - If the dose is not raised too quickly, this effect often wears off.
- Impaired driving

- This problem may not go away with continued use.
- Have someone else drive with patient to be sure that driving skills are not affected.

Benzodiazepines that have been taken in high doses for a few weeks or in low doses for a few months can cause serious and sometimes dangerous withdrawal syndromes if they are stopped abruptly. Some of these syndromes may last for months after the medication is discontinued.

- Benzodiazepines should be withdrawn gradually.
- Withdrawal from alprazolam can be particularly troublesome.

### Buspirone

- Should be taken three times per day.
- If patient has been taking benzodiazepines, same rapid benefit will not be experienced with buspirone.
  - Wait a month before deciding whether the medication is working.
- Side effects include
  - Headache
  - Nausea
  - Insomnia
  - Agitation

### Propranolol

- Take this medication three or four times per day.
  - Single doses are helpful for performance anxiety.
- Propranolol can cause sedation and tiredness.
  - If patient plans to use for performance anxiety, take a test dose to be sure that it will not be too sedating.
- Propranolol also can cause
  - Sexual dysfunction
  - Difficulty concentrating
  - Depression (sometimes)
- Do not stop propranolol abruptly.

### Clonidine

- Common side effects include
  - Dry mouth
  - Sedation
  - Low blood pressure

- Do not stop clonidine abruptly.
  - Can cause dangerous elevations of blood pressure lasting a week or more.
  - Taper this medication whenever possible.

Benzodiazepines, but not buspirone, clonidine, and propranolol, severely potentiate the effects of alcohol.

Under most circumstances, meprobamate should not be prescribed for anxiety.

# CHAPTER EIGHT

# Hypnotics, Analgesics, and Treatments for Substance Abuse

Medications acting on the benzodiazepine receptor are useful for insomnia caused by acute stress, such as hospitalization, or by jet lag. Hospitalized patients, however, should be asked if they would like a sleeping pill; do not routinely prescribe these medications. In many cases, chronic insomnia is probably better treated with a sedating antidepressant.

Hypnotics are used to induce sleep. However, many medications used for anxiety (especially the benzodiazepines) can be used as hypnotics, and hypnotics that act on the benzodiazepine receptor can be used for anxiety. The decision to promote a particular benzodiazepine as an anxiolytic or a hypnotic is based not on the pharmacology of the drug but on marketing strategies and the kinds of studies the manufacturer chose to perform to get FDA approval. There is no reason why preparations with similar onset and duration of action (e.g., temazepam, lorazepam, oxazepam) could not be used for the same indication. In addition, many antidepressants (e.g., trazodone) are commonly used for their hypnotic action.

At one time barbiturates and related medications (e.g., chloral hydrate) were first-line treatments for insomnia. However, they disrupt normal sleep, rapidly induce tolerance, are associated with dangerous withdrawal syndromes, and are fatal in overdose. As a result, these medications have largely been replaced by medications acting either nonspecifically (i.e., benzodiazepines) on benzodiazepine receptors or on specific benzodiazepine receptor subtypes.

This chapter focuses on specific and nonspecific benzodiazepine receptor agonists and other sedating medications and concerns, such as

- Insomnia (pp. 427–430)
- Parasomnias (pp. 436–437)
- Amobarbital interview (p. 438)
- Prescription CNS-depressant withdrawal (pp. 441–450)
- Alcohol withdrawal (pp. 450–452)

- Barbiturate tolerance test (pp. 447–449)
- Restless legs syndrome (Stimulants, pp. 436–437)
- Management of alcoholism and other addictions (pp. 452–457, 458–462)
- Chronic pain (pp. 457–458).
- Sleep-phase syndromes (pp. 433–435)

Related topics that are addressed elsewhere include:
- Cataplexy (Antidepressants, Chapter 3)
- Narcolepsy and excessive daytime sleepiness (Stimulants, Chapter 9)
- Night terrors (Antidepressants, Chapter 3)
- Sleep apnea (Antidepressants, Chapter 3)
- Sleepwalking (Antidepressants, Chapter 3)
- Nicotine dependence (Stimulants, Chapter 9)

Table 8.1 provides a basic overview of the drugs discussed in this chapter.

## PHARMACOLOGY

Benzodiazepines induce sleep by facilitating the inhibitory action of GABA on neurons in the reticular activating system and other arousal centers (see pp. 361–313).
- Benzodiazepines act on all benzodiazepine receptors, producing sedation but also cognitive and psychomotor impairment and withdrawal.
- Benzodiazepines increase quality and length of sleep, decrease sleep latency, and slightly reduce REM sleep.
  - However, tolerance develops to the hypnotic effect after 1 or 2 months.
  - Efficacy can be retained by intermittent use
- Benzodiazepines decrease slow-wave sleep.
- Benzodiazepines replaced earlier hypnotics because they
  - Are safer in overdose
  - Do not suppress REM sleep to the same extent
  - Cause less respiratory and CNS depression
  - Are less likely to be abused
- The choice of a benzodiazepine hypnotic is determined by its pharmacology (see Chapter 7).
  - Flurazepam has a short elimination half-life, but its major active metabolite, desalkylflurazepam, has a half-life longer than a day.

## Table 8.1  Names, Dose Forms, Colors

| GENERIC NAMES | BRAND NAMES | DOSE FORMS (MG) | COLORS |
|---|---|---|---|
| | | **BENZODIAZEPINES** | |
| estazolam | Prosom | t: 1/2 | t: white/coral |
| flurazepam | Dalmane | c: 15/30 | c: orange-ivory/red-ivory |
| quazepam | Doral | t: 7.5/15 | t: all light orange-white speckled |
| temazepam | Restoril | c: 15/30 | c: maroon-pink/maroon-blue |
| triazolam | Halcion | t: 0.125/0.25 | t: white/blue |
| | | **IMIDAZOPYRIDINE AND PYRAZOLOPYRAMIDINE**<br>(SELECTIVE BENZODIAZEPINE RECEPTOR AGENTS) | |
| zaleplon | Sonata | c: 5/10 | c: opaque green-opaque pale green/opaque green-opaque light green |
| zolpidem | Ambien | c: 5/10 | c: pink/white |
| | | **CYCLOPYRROLONE**<br>(PARTIAL BENZODIAZEPINE RECEPTOR AGONIST) | |
| zopiclone | N/A* | t: 3.75, 7.5 | |
| | | **BARBITURATES**\*\* | |
| amobarbital | Amytal | p: 50 mg/ml | |
| butabarbital | Butisol | t: 15/30/50/100<br>e: 30 mg/5 ml | t: lavender/green/orange/pink<br>e: green |
| pentobarbital | Nembutal | c: 50/100<br>su: 30<br>p: 50 mg/ml | c: orange/yellow |
| phenobarbital | | Many generic doses | |
| secobarbital | Seconal | c: 100<br>p: 50 mg/ml | c: orange |
| | | **BARBITURATE-LIKE COMPOUNDS**\*\* | |
| chloral hydrate | | c: 250/500<br>e: 500 mg/5 ml | c: red/red |
| ethchlorvynol | Placidyl | c: 200/500/750 | c: red/red/green |
| paraldehyde | Paral | e: 30 g/30 ml | |

\* Not yet released at time of writing
\*\* Not recommended for general use
c = capsules; e = elixir; p = parenteral; su = suppository; t = tablets.

- Persistence of drug effect makes this medication most useful for patients with daytime anxiety, although high lipid solubility also can result in a rapid onset of action.
- Accumulation with repeated dosing often leads to daytime sedation.
- Accumulation is most problematic for older patients.
- Has been said to be more effective on the second or third night than on the first.

- Temazepam is relatively low in lipid solubility, resulting in a slow onset of action. This property, along with an intermediate half-life, make this medication most appropriate for patients with middle or terminal, but not initial, insomnia.
- Triazolam (a triazolobenzodiazepine in the same class as alprazolam) is very lipid soluble and high in potency with a short elimination half-life, resulting in a very rapid onset but short duration of action.
  - No active metabolites
  - Useful for patients who have difficulty falling asleep and who want to avoid daytime impairment.
  - High frequency of withdrawal symptoms, especially amnesia, the next morning.
  - Rebound insomnia may occur the next night.
  - Withdrawal late at night may cause early-morning awakening and anxiety.
  - Concerns have been raised about the efficacy of lower doses (0.125 mg) and the safety of higher doses (0.5 mg).
- Estazolam is also a triazolobenzodiazepine with high potency and lipid solubility and a fairly short half-life (about 2 hours).
- Duration of action of triazolobenzodiazepines is shorter than predicted by half-life because of rapid distribution in adipose tissue.

The receptor-selective benzodiazepine agonists zolpidem and zaleplon act primarily at benzodiazepine-1 ($\Omega$-1) receptors.

- Zolpidem, an imidazopyridine and zaleplon, a pyrazolopyrimidine, are not benzodiazepines in that they lack a diazepine ring.
  - Although it is technically accurate to describe these medications as "non-benzodiazepines," they act on benzodiazepine receptors, and their clinical effect can be blocked by the benzodiazepine receptor antagonist flumazenil.
  - They are selective for the benzodiazepine-1 receptor and have no significant effect on other benzodiazepine receptor subtypes at usual doses.
    - At higher doses they are less selective.

- Selectivity for the benzodiazepine-1 receptor results in a hypnotic and anxiolytic action.
  - No muscle relaxant or anticonvulsant effect.
- Slow-wave sleep is usually not affected.
- Lack of effects on benzodiazepine-3 receptors appears to result in a lower incidence of withdrawal and rebound symptoms.
  - These may occur, especially at higher doses and with more chronic treatment.
- Zolpidem and zaleplon are primarily used to treat insomnia.
  - As is true of other hypnotics, it is usually recommended that these medications not be administered for more than 2–8 weeks. However, one study showed no tolerance during 6 months of treatment with zolpidem (Cavallaro et al., 1993).
- Not as useful as benzodiazepines for anxiety.
- Not as effective for terminal insomnia because of short duration of action.
- Zolpidem now accounts for about one-third of all hypnotic prescriptions, having eclipsed benzodiazepines because of its more favorable side-effect profile.
  - Zolpidem has bioavailability of 70%.
  - Rapidly absorbed after oral administration and reaches peak plasma levels in 2–3 hours.
  - Ingestion with food slows absorption.
  - Zolpidem has an elimination half-life of 2–3 hours and has no active metabolites.
    - In most cases a bedtime dose is completely eliminated during the night, and there is no daytime hangover.
    - The pharmacology of zolpidem predicts greater usefulness for difficulty falling asleep than for interrupted sleep and early-morning awakening.
  - Zolpidem improves sleep latency and total sleep time to an extent similar to benzodiazepines, without reduction of REM or delta sleep or other changes in sleep architecture.
- Zaleplon is very rapidly absorbed but has just 30% bioavailability because of extensive presystemic metabolism.
  - It reaches peak plasma levels 1–2 hours after dosing and has an elimination half-life of around 1.5 hours.
  - Zaleplon is almost entirely metabolized to inactive metabolites.
  - In a 10 mg dose zaleplon reduces sleep latency to an extent similar to 0.25 mg of triazolam.
  - Usual doses increase total sleep time by about 42 minutes.

- At higher doses (40–60 mg) slow-wave sleep increases, and REM percentage decreases.
- Most useful for initial insomnia; usually will not keep patients asleep.
- Quazepam is also selective for the benzodiazepine-1 receptor.
  - Rapid absorption
  - Like fluazepam, quazepam may be less effective on first night than on subsequent nights.
  - Quazepam is metabolized to desalkylflurazepam, a nonselective benzodiazepine metabolite of flurazepam that accounts for 40% of total drug activity.
    - Desalkylflurazepam has a half-life of 47–100 hours.
    - Quazepam and 2-oxoquazepam have combined half-life of 39 hours.
  - With chronic dosing, this medication is similar to other long-acting benzodiazepine hypnotics.
- Zopiclone
  - Zopiclone is a nonselective partial agonist for benzodiazepine receptors
  - High affinity for benzodiazepine receptor but less sedation, psycho-motor impairment, muscle relaxation or additive potential
  - Sedative effect attributable mainly to S-enantiomer
  - Major metabolite (S-desmethylzopiclone) is more potent than parent drug
  - In a study comparing 593 patients with primary insomnia treated for six months with S-zopiclone with 195 treated with placebo, S-zopiclone significantly improved sleep latency, number of awakenings, number of nights awakened per week, total sleep time and quality of sleep, with significantly better daytime functioning, alertness and sense of physical well-being (Krystal, Walsh, Laska, et al., 2003)
    - Improvement was sustained over 6 months of treatment
  - Minimal rebound insomnia after discontinuation
  - A postmarketing survey of 297 admissions to 3 British addiction treatment centers found abuse potential was similar to antidepressants such as trazodone (Jaffe, Bloor, Crome, Carr, Alam, Simmons, & Meyer, 2004)

Most hypnotics decrease slow-wave and, to a lesser extent, REM sleep (Vorona & Catesby, 2000).

Barbiturates and related compounds (especially chloral hydrate) are rapidly absorbed. They have no active metabolites. Although many have elimination half-lives around a day, their duration of action is much shorter because of high lipid solubility

- Barbiturates suppress REM sleep.
  - Discontinuation causes REM rebound, which produces vivid, disturbing dreams.
- Sleep duration is increased and sleep latency is decreased, but sleep architecture is disrupted.
- Respiratory depression is more marked with barbiturates.
- Barbiturates induce their own metabolism as well as metabolism of other medications.
- Current legitimate uses of these medications include
  - Treatment of epilepsy (phenobarbital)
  - Diagnosis/treatment of CNS-depressant withdrawal (pentobarbital, phenobarbital)
  - Occasionally, psychiatric diagnosis (amobarbital)

Over-the-counter sleeping pills usually contain antihistamines; some also contain an analgesic or anticholinergic agent.

- Common examples:
  - Compoz: methapyrilene (antihistamine), pyrilamine (antihistamine)
  - Nytol: methapyrilene, salicylamide (salicylate)
  - Sleep-Eze: mathapyrilene, scopolamine (anticholinergic)
  - Sominex: methapyrilene, scopolamine, salicylamide (salicylate)
- All of these preparations are no better than placebo in improving sleep.
- They can all induce tolerance and rebound insomnia.
- Anticholinergic properties impair cognition in older and cognitively impaired patients.

Table 8.2 summarizes the dosing parameters for hypnotics and barbiturates.

## CLINICAL INDICATIONS AND USE

Insomnia is defined as insufficient sleep that results in daytime sleepiness or impairment.

- People who sleep just a few hours and do not feel tired do not have insomnia.
  - Some people can function well with little sleep ("short sleepers").
  - Bitter complaints of insomnia with good functioning, lack of fatigue, and intense irritability during the day may be a manifestation of mania/hypomania.

**Table 8.2 Doses**

| GENERIC NAMES | USUAL DOSES (MG) | DOSE RANGES (MG) | WHEN TO TAKE BEFORE BEDTIME (HOURS) | GERIATRIC DOSE (MG) |
|---|---|---|---|---|
| SELECTIVE BENZODIAZEPINE RECEPTOR AGONISTS AND BENZODIAZEPINE PARTIAL AGONISTS | | | | |
| zaleplon | 10 | 5–20 | 0.25 | 5–10 |
| zolpidem | 10 | 5–20 | 0.5 | 5 |
| zopiclone | 7.5 | 3.75–15 | 0.5 | 3.75 |
| BENZODIAZEPINES | | | | |
| estazolam | 1 | 1–2 | 0.5 | 0.5 |
| flurazepam | 15–30 | 15–30 | 0.5 | 15 |
| quazepam | 7.5–15 | 7.5–15 | 1.5 | 7.5 |
| temazepam | 15–30 | 15–30 | 1–2 | 15 |
| triazolam | 0.25 | 0.125–0.5 | 0.5 | 0.125 |
| SLEEP HORMONE | | | | |
| melatonin | 1 | 0.5–3 | 0.5–1 | 0.5–1 |
| BARBITURATES* | | | | |
| amobarbital | 150–200 | 65–200 | 0.5 | 65 |
| butabarbital | 50–100 | 50–100 | 0.5 | 50 |
| pentobarbital | 100 | 50–200 | 0.5 | 50 |
| phenobarbital | 100–200 | 15–600 | 1 | 16 |
| secobarbital | 100–200 | 100–200 | 0.25 | 50 |
| BARBITURATE-LIKE COMPOUNDS | | | | |
| chloral hydrate | 500–1500 | 500–2000 | 0.5 | 500 |
| ethchlorvynol | 500–750 | 500–1000 | 0.5 | 500 |
| paraldehyde | 5000–10,000 | 2000–15,000 | 0.5 | 4000 |

\* Use of these agents for insomnia or anxiety is not recommended.

Before using a hypnotic, consider insomnia secondary to

- Medications
  - Especially stimulants, activating antidepressants, and antipsychotics
    - Induction of anxiety or hypomania by antidepressants in the treatment of bipolar depression

- Withdrawal during the night from short-acting sedating medications (e.g., alprazolam) taken at bedtime
- Rebound insomnia is common with chronic use of sleeping pills.
- Substances
  - Caffeine
    - Half-life of about 5 hours can result in insomnia with ingestion of caffeine in the late afternoon.
  - Stimulants
  - Alcohol
    - Patients with insomnia often drink to get to sleep.
    - The sedative effect of alcohol can induce sleep, but withdrawal from alcohol in the middle of the night wakes up the patient.
    - Alcohol use suppresses the normal nighttime increase in melatonin.
    - Alcohol also directly alters sleep architecture, and effects may persist months to 1 year after discontinuation.
- Medical disorders and parasomnias
  - Pain
  - Nocturnal myoclonus
  - Restless legs syndrome
  - Gastroesophageal reflux
  - Sleep apnea
- Psychiatric disorders
  - Major depression
    - Most common cause of insomnia presenting to a sleep disorders laboratory.
  - Bipolar disorder
  - Nocturnal panic attacks
- Sleep-phase disorders
  - Sleep–wake cycle becomes desynchronized from environmental cues.
  - Sleep-phase delay manifested by difficulty falling asleep and difficulty waking up at a normal time.
  - Sleep-phase advance manifested by feeling sleepy early in the evening and early-morning awakening.
  - Jet lag
  - Work shift change
    - Sleep may never normalize for some night-shift workers.

Treatment of the primary condition often reverses secondary insomnia.
- Insomnia may remit weeks to months after remission of depression.

- Early treatment of secondary insomnia may be necessary while anxiety, depression, or mania/hypomania is being treated. Initial choices for treating insomnia include
  - Trazodone in unipolar depression
  - Sedating atypical antipsychotic (e.g., olanzapine, quetiapine)
  - Selective benzodiazepine-1 receptor agonist (e.g., zolpidem)
  - Valproate

For primary insomnia, cognitive–behavior therapy is as effective as pharmacotherapy.
- Benefits of psychotherapy persist after treatment is discontinued.
- Benefit of hypnotics does not persist after medication is discontinued unless a situation causing insomnia is resolved.

Hypnotics are most effective for time-limited insomnia associated with a stressor or sleep-phase change (e.g., jet lag).
- Barbiturates and related medications are rarely appropriate for this indication.
- Over-the-counter sleeping pills are no more effective than placebo and are risky for older patients.
- Benzodiazepine receptor agonists (zolpidem, zaleplon, and benzodiazepines) are now first choices for transient insomnia.

Common problems with hypnotics include:
- High-potency, highly lipid-soluble short half-life benzodiazepines (e.g., triazolam) induce sleep rapidly but have a high incidence of amnesia the next day (withdrawal).
- Medications with longer half-lives can cause daytime impairment and can accumulate with repeated dosing.
  - Risk of falls and confusion in older patients
- Total sleep time increased by less than 1 hour.
  - The perception of increased sleep is > actual increased sleep time.
- Tolerance may develop in a few weeks.
- Receptor-selective agents may not be as effective as benzodiazepines.
- Rebound insomnia:
  - Discontinuation syndrome that can occur after prolonged treatment with any hypnotic.
  - As with other discontinuation syndromes, risk of rebound insomnia is a function of half-life, potency, and lipid solubility, with higher risk for
    - Triazolam
    - Estazolam

- Temazepam
- Flurazepam
- Quazepam
- Rebound insomnia can lead to escalation of both dose and frequency of treatment, which then makes the problem worse.
- Management of rebound:
  - Withdraw medication very slowly.
  - Switch to longer-acting benzodiazepine and then withdraw that gradually.
  - Add trazodone before withdrawing the other hypnotic.

## Choosing a Hypnotic

The nature of the insomnia and associated symptoms should dictate the choice of a hypnotic, as should comorbid disorders.

- Primarily, difficulty falling asleep
  - Estazolam
  - Triazolam
  - Zaleplon
  - Zolpidem
  - Alprazolam
  - Diazepam
- Middle insomnia
  - Zolpidem
  - Temazepam
  - Oxazepam
  - Lorazepam
- Late (terminal) insomnia
  - Quazepam
  - Temazepam
  - Flurazepam
  - Clonazepam
- Daytime anxiety
  - Flurazepam
  - Chlordiazepoxide
  - Clonazepam
- Need for chronic treatment or concern about substance dependence
  - Trazodone
    - Rapid absorption

- Peak levels in 20–30 minutes
- Half life 5–8 hours; daytime sedation in about 20%
- No studies of long-term efficacy, but many clinicians find it to be useful.
- Low bedtime doses can cause priapism.
  - Sedating TCA (doxepin, trimipramine, amitriptyline)
    - Low doses can be used to augment SSRI that causes or does not help insomnia.
    - Half-life > 24 hours can result in accumulation.
    - Hypotension, slowed cardiac conduction, and anticholinergic side effects can be problematic for older patients.
  - Sedating atypical antipsychotic
    - Especially useful for insomnia associated with severe or psychotic depression.
    - Sometimes helpful for nonpsychotic patients, especially if they are depressed.
    - First choices are quetiapine or olanzapine.
  - Melatonin (see pp. 507, 512–513)
    - Melatonin levels decrease with age.
    - More likely to correct reduced sleep than to improve normal sleep.
    - Doses of 1 mg produce physiological levels.
    - Peak hypnotic effect occurs 2 hours after taking higher doses (e.g., 5 mg oral, 1.7 mg sublingual).
    - May be indicated for insomnia associated with alcohol dependence.
  - Tryptophan and 5-hydroxytryptophan
    - Most useful for multiple partial awakenings without full awakening.
    - Not as effective as benzodiazepines and related compounds.
    - Eosinophilia-myalgia syndrome with tryptophan traced to manufacturing problem that has been corrected.
    - Hypnotic dose 1–2 gm L-tryptophan

Insomnia associated with bipolar disorder
- Valproate
  - Often requires a daytime dose as primary thymoleptic, but can improve sleep in moderate doses.
- Atypical antipsychotic
  - Olanzapine best studied for mania.
    - May be helpful chronically, but occasionally becomes over-stimulating.

- Quetiapine
  - Less antidepressant effect at lower doses makes sedative effect predominate without risk of destabilizing mood.
- Both may produce daytime sedation.
- Neuroleptic
  - May reduce insomnia caused by dysphoric overstimulation associated with not being able to shut off one's mind.

## Night Terrors

- Result from a disturbance of stage-4 sleep.
- Benzodiazepines can be useful.
- SSRIs are sometimes helpful.

## Sleep-Phase Disorders

Desynchronization of the sleep–wake cycle from circadian cues can be caused by
- Sleep-phase syndromes
  - Amount of sleep is normal if patient is allowed to fall asleep and wake up in accordance with time of feeling sleepy and alert rather than with environmental zeitgebers.
  - Sleep-phase delay
    - Initial insomnia, with difficulty getting out of bed in the morning
  - Sleep-phase advance
    - Feeling tired early in the evening, with early-morning awakening
- Mood disorders
  - Sleep-phase advance in depression with typical symptoms
  - Sleep-phase delay more common in atypical and bipolar depression and in seasonal affective disorder (SAD)
- Jet lag
  - Traveling east across time zones can cause sleep-phase delay in new time zone.
  - Traveling west can cause sleep-phase advance in new time zone.
- Work shift change
  - Many jobs (e.g., police, fire fighters) rotate shifts every few weeks.
    - May make it impossible to accommodate to any sleep schedule.
    - Workers function in a chronically impaired state.
  - Some workers never accommodate to permanent night shift.

TREATMENT

### General principles

- The best cue to an abnormal sleep–wake cycle is exposure to bright light at the time of waking up (see pp. 157–158).
- Sedating medications at bedtime may promote sleep but do not reset the sleep–wake cycle.
- Because the normal sleep–wake cycle is longer than the 24-hour day, it is easier to extend it than to shorten it.
  - More difficult to voluntarily move sleep earlier than to phase-delay sleep.
- For change to endure, sleep should not be shifted by more than an hour/night.

### Sleep-phase advance

- Patient starts going to bed when first feels sleepy, even if this is in late afternoon or early evening, and wakes up naturally, even if it is in the middle of the night.
- Patient starts going to bed 30–60 minutes later each night.
  - Sleeping pill often not necessary because patient is already sleepy.
- Wake up in morning 30–60 minutes later with each corresponding change in bedtime.
  - Use artificial bright light (10,000 lux) for at least 30 minutes on awakening.
- Continue gradually delaying time of going to sleep and waking up until these are in phase with environmental cues.
- Morning bright light may have to be continued.
- Taking melatonin early in the morning may help to phase-delay sleep.

### Sleep-phase delay

- Patient tries to go to bed and wake up 30 minutes earlier each day.
  - Attempts to phase-advance sleep can be facilitated by taking melatonin at bedtime and using bright light at the time of waking.
  - Bedtime hypnotic may facilitate moving sleep earlier.
- If sleep cannot be advanced, it may be necessary to phase delay it progressively.
  - Difficult for patients who must work during the day.
  - Patient starts going to bed when sleepy, even if very late at night, and sleeps until he or she feels like waking up, even if during the afternoon.
  - Starts going to bed and waking up 30–60 minutes later each day.

- Hypnotic usually not necessary, because patient feels sleepy at time of going to bed.
- Use artificial bright light at time of waking up.
- Continue to make sleep later, until it has gone around the clock to time that is synchronized with the environment.

## SPECIFIC CONDITIONS

Jet lag
- Traveling east across multiple time zones
  - On airplane, go to sleep at time that corresponds to bedtime at destination.
    - Skip meal and movie, if necessary.
    - Take melatonin or hypnotic.
  - Upon arrival, go outside in sunlight or use artificial bright light.
  - Do not go to sleep until the normal bedtime at the destination.
- Traveling west across multiple time zones
  - Go to sleep as soon as airplane takes off.
    - Take melatonin or hypnotic, if necessary.
  - Wake up at time corresponding to time of awakening at destination.
    - May be a just few hours later.
  - Do not take a nap the first day
  - Go to sleep at normal bedtime for destination.
    - Hypnotic necessary only if patient is not sleepy or has taken a brief nap before bedtime.
  - Go out into daylight or use artificial bright light the next morning.

Work shift change
- Rotating shifts more frequently than every 3 weeks results in chronic sleep-phase desynchronization.
- Use artificial bright light at time of awakening that corresponds to work schedule.
- Ambient bright light (>10,000 lux) in workplace helps to promote alertness and synchronize sleep–wake schedule to work shift.

Insomnia in demented patients with agitation at night and confusion during the day is often caused by reversal of the sleep–wake cycle.
- Hypnotics increase cognitive impairment and cause more confusion.
- Morning bright light may correct the sleep-phase reversal and reduce difficulty falling asleep at night as well as nighttime wandering and daytime impairment.

### Sleep Movement Disorders

Restless legs syndrome and nocturnal myoclonus are common causes of insomnia.

Signs and symptoms of restless legs syndrome (RLS)
- Restlessness in both legs, sometimes also in arms and other regions
- Irresistible urge to move legs, often with uncomfortable sensation within legs
- Symptoms worse when body at rest.
  - Temporarily relieved with motor activity, especially walking.
- Milder symptoms are more frequent earlier in the evening.
  - More severe symptoms do not have a circadian pattern.
- Usually associated with periodic limb movements of sleep.
- Symptoms worsened by drowsiness and improved by alertness.


RLS may be secondary to
- Iron deficiency
  - Symptoms can be treated with 40–50 µg/L ferratin.
- End-stage renal disease
  - 20–62% have RLS.
  - May be secondary to anemia.
    - Relieved by erythropoietin or other measures to treat anemia.
    - Dialysis does not relieve RLS.
- Pregnancy
  - Iron deficiency anemia in pregnancy causes RLS.
  - About 10–25% of pregnant women have it.
  - Most common in third trimester and postpartum period.
- Treatment with SSRIs
- Arthritis


Treatment of RLS
- Dopaminergic agents are most predictably useful (see pp. 467–473).
- Bedtime hypnotics
  - Clonazepam 0.25–2 mg
  - Oxazepam 10–40 mg
  - Zaleplon 5–20 mg
  - Zolpidem 5–20 mg
  - Triazolam 0.125–0.5 mg

- Anticonvulsants
  - Gabapentin
    - Start with 300 mg.
    - Increase to 3600 mg/day, given on tid basis.
- Some opioids reduce RLS symptoms
  - Propoxyphene
    - Start with 100–200 mg.
    - Increase to 600 mg/day in two or three doses.
  - Hydrocodone
    - Start with 5 mg.
    - Increase to 20–30 mg/day in two or three doses.
  - Oxycodone in same doses as hydrocodone
  - Codeine
    - Start with 30 mg.
    - Increase to 180 mg/day in two or three doses.
  - Methadone
    - Start with 5 mg at least 2 hours before bedtime.
    - Increase to 20 mg/day in two doses.
  - Tramodol
    - Start with 50 mg.
    - Increase to 300 mg/day in two or three doses.
  - Subcutaneous apomorphine
- Sequence of treatments
  - If symptoms occur every night, start with dopamine agonist, then try opiate, then gabapentin or hypnotic.
  - If occasional symptoms, start with levodopa, then hypnotic, then opiate.
  - If symptoms are painful, start with gabapentin or opiate, then dopaminergic agent, then hypnotic.

## Periodic limb movements of sleep (PLMS)

- The majority of patients with RLS also have PLMS.
- Treatment is the same as for RLS.
- Nocturnal myoclonus can be side effect of SSRIs.
  - Treat with dopaminergic agent such as bupropion.
    - May disrupt sleep if taken in the evening.

### Amobarbital Interview

IV amobarbital is occasionally used to
- Distinguish between psychogenic and neurological confusion/memory loss
  - Neurological causes get worse, whereas psychogenic syndromes may improve.
- Facilitate diagnosis of conversion disorder
  - Functional symptoms may remit with amobarbital.

Use of amobarbital is *not* recommended
- To facilitate recall of repressed memories
- To diagnose malingering or lying
- For ongoing treatment

Use of the amobarbital interview
- Examine for papilledema.
  - Increased intracranial pressure is a contraindication to barbiturates.
- Those administering interview should be able to resuscitate patient, if necessary.
  - Certification in advanced or, at least, basic cardiac life support is recommended.
  - Resuscitation equipment should be available.
- Mix 500 mg sodium amobarbital in 10 mL sterile water.
- Open intravenous line through 21-gauge butterfly needle.
- Administer 50 mg/minute, up to 100–150 mg.
- Wait 2–5 minutes between subsequent dosage increases of 50 mg.
- Dose to mild intoxication level.
  - Slight dysarthria and nystagmus
- Use brief, concrete sentences.
- If patient falls asleep, attempt to awaken and continue interview.
  - If patient cannot wake up or is not fully coherent, let the patient sleep.
  - Observe for respiratory depression until the patient is fully awake.

## SIDE EFFECTS

Side effects of benzodiazepine hypnotics are the same as those for benzodiazepine anxiolytics (pp. 393–398).

Time course of side effects depends on pharmacology of medication and age of patient.

- Older patients have more severe side effects with lower doses.
- Long-acting medications accumulate with repeated dosing, leading to daytime sedation, cognitive impairment, hypotension, and falls after a few weeks of treatment.
- Benzodiazepine receptor-selective agonists produce side effects that are similar to benzodiazepines but are attenuated.

### Cardiovascular/Respiratory Side Effects

RESPIRATORY DEPRESSION

- Benzodiazepines and other CNS depressants can aggravate chronic obstructive lung disease, asthma, and sleep apnea.
- For patients with risk factors for respiratory depression who need a hypnotic, safer medications include
  - Trazodone
  - Quetiapine
  - Zolpidem or zaleplon *not* entirely safe.

### Central Nervous System Side Effects

AMNESIA

- Anterograde amnesia is most frequently caused by withdrawal from a single bedtime dose of a high-potency, short half-life benzodiazepine hypnotic, especially triazolam.
  - More likely with higher doses (e.g., 0.5 mg)
  - Multiple reports of amnesia occurring when triazolam is taken to prevent jet lag and the traveler has had a few drinks.
  - No memory of events occurring within 6–11 hours of ingesting medication.
  - Does not necessarily recur following a second dose the next night.
  - Has also been reported with 20 mg or more of zolpidem or zaleplon.
    - Amnesia only for about 1–3 hours

FALLS

- Can be caused by ataxia or confusion when getting up in the middle of the night.
- Can occur at night with any hypnotic.
- May occur during the day with hypnotics that accumulate.
  - Long-acting benzodiazepines should be avoided in older patients.

HANGOVER

- More common with long-acting benzodiazepine hypnotics
- Sometimes occurs with trazodone and quetiapine.
- Aggravated by
  - Alcohol intake
  - Decreased fluid intake
- Management:
  - Change to a shorter-acting agent.
  - Take medication earlier in the evening.

RENAL/URINARY

- Interstitial nephritis has been reported with zopiclone

## PREGNANCY AND LACTATION

- Insomnia is common during pregnancy.
- Necessary to balance risk of medication with risk of sleep deprivation.
- If insomnia is caused by physical discomfort or anxiety about the pregnancy, addressing these issues is more effective than giving a sleeping pill.
- "Natural" hypnotics such as melatonin (see pp. 512–573) have not been proven to be safe during pregnancy.

### Teratogenicity

- Amobarbital is teratogenic.
  - Ethchlorvynol also may cause fetal malformations.
  - No data on chloral hydrate and other barbiturates.
- Benzodiazepine teratogenicity discussed on pages 398–399.
- Insufficient data on receptor-selective benzodiazepine agonists.

### Direct Effects on Newborn

- Withdrawal may occur in newborns who experience in utero exposure to CNS depressants.
  - Withdrawal from barbiturates and related medications is more severe.
- Newborn may be overly sedated with CNS depression and manifest
  - Hypotonia
  - Poor feeding

- Impaired early attachment
- More common with longer-acting medications.
- Usually advisable to discontinue hypnotics a few weeks before anticipated date of delivery, unless they are absolutely necessary.

### Lactation

- All hypnotics enter breast milk.
- Infant exposure to hypnotics in breast milk can cause
  - Sedation
  - Respiratory depression
  - Poor feeding
  - Impaired temperature regulation
  - Withdrawal syndromes if breast milk levels are inconsistent
- Effects may persist for weeks after exposure to long-acting benzodiazepines.
- If hypnotics must be used during lactation
  - Use shorter-acting preparation.
  - Tell mother to nurse before taking medication.
  - Assess infant plasma benzodiazepine level.
  - Monitor infant closely.

Table 8.3 summarizes interactions between hypnotics and other drugs.

Table 8.4 presents the effects on laboratory tests.

### WITHDRAWAL

Three types of discontinuation syndromes may occur with abrupt or rapid cessation or decrease in dose of CNS-depressant hypnotics.

- *Relapse:* return of insomnia suppressed by the hypnotic
- *Rebound:* increased insomnia caused by stopping medication
- *Withdrawal:* New signs and symptoms that are not a component of insomnia, such as
  - Agitation
  - Confusion
  - Myoclonus
  - Hyperreflexia
  - Increased blood pressure
  - Agitation
  - Delirium
  - Seizures

**Table 8.3  Drug–Drug Interactions**

| DRUGS (X) INTERACT WITH: | CHLORAL HYDRATE (C) | COMMENTS |
|---|---|---|
| alcohol | X↑ C↑ | This "Mickey Finn" combination yields CNS depression. Patients can have fainting, sedation, flushing, tachycardia, headache, hypotension, and amnesia. Avoid mixture, especially in cardiovascular problems. |
| dicumarol | X↑ | Chloral hydrate may briefly accelerate hypoprothrombinemic response to dicumarol, but effect quickly disappears. Adverse clinical responses are uncommon, but bleeding may occur. Benzodiazepine hypnotics are preferred. *Don't* give chloral hydrate to patients on anticoagulants. |
| furosemide | X↑ | Diaphoresis, hot flashes, and hypertension occur with IV furosemide. Give IV furosemide with caution to any patient on chloral hydrate in past 24 h. |
| sedatives and sedating drugs | X↑ C↑ | Increased sedation, confusion. |
| TCAs | X↓ | Decreased antidepressant effect. |
| warfarin (*see* dicumarol) | | |

| DRUGS (X) INTERACT WITH: | DISULFIRAM (D) | COMMENTS |
|---|---|---|
| alcohol | D↑ | (*See* pages 453–455.) |
| amitriptyline | X↑ | Avoid combination until more information. When amitriptyline was added to disulfiram, 2 cases of a CNS cognitive disorder were reported with confusion, hallucinations, and memory loss in 1–4 weeks. Rapid improvement when one or both agents stopped. |
| anticonvulsants | X↑ | Excessive sedation. |
| barbiturates | X↑ | Excessive sedation. |
| benzodiazepines | X↑ | Disulfiram increases most benzodiazepine levels (not 3-hydroxy compounds, lorazepam, oxazepam, temazepam, and, partially, clonazepam); more sedation. Lower benzodiazepines or switch to 3-hydroxy compounds. |
| cephalosporins | D↑ | Disulfiram reaction. |
| cocaine | D↑ | Increased disulfiram effect. |
| dicumarol (*see* warfarin) | | |

(*continues*)

## Table 8.3 Continued

| DRUGS (X) INTERACT WITH: | DISULFIRAM (C) | COMMENTS |
|---|---|---|
| isoniazid | D↑ | Combination produces ataxia, irritability, disorientation, dizziness, and nausea. Frequency unclear, but combine cautiously. Reduce or stop disulfiram. |
| metronidazole | D↑ | Combination produces CNS toxicity, psychosis, and confusion. |
| MAOIs | D↑ | Severe CNS reactions. |
| paraldehyde | X↑ | Disulfiram may inhibit paraldehyde's metabolism, leading to toxicity. |
| perphenazine | X↑ | Decreases perphenazine's metabolism, risking toxicity. |
| phenytoin | X↑ | Disulfiram consistently increases phenytoin, inducing phenytoin toxicity (e.g., ataxia, mental impairment, nystagmus). Often occurs about 4 h after disulfiram's initial dose. After stopping disulfiram, symptoms may persist for 3 weeks. Monitor for reduced phenytoin response when disulfiram is stopped. |
| theophylline | X↑ | Disulfiram increases theophylline, which may prompt toxicity. Lower theophylline may be needed. If disulfiram is changed, monitor patient's theophylline level. |
| warfarin | X↑ | Disulfiram increases response to warfarin, which prompts bleeding. If disulfiram is started or stopped in patients taking oral anticoagulants, monitor carefully. Similar interaction with dicumarol likely but not reported. |

| DRUGS (X) INTERACT WITH: | ETHCHLORVYNOL (E) | COMMENTS |
|---|---|---|
| amitriptyline | X↑ E↑ | Transient delirium noted in patient taking 1 g of ethchlorvynol and amitriptyline. |
| anticoagulants | X↓ | Ethchlorvynol may inhibit response to dicumarol and possibly warfarin. May need to adjust oral anticoagulants or, preferably, replace ethchlorvynol with a benzodiazepine. |

↑ Increases; ↓ Decreases.

After reviewing the benzodiazepine interactions on pages 401–404, examine these other interactions specific to hypnotics. All of these are potentiated by other sedatives and sedating drugs. All CNS depressants, including agents selective for benzodiazepine-1 receptors and benzodiazepine partial agonists, have additive interactions with alcohol.

Table 8.4 **Effects on Laboratory Tests**

| GENERIC NAMES | BLOOD/SERUM TESTS | URINE TESTS |
|---|---|---|
| Benzodiazepines | WBC ↓, RBC ↓, LFT ↑ | None |
| Chloral hydrate | WBC ↓ | Ketones ↑<br>Glucose*** ↑<br>Catecholamines**** ↑↓<br>17-hydroxycorticosteroids† ↑ |
| Disulfiram | Cholesterol ↑ | VMA ↓ |

↑ Increases, ↓ Decreases

Rebound and withdrawal are more likely to occur with

- Rapid medication discontinuation of usual doses taken for just a few months
- Discontinuation of higher doses
- Longer duration of treatment
- CNS depressants that are
  - Shorter acting
  - More potent
  - More lipid soluble
- Dependence (tolerance or withdrawal) can occur
  - After 4–6 weeks at three to four times the therapeutic dose
  - After several months at usual therapeutic doses
- In general, withdrawal
  - Appears sooner, is more intense, but does not last as long with short-acting medications that do not have active metabolites (e.g., triazolam, alprazolam).
    - Interdose withdrawal is common with short-acting, high-potency benzodiazepines such as alprazolam.
    - Withdrawal after a single dose is common with midazolam.
  - Appears later, is attenuated, but lasts much longer with long-acting medications and medications with active metabolites (e.g., flurazepam, diazepam).
- CNS-depressant withdrawal usually begins
  - 12–16 hours after discontinuing barbiturates
  - 12 hours–3 days after discontinuing alprazolam
  - 5 days–2 weeks after discontinuing diazepam
- Withdrawal may appear weeks after discontinuation of long-acting benzodiazepines and may persist for months.

- Signs and symptoms are attenuated but prolonged and include anxiety, insomnia, myoclonus, hyperesthesias, paresthesias, and hypervigilance.
- Benzodiazepines > placebo in controlled trials of CNS-depressant withdrawal for reducing withdrawal symptoms and preventing seizures (Kosten & O'Connor, 2003).

Alcohol withdrawal syndromes, described in the section below, are a group of CNS-depressant discontinuation syndromes that occur more frequently with alcohol than other agents but that overlap with other CNS depressants, especially barbiturates.

## Withdrawing Benzodiazepines and Selective Benzodiazepine Receptor Agonists

There are a number of situations in which benzodiazepines are withdrawn electively.

- An alternative medication that is not a CNS depressant (e.g., an antidepressant for GAD or panic disorder) is substituted for a benzodiazepine.
  - The new medication will not prevent benzodiazepine withdrawal, but it will prevent relapse and may reduce rebound of the underlying disorder.
  - Add the new medication first and determine whether it is effective.
  - Slowly withdraw the benzodiazepine.
    - If necessary, first switch from a shorter- to a longer-acting benzodiazepine (see below).
- A patient who has been taking a low dose of a benzodiazepine or other hypnotic for a few weeks no longer is experiencing the same stress, and the medication is being discontinued.
  - Reduce the dose by 10–25% every few days.
- A patient who has been taking a high dose of a benzodiazepine for a short period of time or a lower dose for months or longer wants to discontinue the medication.
  - Decreasing the dose by 10% every week or so produces a more comfortable, if longer, withdrawal.
  - Decreasing the dose by 25% every week can produce withdrawal symptoms but is unlikely to cause a seizure.
- A patient discontinuing a short-acting benzodiazepine develops significant withdrawal or rebound symptoms, even if the dose is being reduced very slowly.
  - Switch over gradually to a longer-acting benzodiazepine.

- Changing immediately from the shorter- to the longer-acting medication may be poorly tolerated, because the short-acting drug is already at a steady state, whereas it will take four to seven half-lives for the new medication to achieve steady state.
- Add the new medication at a dose equivalent to 25% of the existing medication.
- Decrease the dose of the short-acting medication by 25%.
- Exchange 25% of the total dose at a rate equivalent to the time to steady state of the new medication.
- Then withdraw the long-acting medication at a rate of 10% every 4–7 days.
- Faster withdrawal may be possible
- Add carbamazepine.
  - May reduce withdrawal symptoms with short-acting benzodiazepines.
  - Carbamazepine is better than placebo and comparable to benzodiazepines (Kosten & O'Connor, 2003).
  - Mostly useful for preventing seizures
  - Usual dose around 600 mg/day
  - Continue carbamazepine for 4 weeks after benzodiazepine has been withdrawn.
- Add valproate.
  - No controlled studies, but GABAergic action may help to attenuate receptor changes associated with withdrawal.
  - Valproate has antianxiety actions that may be useful.
- After reducing an initially high dose, attempts to discontinue the last 1–1.5 mg of alprazolam results in intolerable withdrawal symptoms.
  - Chronic use of benzodiazepines results in down-regulation of benzodiazepine receptors and up-regulation of an endogenous benzodiazepine inverse agonist that increases arousal.
  - Normally, benzodiazepine receptors gradually up-regulate as the number of benzodiazepine molecules decreases.
  - Alprazolam withdrawal is associated with paradoxical down-regulation of benzodiazepine receptors at lower doses.
    - Because more molecules of the inverse agonist compete with fewer benzodiazepine receptors for a small number of receptors, arousal increases.
  - Add a longer-acting benzodiazepine in equivalent doses (e.g., 0.5–2 mg clonazepam), withdraw the remainder of the alprazolam more slowly, then withdraw the other benzodiazepine.

- Benzodiazepines also may be discontinued using the barbiturate protocol described below.

### Barbiturate Tolerance Test

CNS depressants, including benzodiazepines, barbiturates, and alcohol, are all cross-reactive because they act at one or another site on the GABA–benzodiazepine receptor complex. One such agent therefore can be substituted for another to treat abstinence syndromes. When the substance is known and the patient is relatively reliable, a long-acting benzodiazepine can be substituted and slowly withdrawn. However, when the clinical picture is complicated, the diagnosis is unclear (e.g., delirium of unknown etiology), multiple CNS depressants are being used, or substances with unpredictable abstinence syndromes (e.g., glutethimide) are suspected, a barbiturate tolerance test can be used to diagnose a withdrawal syndrome. The barbiturate can then be used for withdrawal. Phenobarbital is used in 10% of substance abuse programs in the U.S., but only a few controlled studies have been published (Kosten & O'Connor, 2003). Barbiturates are more likely to cause respiratory depression than benzodiazepines.

- The patient should be exhibiting signs of withdrawal, usually with a negative toxicology screen.
- Be certain that patient does not have increased intracranial pressure, porphyria, or hypersensitivity to barbiturates.
- Administer a test dose of pentobarbital or phenobarbital and examine 1 hour later for signs of intoxication or withdrawal (Smith & Wesson, 1999).
  - Confusion, dysarthria, postural hypotension, and even somnolence may occur in either state.
  - Manifestations specific to withdrawal include
    - Hyperreflexia
    - Hypertension
    - Tachycardia
    - Fever
    - Tremor
  - Manifestations specific to intoxication include
    - Ataxia
    - Depressed reflexes
    - Nystagmus
    - Positive Romberg test

- Patients who develop obvious intoxication are not tolerant to a barbiturate, are not likely to be experiencing an abstinence syndrome, and do not require further treatment.
- The pentobarbital tolerance test is based on the patient's response to a standardized dose of pentobarbital.
  - Administer 200 mg pentobarbital during signs of withdrawal.
  - Estimated 24-hour dose of pentobarbital equivalent is based on response 1 hour after test dose, as summarized in Table 8.5.
  - If patient has no evidence of tolerance, give additional 100 mg of pentobarbital every 2 hours, until patient is intoxicated or total pentobarbital dose administered is 500 mg in 6 hours.
    - The total test dose needed to produce signs of intoxication is the 6-hour pentobarbital requirement.
  - The estimated total daily dose is then divided into four equal doses and given every 6 hours for 1–2 days.
  - The total dose is reduced by 10%/day.
  - Increase the rate of dosage reduction if intoxication develops.
  - Reduce the rate of dosage reduction if withdrawal recurs.
  - Phenobarbital can be substituted for pentobarbital and withdrawn instead (30 mg phenobarbital = 100 mg pentobarbital).

Phenobarbital has advantages over pentobarbital.
- Longer half-life
- Better anticonvulsant
- Available in injectable form

Phenobarbital test utilizes a similar approach to a test dose.
- Keep a table of specific signs and symptoms recorded 1 hour after, and just before, each dose.

Table 8.5  Pentobarbital Tolerance Test

| DEGREE OF TOLERANCE | SIGNS | ESTIMATED 24-HOUR PENTOBARBITAL DOSE (MG) |
|---|---|---|
| None | Asleep | None |
| Mild–moderate | Drowsy, gross ataxia, coarse nystagmus, positive Romberg | 300–450 |
| Definite | Dysarthria, mild ataxia, fine nystagmus | 450–700 |
| Marked | Nystagmus only | 700–850 |
| Severe | No response or patient wakes up | ≥ 850 |

- Give 100 mg when patient has evidence of withdrawal and assess response 1 hour later.
  - Consider lower initial dose (30–60 mg) for older patients.
- The next dose depends on the patient's response.
  - Patient falls asleep or is grossly intoxicated:
    - No further treatment needed.
  - Patient shows signs of moderate intoxication (e.g., drowsiness, dysarthria, nystagmus):
    - Give another 100 mg dose in 2–4 hours and reassess an hour later.
  - Patient has mild intoxication (e.g., nystagmus only):
    - Give 100 mg phenobarbital in 1 hour and reassess.
  - Patient has no intoxication or wakes up:
    - Give 100–200 mg in 1 hour and reassess.
  - Based on response to each dose, give additional doses of phenobarbital until patient is clearly intoxicated or has had about 500 mg.
    - If moderate intoxication after subsequent doses, give 100 mg doses every 2–4 hours.
    - If no intoxication with subsequent doses, give 100–200 mg every 1–4 hours.
  - Divide the total dose necessary to produce intoxication into three or four daily doses and give every 6–8 hours for 2 days.
  - Decrease dose by 10% or 30 mg (whichever is less) per day.
  - Slow rate of discontinuation if withdrawal reemerges.
  - Phenobarbital often accumulates with repeated dosing, producing intoxication after 4 days or so.
    - If this occurs, increase rate of dosage reduction.
  - Withdrawal from glutethamide, which is recirculated in the enterohepatic circulation, can produce alternating withdrawal and intoxication as the blood level varies.

### Withdrawing Alcohol

Withdrawal from alcohol peaks within 72 hours after last drink. Withdrawal syndromes are caused by decreased GABA neurotransmission, increased inverse agonism, and increased NMDA neurotransmission. Severity of alcohol withdrawal can be measured with the Clinical Institute Withdrawal Assessment for Alcohol (Table 8.6; Kosten & O'Connor, 2003).

- Severe withdrawal (total score > 15) predicts seizures and delirium.

Table 8.7 summarizes the characteristics of alcohol withdrawal syndromes.

**Table 8.6  Clinical Institute Withdrawal Assessment for Alcohol**

| FEATURE | RANGE OF SCORES | EXAMPLES |
| --- | --- | --- |
| Agitation | 0–7 | 0 = Normal<br>7 = Constant thrashing |
| Anxiety | 0–7 | 0 = No anxiety<br>7 = Panic |
| Auditory hallucinations | 0–7 | 0 = None<br>7 = Constant auditory hallucinations |
| Clouded sensorium | 0–4 | 0 = Clear sensorium<br>4 = Disorientation |
| Headache | 0–7 | 0 = Not present<br>7 = Severe |
| Nausea/vomiting | 0–7 | 0 = None<br>7 = Constant nausea or vomiting |
| Sweating | 0–7 | 0 = None<br>7 = Drenching sweats |
| Tactile disturbances | 0–7 | 0 = None<br>7 = Continuous tactile hallucinations |
| Tremor | 0–7 | 0 = None<br>7 = Severe |
| Visual hallucinations | 0–7 | 0 = None<br>7 = Constant visual hallucinations |

From Kosten & O'Connor (2003).

Treatment of alcohol withdrawal usually involves benzodiazepine agonists. A barbiturate protocol can be used for detoxification from alcohol, especially if alcohol combined with other CNS depressants is causing mixed withdrawal. For uncomplicated alcohol withdrawal, a standardized benzodiazepine protocol can be used.

- Most protocols use chlordiazepoxide or clorazepate.
  - Chlordiazepoxide is long acting and can be tapered easily.
  - Clorazepate has a short elimination half-life, but like chlordiazepoxide, it is converted to desmethyldiazepam.
- These medications may accumulate in older patients and patients with hepatic impairment.
  - Lorazepam may be preferable.

BENZODIAZEPINE DOSING STRATEGIES IN ALCOHOL WITHDRAWAL

- Fixed dose
  - Used for patients without past history or other risk factors of severe withdrawal syndrome.

**Table 8.7 Alcohol Withdrawal Syndromes**

| SYNDROME | % OF PATIENTS | STARTS AFTER LAST DOSE | DURATION | SIGNS AND SYMPTOMS |
|---|---|---|---|---|
| Shakes | 80 | 5–10 hours | 3 days–2 weeks | Tremulousness, insomnia, bad dreams, anxiety, blepharospasm, agitation, labile blood pressure, nausea, vomiting, transient illusions or hallucinations |
| Seizures | 10–25 | 6–48 hours | Days | Single or multiple major motor seizures that do not recur |
| Delirium tremens | 5–15 | 2–4 days | 4–7 days | Delirium, flagrant hallucinations, autonomic hyperactivity, unstable delusions, ataxia, coarse tremor |
| Hallucinosis | 5–25 | 12 hours–7 days | 1 week–2 months | Threatening auditory hallucinations in a clear sensorium, fear, agitation |

- Start with chlordiazepoxide 50–100 mg qid.
  - Add 25–50 mg prn.
  - Give 200–400 mg chlordiazepoxide/day for 2 days, then decrease dose by 25%/day over days 4–7.
- Substitute equivalent dose of lorazepam for patients with hepatic impairment.
- Loading dose, for example:
  - Diazepam 20 mg initially, with level allowed to self-taper
- Symptom-triggered (see below)
- For delirium tremens use IV diazepam 5–10 mg every 2–3 hours.

SYMPTOM-TRIGGERED ALCOHOL WITHDRAWAL

- Used when patient is not at high risk for major withdrawal syndrome.
- Keep chart of specific signs of withdrawal and intoxication.
- Record vital signs at least hourly.
- Give 5 mg diazepam or 25–50 mg chlordiazepoxide equivalent for emerging signs of withdrawal such as agitation, hypertension, tachycardia, hallucinations, disorientation, or score of ≥ 8 on the Clinical Institute Withdrawal Assessment for Alcohol scale.
  - Repeat every 1–8 hours for score ≥ 8.
- Protocol is not reliable if patients are taking medications that may mask signs of withdrawal (e.g., beta-blocker).

Outpatient Protocol

- Most patients can be withdrawn from alcohol as outpatients or in partial care setting.
- Indications for hospitalization
  - Medical complications
  - Delirium tremens
  - Suicide risk
  - Psychosis
  - Lack of support with high risk of noncompliance
- For well-motivated patients with adequate support and monitoring at home, give chlordiazepoxide 25 mg every 4–6 hours on first day.
- Then reduce dose by 25%/day.
- Use higher initial dose for patients who are very tremulous.

All patients experiencing alcohol withdrawal should receive thiamine to prevent Wernicke's encephalopathy, which may be precipitated by glucose administration in alcohol withdrawal.

- Give 100 mg po or IM for 3 consecutive days.

Other adjunctive treatments for alcohol withdrawal include:

- Beta-blockers (e.g., propranolol, atenolol) can be useful for autonomic arousal and craving.
- Clonidine can decrease severity of withdrawal symptoms.
  - Does not treat delirium or seizures.
- Valproate 100–1200 mg for 4–7 days reduced withdrawal symptoms and seizures in two double-blind randomized trials (Kosten & O'Connor, 2003).
- Antipsychotics may reduce associated psychotic symptoms.
- NMDA antagonist might be helpful.

## Medications for Alcoholism

The treatment of alcoholism and most other forms of substance dependence is primarily psychosocial. However, medications can be used adjunctively.

Alcoholism and Comorbid Bipolar Disorder

- Lithium may reduce craving for alcohol.
  - Alcohol does not accelerate metabolism of lithium.

Alcoholism and Comorbid Unipolar Depression

- Alcohol causes mental depression as a side effect.
  - May persist for several months after abstinence.

- Some patients first become aware of primary depression after they discontinue heavy drinking.
- Comorbid primary mood disorder suggested by
    - Clear onset of depression prior to onset of alcohol use.
    - Depression persists during prolonged sobriety.
    - Later-onset depression
    - Family history of depression but not substance abuse
- Continued use of alcohol interferes with action of antidepressants.
    - Counteracts central effect of antidepressant.
    - Accelerates antidepressant metabolism.
    - Persistent drinking, despite knowledge it is aggravating depression, may indicate minimal motivation for treatment.
- Continued depression interferes with treatment for alcoholism (and other forms of substance dependence).
- Initiate treatment of both depression and alcoholism at the same time.
- SSRIs are initial treatments for depression in alcoholic patients.
    - Lower toxicity
    - Fewer interactions with alcohol
    - SSRIs may reduce substance craving.

## ALCOHOL-INDUCED AGGRESSION/HALLUCINATIONS

- Responds to high-potency antipsychotics such as haloperidol 2–5 mg, risperidone 1–5 mg, aripiprazole 5–15 mg.
- Low-potency antipsychotics may potentiate hypotension associated with alcohol use and withdrawal.

## FOR PREVENTION OF RELAPSE OF ALCOHOL USE

- Disulfiram
    - Inhibits acetaldehyde dehydrogenase, leading to accumulation of acetaldehyde when alcohol is consumed.
        - It also inhibits dopamine β-hydroxylase.
    - Disulfiram may interact with small amounts of alcohol in aftershave lotion, foods, and cough syrup.
    - Explain interaction of alcohol and disulfiram in detail to patient.
    - More effective if monitored
    - Alcohol-disulfiram reaction causes
        - Flushing
        - Sweating
        - Headache and neck pain
        - Palpitations

- Dyspnea
- Hyperventilation
- Tachycardia
- Hypotension
- Nausea
- Vomiting
- More serious reactions include
  - Chest pain
  - Dyspnea
  - Severe hypotension
  - Sleep
  - Disulfiram reactions are rarely fatal.
- Severity of interaction is greater with higher disulfiram dose (> 500 mg/day) and heavier alcohol use.
- Disulfiram reactions may occur up to 14 days after the last drink.
- Avoid disulfiram in
  - Suicidal or self-destructive patients
  - Demented and confused patients
  - Patients with severe cardiac disease
  - Renal failure
  - Pregnancy
  - Allergy to thiuram derivatives in pesticides or vulcanized rubber
- Obtain baseline LFTs, EKG, physical examination.
  - Liver disease requires closer monitoring of LFTs, but risk of alcohol use is > risk of disulfiram to liver.

## USE OF DISULFIRAM

- Wait at least 12 hours after last drink and ideally 2 weeks.
- Begin 250 mg hs for 1–2 weeks.
  - Continue that dose for patients > 170 lbs.
  - Consider reducing dose to 125 mg hs for smaller patients.
- Rapid loading for patients who tolerate initial 250 mg dose can be considered.
  - 250 mg bid or 500 mg hs for 2 days
  - Then 250 mg hs
- Common side effects
  - Drowsiness, sedation, fatigue, dizziness
  - Halitosis, bad taste, body odor
  - Headache

- Tremor
- Sexual dysfunction
- Rare hepatotoxicity, neuropathy, psychosis
- Management of disulfiram–alcohol reactions:
  - Diphenhydramine 50 mg IV
  - Treat hypotension, shock, arrhythmias.
  - Administer oxygen for patients with respiratory disease.
  - High dose of vitamin C may reduce reaction.

## ALTERNATIVE TREATMENTS

- Naltrexone
  - Naltrexone 50 mg/day has been investigated in 10 controlled studies involving 1,500 patients.
  - In most studies, naltrexone has been superior to placebo in reducing craving, risk of relapse to heavy drinking as well as the number of days drinking.
    - However, in a double-blind multicenter VA trial in 627 alcohol-dependent patients who had been sober for at least 5 days, there was no difference after 13 weeks in days to relapse between naltrexone and placebo (Krystal, Cramer, Krol, Kirk, & Rosenheck, 2001).
    - After 1 year, there were no significant differences in percentage of days drinking or number of drinks consumed per drinking day.
  - A review of 19 randomized trials found that the number of patients who returned to drinking and percentage or number of drinking days were significantly lower with naltrexone than placebo, but differences were not great, and short-term treatment discontinuation rates were similar with naltrexone and placebo (Srisurapanont & Jarusuraisin, 2002).
    - There were no differences between naltrexone and placebo in abstinence after 3–6 months of treatment, although patients who took naltrexone regularly drank less alcohol.
  - Use of naltrexone
    - Patient must be opiate free for at least 7–10 days.
    - Avoid in patients with hepatic impairment.
    - Usual dose 50 mg/day.
  - Side effects
    - Abdominal pain
    - Anxiety
    - Fatigue
    - Headache

- Insomnia
- Joint, muscle pain
- Nausea, vomiting
- Anorexia
- Chills
- Constipation
- Sexual dysfunction
- Diarrhea
- Dizziness
- Depression
- Irritability
- Increased thirst
- Skin rash
- Side effects at doses > 250 mg/day: Increased LFTs; Hepatotoxicity in morbidly obese patients; Hepatotoxicity when high doses combined with NSAIDs; Lymphocytosis.

More predictably useful for

- Repetitive self-injurious behavior (e.g., cutting, biting, head banging) in patients with
  - Brain damage
  - Congenital disorders
  - Personality disorders

An open study of naltrexone at an average dose of 145 mg/day in 10 patients with kleptomania found significant improvement over 11 weeks.

- 7 patients very much improved
- 2 patients much improved at the end of the study (Grant & Kim, 2002).
- Acamprosate
  - A calcium acetyl homotaurinate that acts on NMDA receptors and has been studied in 14 published trials involving about 4,000 patients (Anton & Swift, 2003).
  - Reported to increase time to relapse of drinking, decrease drinking days, and increase complete abstinence in alcohol-dependent patients.
    - Two studies were negative.
  - Effect size equivalent to naltrexone (0.1–0.4).
  - After detoxification, 160 patients with alcoholism were randomly assigned to 12 weeks treatment with naltrexone (50 mg), acamprosate (1998 mg), a combination of the two, or placebo (Kiefer et al., 2003).

- Both medications and the combination were significantly better than placebo in reducing relapse to heavy drinking.
- There was no difference between acamprosate and naltrexone, but the two together were better than either one alone.
- The same results were obtained for time to the first drink.
- Relapse rate in the combination group was 25%, which is lower than in trials of either agent.
  - Side effects of acamprosate
    - Diarrhea
    - Abdominal discomfort
    - Headache
- Serotonin 5HT$_3$ antagonists
  - Ondansetron, granisetron
  - Limbic dopamine release is mediated by 5HT$_3$ heteroreceptors.
    - Antagonizing these receptors attenuates reward from substance use and decreases craving.
  - Usual ondansetron dose 2–8 mg bid–qid
  - Patients with early-onset alcoholism have been found to have reduced drinking with low doses of ondansetron (2–32 μg/kg/day; Anton & Swift, 2003).
  - Granisetron not as well studied but probably equally effective.
    - Usual dose 1–2 mg bid.

## Medications for Chronic Pain

Narcotics generally have been considered inappropriate for chronic benign (non-cancer) pain, but recent experience suggests that these medications can be helpful in moderate doses. However, tolerance to the analgesic effect and rebound pain between doses are common problems. Higher doses are more effective but have more side effects. A number of psychotropic medications have been used adjunctively for chronic pain.

- At best, a single agent will reduce chronic pain by about 50%.
  - Polytherapy may be indicated for some patients (Mendell & Sahenk, 2003).
- Antidepressants
  - About one-third of patients achieve a 50% reduction of neuropathic pain with TCAs (Mendell & Sahenk, 2003).
    - Side effects can be problematic, especially in the elderly.
  - Efficacy of SSRIs is less than that of TCAs (Mendell & Sahenk, 2003).

- Venlafaxine was effective in a small randomized trial in painful sensory neuropathy associated with cancer (Tasmuth, Hartel, & Kalso, 2002).
- Bupropion for 6 weeks reduced neuropathic pain by 30% in 41 patients (Semenchuk, Sherman, & Davis, 2001).
- Nefazodone and duloxetine have some potential for treatment of chronic pain.
- Anticonvulsants
  - Carbamazepine effective for trigeminal neuralgia.
    - A placebo-controlled trial in 30 subjects suggested benefit in diabetic neuropathy (Rull, Quibrera, Gonzalez-Millan, & Lozano Castenada, 1969).
    - Oxcarbazepine seems to have efficacy similar to carbamazepine for trigeminal neuralgia (Mendell & Sahenk, 2003).
  - Gabapentin was equal to amitriptyline in neuropathic pain reduction (Morello, Leckband, & Stoner, 1999).
    - Doses > 1600 mg/day are usually necessary.
  - Lamotrigine (400–600 mg/day) was useful in a single small trial of pain associated with HIV neuropathy (Simpson et al., 2000).
  - Tiagabine, topiramate, levetiraceram and oxcarbazepine are sometimes helpful for neuropathic pain.
- NMDA antagonists
  - NMDA receptor activation stimulates pain neurons and fosters neuronal remodeling
  - Memantine may be helpful

## Medications for Narcotic Withdrawal and Abuse

Signs and symptoms of opioid withdrawal resemble severe case of influenza:

- Dilated pupils
- Lacrimation
- Yawning
- Sneezing
- Anorexia
- Nausea
- Vomiting
- Diarrhea
- Seizures and delirium do not occur.
- Life threatening only in patients who are dehydrated or debilitated.

The time course of withdrawal varies with the drug.

- Heroin withdrawal peaks in 36–72 hours and lasts 7–10 days.
- Methadone withdrawal peaks in 72–96 hours and lasts 2 weeks.
- Buprenorphine withdrawal peaks in about 3–4 days and lasts about 1 week.
  - Less severe than withdrawal from other narcotics.

### OPIOID DETOXIFICATION

- The standard approach to withdrawing narcotics is to substitute a dose of methadone that suppresses withdrawal symptoms and then either maintain or slowly withdraw methadone.
  - Methadone detoxification usually takes 10–21 days.
  - Usual dose 20–50 mg/day in divided dose
  - Reducing the dose of methadone by 3%/week is associated with fewer dropouts, less severe withdrawal, and less illicit opioid use than when dose is decreased by 10%/week.
    - Abstinence after detoxification is only 40% with any protocol (Kosten & O'Connor, 2003).
  - Methadone can be prescribed by any physician for pain, but it can only be used for narcotic detoxification or withdrawal in a federally qualified setting.
- Adjunctive use of alpha-2 adrenergic agonists
  - Clonidine and lofexidine used to reduce noradrenergic hyperactivity in withdrawal.
- Naloxone and naltrexone accelerate opiate withdrawal because dosage reduction is not gradual.
  - 89 patients with DSM-IV opiate dependence were stabilized for 3 days on methadone titrated against signs and symptoms of opiate withdrawal and then randomly assigned to lofexidine 1.4–2.0 mg plus injections of 0.8 mg naloxone or placebo (Beswick et al., 2003).
    - Compared with placebo, naloxone was associated with less withdrawal and craving.
    - There was no difference in compliance or likelihood of completing treatment.
- In six controlled studies involving 357 patients, buprenorphine ameliorated opioid withdrawal, and 65–100% of patients completed withdrawal (see next section, pp. 460–461; Gowing, Ali, & White, 2002a).
  - A randomized trial is underway comparing buprenorphine and methadone detoxification.
    - Most adverse effects are related to withdrawal or consequences of addiction rather than the medication.

Detoxification using various narcotic antagonists under general anesthesia or heavy sedation has been popularized. However, a review of published data on this approach found insufficient evidence of efficacy or safety (Gowing, Ali, & White, 2002b). The risks of aspiration, respiratory depression, and cardiac arrhythmias mandate careful intensive monitoring.

### MAINTENANCE THERAPY FOR NARCOTIC ADDICTION

#### Methadone
- Clearly reduces relapse in narcotic addiction.
- Average doses are 20–100 mg/day.

#### L-alpha-acetylmethodol acetate (LAAM)
- Long-acting opiate with properties similar to methadone
- Equal to or better than methadone in reducing IV narcotic use
- Can be administered three times per week.
- Starting dose 20 mg three times/week
  - Increased by 10 mg/week, up to 80 mg three times/week
- A meta-analysis of 12 controlled studies found that abstinence was more likely with LAAM than with methadone.
  - Patients were more likely to discontinue LAAM and switch to methadone (Clark et al., 2002).
- LAAM is scheduled for withdrawal from the market.

#### Buprenorphine
- Partial μ-opioid agonist and a κ-opiate receptor antagonist
- Because it has high affinity for opioid receptors, high doses block subjective and physiological effects of administered opioids.
- Daily treatment is effective for maintenance treatment of narcotic abuse.
  - Dosing less frequently than once a day may be effective.
- Supplied in 2 and 8 mg sublingual tablets
- Starting dose in opioid dependence is 2–4 mg sublingually.
  - Increased gradually to 8–16 mg/day.
  - Average maintenance dose is 4–16 mg/day.
- 14 heroin-dependent outpatients received double-blind treatment for 2 weeks with 2 mg/day of buprenorphine, 4 mg/day alternating with placebo on alternate days, 16 mg/day, and 32 mg on 1 day and placebo the next (Greenwald, Schuh, Hopper, Schuster, & Johanson, 2002).
  - On each regimen, patients chose between money and injections of hydromorphone.

- Buprenorphine 16 mg/day and alternating 32 mg/placebo reduced heroin craving and opioid withdrawal.
- The 16 and alternating 32 mg doses of buprenorphine reduced the choice of hydromorphone over money.
- The alternating placebo day schedule at the higher dose (i.e., active drug every other day) seems as effective as daily dosing, and daily 16 and alternating 32/placebo schedules were more effective than 2 mg and 4 mg/placebo schedules.
- Naltrexone is an opioid antagonist used alone or combined with buprenorphine.
  - Combining buprenorphine with naloxone reduces potential for abuse of buprenorphine
  - Combination of buprenorphine and naloxone (Suboxone) is approved for outpatient maintenance treatment of heroin addiction.
  - Buprenorphine and buprenorphine–naloxone can be used for other purposes by any physician, but they can only be prescribed for treatment of narcotic addiction if the clinician has passed addiction subspecialty boards or a postgraduate course in outpatient treatment of narcotic abuse.
  - A careful review of 11 studies of naltrexone maintenance treatment for preventing relapse of opioid dependence after detoxification found that there was a statistically significant reduction in reincarceration with naltrexone + behavior therapy vs. behavior therapy alone.
    - Because the studies were of such poor quality, no other conclusions could be drawn (Kirchmayer, Davoli, & Verster, 2002).
- In a 4-week randomized controlled trial of a sublingual tablet of buprenorphine + naloxone in a ratio of 4:1 (16 mg/4 mg), 323 patients with opiate dependence were followed by an open-label safety phase of 48 weeks for patients in the double-blind phase and 52 weeks for patients who had not been in the first trial and who openly took a 24:6 mg ratio of buprenorphine and naloxone (N = 268 and 193, respectively; Fudala et al., 2003).
  - The controlled trial compared buprenorphine–naloxone with buprenorphine alone and with placebo.
    - This study was terminated early because of superiority of both active treatments to placebo.
    - 243 of 323 patients completed the study.
    - Percentages of urines negative for opiates were 18% for buprenorphine–naloxone, 21% for buprenorphine alone, 6% for placebo ($p < 0.001$).
    - Both active treatments produced significantly more reduction in craving than placebo.

- In the open-label trial
  - Percentages of opiate-negative urines ranged from 35 to 67%, depending on the week.
  - Overall rate of opiate use was lower than in double-blind trial.
  - Use of cocaine and benzodiazepines did not change.
  - Most adverse events were related to drug withdrawal or concomitant hepatitis.

## TOXICITY AND OVERDOSE

### Benzodiazepines

- Benzodiazepine overdose is discussed in Chapter 7.
- Lethality of zopiclone overdose equivalent to that of benzodiazepines

### Barbiturates and Related Hypnotics

Overdose of these medications can be fatal.
- $LD_{50}$ is about 10 times daily dose.
- About 0.5–12% of barbiturate overdoses are fatal.
- Barbiturate overdoses occurring in dissociated state caused by the first dose have been reported.
  - Patient apparently forgets previous dose and has no memory of overdose.
  - Genuine "autonomous" overdoses are less frequent than is commonly reported.
- Management involves supportive measures discussed in Chapter 7, alkalinization of urine to increase excretion, and dialysis in severe cases.

### Chloral Hydrate

- Lethal dose is about 5–10 times the hypnotic dose.
- Common signs of overdose include
  - Abdominal distress
  - Hypotension
  - Hypothermia
  - Respiratory depression
  - Cardiac arrhythmias
  - Coma

- Less common are
  - Miosis
  - Vomiting
  - Areflexia
  - Muscle flaccidity
- Rare signs are
  - Esophageal stricture
  - Gastric necrosis/perforation
  - GI hemorrhage
  - Transient hepatotoxicity
- Management:
  - General management, as noted for benzodiazepines (pp. 412–413)
  - Hemodialysis eliminates metabolite trichloroethanol.
  - Peritoneal dialysis also helpful.

### Ethchlorvynol

- Signs include
  - Hypotension
  - Bradycardia
  - Hypothermia
  - Mydriasis
  - Areflexia
  - Pulmonary edema
  - Pancytopenia
  - Hemolysis
  - Cardiorespiratory depression
  - Coma
    - Lying in one position during prolonged coma can cause peripheral neuropathy.
- Management:
  - Provide support for blood pressure and pulmonary function.
  - Hemodialysis benefit uncertain.
  - Urinary alkalinization does not increase drug excretion.

## PRECAUTIONS

All hypnotics can aggravate sleep apnea. This is less of a problem with trazodone. Since hypnotics have CNS-depressant properties, they can cause delirium in demented patients. Insomnia in these patients may respond to morning artificial bright light (see pp. 157–158).

Contraindications to barbiturates and related medications include

- Hypersensitivity to the medication
- Pregnancy
- Porphyria
- Significant suicide risk
- High risk of drug dependence
- Increased intracranial pressure
- Chronic pulmonary disease

## ADVICE FOR CARETAKERS

Patients taking hypnotics should be observed for

- Dizziness or confusion
- Trouble finding bed after taking medication
- Skin rash
- Weakness
- Symptoms of intoxication or withdrawal

Most of the time, use of hypnotics should be short term.

- Changes in sleep phase treated with artificial bright light and gradual sleep-phase changes.
- Psychophysiological insomnia treated with cognitive–behavioral techniques.

## NOTES FOR PATIENT AND FAMILY

Hypnotics are most appropriately used for the short-term treatment of initial or middle insomnia associated with a stressor. These medications all usually lose their efficacy with chronic dosing. Nonpharmacological techniques are often more successful in the long run. Consider the following precautions.

- Do not combine hypnotics with alcohol.
- Avoid barbiturates and related medications.
    - If one of these medications is prescribed, ask whether a benzodiazepine selective agent such as zolpidem or zopiclone might work as well.
- If sleeping pills have been taken for a long time, do not stop them abruptly.
    - Abrupt withdrawal of CNS depressants can cause seizures.

- Avoid driving or working around machinery within 6 hours of taking a sleeping pill.
  - Benzodiazepines and barbiturates can impair driving significantly.
- Sleeping pills can be taken with food, but this may slow absorption of the medication and delay the onset of sleep.
- If a dose is forgotten, it can be taken within 4 hours; otherwise, wait until the next night.
  - Do not double the dose.

# CHAPTER NINE

# Stimulants and Related Medications

Stimulants are the most widely prescribed psychotropic medications for children. They activate the central nervous system through dopaminergic mechanisms; some newer medications, such as atomoxetine and modafinil, have different mechanisms of action.

The ability of stimulants to reduce hyperactivity and improve academic performance was first noted in 1937. By 1966, 161 randomized trials had been published of 5,899 children, adolescents, and adults showing improvement in ADHD (65–75% on stimulants vs. 5–30% on placebo; Greenhill, Pliszka, Dulcan, & AACAP, 2002). Evidence is greater for efficacy in school-age children than in both younger children and adults. More than 10 million methylphenidate prescriptions were written in 1996. At the same time that only a minority of children with ADHD are reported to receive treatment (1/8, in a 1999 survey of four communities; Greenhill, Pliszka, et al., 2002), another study showed that the majority of children taking stimulants did not meet criteria for ADHD (Greenhill, Pliszka, et al., 2002). This chapter addresses

- Attention-deficit disorder (ADD) and attention-deficit/hyperactivity disorder (ADHD)
- Adult ADD
- Narcolepsy and other sleep disorders
- Treatment-resistant depression
- Depression and debilitation associated with chronic medical illness
- Obesity
  - Eating disorders are discussed on pages 131–132.
- Sedative side effects of other medications
- Stimulant misuse and withdrawal

**Table 9.1 Names, DEA Schedule, Dose Forms, Colors**

| GENERIC NAMES (DEA SCHEDULE #) | BRAND NAMES | DOSE FORMS (MG) | COLORS |
|---|---|---|---|
| dextroamphetamine[(II)] | Dexedrine | t: 5<br>e: 5 mg/5 ml | t: orange[†]<br>e: orange |
| | Spansule | sr-sp: 5/10/15 | sr-sp: all brown—clear |
| methylphenidate[(II)] | Ritalin<br>Methylin | t: 5/10/20 | t: yellow/pale green/pale yellow[†] |
| methylphenidate SR | Ritalin-SR | sr-t: 20 | sr-t: white |
| methylphenidate extended release | Metadate | sr-c: 10/20/30 | c: white |
| methylphenidate controlled release | Concerta | sr-t: 18/27/36/54 | sr-t: multicolored |
| pemoline[(IV)] | Cylert | t: 18.75/37.5/75<br>ct: 37.5 | t: white/orange/tan<br>ct: orange |
| madafinil[(IV)] | Provigil | t: 100/200 | t: white[†] |
| phendimetrazine[(IV)] | Plegine | t: 35 | t: beige |
| | Prelu-2<br>(timed release) | sr-c: 105 | sr-c: celery-green |

c = capsule; ct = chewable tablet; e = elixir; sp = spansule; sr = sustained-release; t = tablets.
[†] = scored.

## PHARMACOLOGY

Actions of stimulants include

- Direct release of the catecholamines dopamine and norepinephrine
- Catecholamine reuptake inhibition
- Inhibition of MAO, slowing catecholamine breakdown
- Direct agonism of dopamine receptor
- Enhancement of central dopaminergic and noradrenergic pathways crucial to frontal lobe function may enhance executive functions such as planning and impulse control.
  - Primary actions are on mesocorticolimbic and nigrostriatal dopamine systems.
  - Inhibition of dopamine transporter in striatum may further improve executive function.
- All stimulants improve alertness, attention, wakefulness, vigilance, fatigue, and psychomotor performance.

- Improvement of attention occurs later after dosing than improvement of behavior.
- Stimulants can induce euphoria.
  - Uncommon in patients with ADHD
  - Most marked with methamphetamine and cocaine
- Benefits of immediate-release stimulants in children last 3–5 hours and include
  - Decreased interrupting and fidgeting
  - Increased on-task behavior
  - Reduced impulsivity
  - Increased compliance
  - Improved attention, short-term memory, reaction time, and problem solving
- Effects of stimulants in adults
  - Prolonged performance of repetitive tasks
  - Decreased fatigure
  - Elevated mood
  - Increased rate of speech
  - Increased alertness on tasks requiring prolonged vigilance
  - Reduced impulsive responses on cognitive tasks
  - Improved short-term memory, reaction time, and problem solving
- Pharmacokinetics of stimulants as a class
  - Rapid absorption
    - Prompt concentration peak
  - Low plasma protein binding
  - Rapid metabolism
  - Absorption and bioavailability may increase if taken with food.
  - Once dose is weight adjusted, there is no effect of age on dose.
  - Long-term tolerance to effect in ADHD is rare.
- Sensitization with long-term stimulant treatment has been thought to predispose to later substance abuse, but animal studies only demonstrate behavioral sensitization with high doses, intermittent dosing, and nonoral dosage.
- Rebound as short-acting stimulants wear off occurs in about 30% and is significant in < 10%.

Stimulants are clearly effective for
- Childhood ADHD
- Narcolepsy
- Augmentation of antidepressants in refractory depression

Stimulants are probably effective for

- Adult ADD
  - Hyperactivity component often improves or remits in adulthood.
- Acute treatment of bipolar depression
- Depression in medically ill patients
- Apathy and withdrawal associated with chronic medical illness
  - Possible usefulness for low motivation and depression in AIDS patients
- Chronic fatigue syndrome

## Dextroamphetamine

- Rapidly absorbed
- Peak level in 2 hours
- Half-life 11 hours
- Produces
  - Increased pulse and blood pressure
    - Not clinically significant unless patient has cardiac disease
    - More cardiovascular effects than methylphenidate
  - Initial insomnia

## Methamphetamine

- Rapidly absorbed
- Peak level in 1 hour
- Half-life 3 hours
- Clinical action may end before medication is eliminated (clockwise hysteresis).
- High addiction potential

**Table 9.2 Attention-Deficit Hyperactivity Stimulant Doses in Children**

| GENERIC NAMES | SINGLE USUAL STARTING DOSE (MG) | DAILY DOSE RANGE (MG/KG/DAY) | USUAL DOSE RANGE (MG/KG/DAY) | EXTREME DOSE RANGE (MG/DAY) |
|---|---|---|---|---|
| adderall | 5–10 mg bid | 0.15–0.5 | 0.3–0.9 | 1–1.5 |
| dextroamphetamine | 5–10 qd | 0.15–0.5 | 0.3–2.0 | 5–60 |
| methylphenidate | 2.5–5 bid | 0.3–0.7 | 0.3–2.0 | 10–80 |
| pemoline | 18.75–37.5 qd | 0.5–2.5 | 0.5–3.0 | 37.5–112.5 |

### Methylphenidate

- Rapidly absorbed
    - Generic is absorbed more rapidly than brand-name preparation.
- Effect persists for 2–4 hours with immediate-release and 3–5 hours after sustained-release tablet.
    - Sustained-release methylphenidate absorbed more slowly, with lower plasma level than immediate-release preparation.
- Short-term tolerance develops by second dose of the day.
    - Requires increasing levels throughout the day to maintain efficacy.
- Lower incidence of anorexia, cardiovascular effects, and dependence than dextroamphetamine.

### Long-Acting Stimulants

- Problems with immediate-release stimulants
    - Peak level occurs at unstructured times (e.g., lunch, recess).
    - Interdose rebound or loss of efficacy occurs.
    - Need to administer midday dose at school.
    - Reduced compliance
- Slow-release preparations vary in method of medication release into bloodstream

### Sustained-Release Methylphenidate

- Ritalin-SR
    - Wax-matrix vehicle provides slow release.
    - Methylphenidate-SR, Metadate, and Methylin-SR use same mechanism as Ritalin-SR.
    - Action begins in 90 minutes (vs. 30 minutes for immediate-release version).
        - Peak benefit occurs at 3 hours.
    - Peak plasma level lower than with comparable dose of immediate-release version.
- In a 3-week study of Metadate CD (controlled-release methylphenidate) in 308 ADHD patients ages 6–17, 65% were rated very much or much improved (Dirksen, D'Imperio, Birdsall, & Hatch, 2002).
- However, slow-release methylphenidate is generally thought to be less effective than immediate-release preparation (Greenhill, Pliszka, et al., 2002).

- Immediate release methylphenidate produces higher peak plasma concentrations and steeper absorption phase slopes.
- Gradually decreasing blood level after peak at 3 hours may result in reduction of symptom control (afternoon attenuation).

OROS method sustained-release methylphenidate (OROS methylphenidate, Concerta)

- Constant blood level over the day may result in tachyphylaxis, with loss of efficacy of each dose.
- Gradual increase in methylphenidate concentration provides same symptom reduction as sharp peaks from three increasing doses/day.
- Osmotic pump in capsule containing small medication particles releases increasing amounts of methylphenidate throughout day to overcome tolerance that develops after each dose.
- Once daily Concerta at 18, 36, or 54 mg/day was compared to 15, 30, or 45 mg/day (tid schedule) immediate-release methylphenidate in children with ADHD ages 7–13 (Swanson, 2003).
  - Both immediate-release methylphenidate and the new sustained-release preparation were significantly better than placebo and similar to each other on a variety of measures, with effect sizes as high as 1.53.
    - Effect size greater than that seen with standard sustained-release preparations.
  - Effectiveness maintained at 12 months in 289 of 407 children ages 6–13 who completed an open trial (Wilens et al., 2003).
    - No meaningful changes in blood pressure, pulse, or height.
- Concerta was as effective as tid immediate-release methylphenidate in a double-blind placebo-controlled multisite study (Greenhill, Pliszka, et al., 2002).

### Dexedrine Spansules

### Mixed Amphetamine Salts (Adderall)

- Consists of 25% levoamphetamine + 75% dextroamphetamine.
- Effective in two daily doses in most patients.
  - Methylphenidate effective in two daily doses in a minority of patients.
- Adderall XR
  - Sustained-release preparation of mixed amphetamine salts
  - Time to maximum concentration is 3 hours longer than with Adderall.
  - Permits once daily dosing.
- Not demonstrated to be more effective than dextroamphetamine.

### Pemoline

- Rapidly absorbed
- Clinical effect appears in 2 hours.
- Effect lasts up to 6 hours.
- 50% bound to plasma protein
- Reaches steady state in 2–3 days.
- Despite slow dosage increase and long half-life, effective after first dose.
- Less activating than methylphenidate, Dexedrine, and related medications.
  - Impairs sleep and decreases appetite in 30% of patients.
  - No abuse potential
  - Most appropriate for patients at risk of substance misuse
- Most important problem is hepatotoxicity.
  - Altered liver function tests reported in 44 children.
    - Since pemoline released, 13 children had total liver failure; 11 required transplantation or died within 4 weeks.
  - Appears 10–12 months after beginning treatment.
  - Elevated bilirubin, transaminases
  - Clinically significant allergic hepatitis in 3%
  - Liver function tests must be obtained at baseline and every 4–6 months during treatment.
  - Do not combine with other medications that can cause hepatotoxicity.
  - Do not administer to patients with liver disease.
  - Risk of hepatotoxicity and need for monitoring make pemoline a third-line treatment, at best.

### Stimulant Dosing

Methylphenidate and dextroamphetamine/mixed Amphetamines
- Starting dose in children is 5 mg methylphenidate or 2.5 mg dextroamphetamine or mixed amphetamine salts.
  - Cognitive effects at 0.3 mg/kg
  - Behavioral response at 1 mg/kg
  - Give methylphenidate after breakfast and lunch.
    - Give third dose after school if necessary for homework.
  - Give dextroamphetamine or mixed amphetamine salts in the morning and at noon if effect wanes.
    - Increasing the morning dose may extend duration of action.

- Maximum total daily dose for children
  - 60 mg methylphenidate or up to 1 mg/kg
  - 40 mg for amphetamines or 0.9 mg/kg of dextroamphetamine
  - Children who weigh < 25 kg should not take single doses > 15 mg methylphenidate or 10 mg dextroamphetamine/mixed amphetamines.
- Dosing in preschool children
  - Most studies show methylphenidate > placebo.
  - No dose-finding studies
  - Starting dose no more than 0.5 mg/kg
    - 1.25 mg methylphenidate bid recommended
- Dextroamphetamine is usually taken bid–tid.
  - Clinical effects begin within 30 minutes of each dose, peak in 1–3 hours, and are gone by 4–6 hours.
- Methylphenidate is usually taken bid–qid.
- Doses are usually spaced 4 hours apart.
- Sustained-release forms are taken once or twice a day.
- Dose generally increased once a week by 5–10 mg methylphenidate or 2.5–5 mg dextroamphetamine/mixed amphetamines.
- Forced titration method
  - Give daily doses of 5, 10, 15, and 20 mg methylphenidate, or 2.5, 5, 7.5, or 10 mg dextroamphetamine for 1 week at each dose.
    - Give patient dose that produced best improvement of rating scale scores with fewest side effects.
- Dosing of methylphenidate-SR and Dexedrine Spansules
  - Start patient on immediate-release preparation.
  - Add morning and noon doses together for dose of sustained-release form.
  - A midday dose of immediate-release form can be added if effect of morning sustained-release dose wanes.

**Table 9.3 Other Stimulant Doses**

| GENERIC NAMES | ADULT ADHD (MG/DAY) | ADULT DEPRESSION (MG/DAY) | ADULT NARCOLEPSY (MG/DAY) | GERIATRIC PATIENTS (MG/DAY) |
|---|---|---|---|---|
| adderall | 10–30 mg bid | — | — | — |
| dextroamphetamine | 10–60 qd or bid | 5–40 | 20–30 | 10–15 |
| methylphenidate | 10–80 qd or bid | 10–80 | 10–30 | 10–30 |
| pemoline | 37.5–75 qd or bid | 18.75–150 | 37.5–75 | — |

- Dosing of OROS methylphenidate
  - 36–54 mg daily
- Medication should be taken after meals to reduce impact of appetite suppression.
  - Absorption not affected by taking medication with meals.
- No correlation between response and serum or saliva level.

Pemoline
- Taken once daily
  - Titrate up to 56 mg/day.
    - Dose can be increased in 18.75 mg increments to 112.5 mg/day.
  - Discontinue if no improvement seen after 3 weeks.
  - Discontinue if ALT increases to twice normal.

## Atomoxetine

- Selective norepinephrine reuptake inhibitor
- Rapidly absorbed
- Peak plasma concentration 1–2 hours after dosing
- Elimination half-life 3–5 hours
- Duration of action 8 hours
- Twice daily dosing
  - In a 6-week double-blind placebo-controlled study of 171 children and adolescents with ADHD, once daily atomoxetine was more effective than placebo and about as effective (effect size 0.71) as twice daily atomoxetine (Michelson et al., 2002).
- Similar pharmacokinetics in children and adults, correcting for weight.
- Improves inattention, hyperactivity, and impulsivity.
  - In four randomized controlled trials, reduction in ADHD scores was 34–38% with atomoxetine vs. 13–16% with placebo (Simpson & Perry, 2003).
- No abuse potential
- Atomoxetine dosing
  - Taken once in the morning or once in morning and once in the late afternoon.
  - Food does not affect absorption.
  - Usual initial dose 40 mg or 0.5 mg/kg
    - Increase after 3–7 days to 80 mg.
    - Increase to maximum of 100 mg or 1.2 mg/kg after 2–4 additional weeks.

- Doses > 100 mg, or 1.4 mg/kg, do not result in additional benefit.

### Modafinil

- Hypocretin (orexin) is a central excitatory neurotransmitter.
  - Located in lateral hypothalamus and projecting to sleep areas.
  - Mutation of hypocretin-2 receptor and low hypocretin activity implicated in narcolepsy.
- Modafinil activates orexin-containing neurons in lateral hypothalamus.
  - Requires intact adrenergic system but does not act on this system.
  - No direct dopaminergic action
- Benzhydrylsulfinylacetamide structure
- Schedule IV drug (amphetamines and methylphenidate are schedule II).
- Peak plasma level in 2–4 hours.
- Eliminated by hepatic metabolism and renal excretion.
  - Induces its own metabolism.
  - Inhibits CYP 2C19.
  - Hepatic impairment reduces oral clearance by 60% and doubles steady-state concentration.
- Elimination half-life in chronic dosing is ~ 15 hours.
- Induces CYP450 2C19 and 2C9.
  - May reduce levels of carbamazepine, phenobarbital, and phenytoin.
- Modafinil dosing
  - Start with 100 mg in morning
  - Increase to 200–400 mg, if necessary.
    - 400 mg has not been shown to be > 200 mg.
  - Food delays but does not alter absorption.

### Sibutramine

- Serotonin and norepinephrine reuptake inhibitor
  - Does not induce serotonin release.
- Approved for treatment of obesity.
- Induces satiety and stimulates thermogenesis.
- No reports of valvular heart damage or primary pulmonary hypertension.
- Usual dose 10 mg/day

- Can be increased to maximum of 15 mg if tolerated
- Reduce to 5 mg if poorly tolerated

### Antidepressants

Antidepressants with noradrenergic and dopaminergic properties have been found to be potentially effective alternatives to stimulants in the treatment of ADHD. These medications have the advantage of much lower abuse potential, but they are probably not as effective as stimulants.

- Tricyclic antidepressants
  - Desipramine and nortriptyline have been found to be more effective for hyperactivity than attention.
  - Do not aggravate tics.
  - Children are more likely to experience hypertension than hypotension with TCAs.
  - Unexplained sudden death has been reported in several children taking desipramine.
    - Desipramine also has higher risk of death in overdose.
- Venlafaxine
  - Open experience suggests improvement of inattention.
  - Concern has been raised about risk of inducing suicidality in depressed children.
- Bupropion
  - Most frequently used antidepressant for ADHD
  - Greater reduction in ADHD scores than atomoxetine
  - More likely than stimulants to cause a rash
- SSRIs
  - Helpful for impulsivity
  - Not particularly useful for inattention or hyperactivity
- Selegiline
  - Stimulant properties could be useful for ADD with comorbid neurological illness or depression.
    - Metabolized to amphetamine and methamphetamine-like compounds.
  - Double-blind study of 28 children with DSM-IV ADHD randomized to methylphenidate 1 mg/kg/day or selegiline 5 mg/day (under 5 years old) or 10 mg/day (over 5 years old; Akhondzadeh, Tavakolian, Davari-Ashtiani, Arabgol, & Amini, 2003).
    - Both were equally effective.
    - Selegiline was better tolerated.

## Alpha-2 Agonists

- Clonidine
  - Binds to alpha-adrenergic 2A, 2B, and 2C receptors.
- Guanfacine
  - Specific agonist for $\alpha_{2A}$ receptor, which exists primarily in brain.
- Both drugs are more effective for hyperactivity and irritability than inattention and impulsivity.
- Children ages 6–14 with ADHD and comorbid oppositional defiant disorder had placebo (N = 29) or clonidine syrup (N = 38) 0.1–0.2 mg day added to ongoing treatment with stimulants (Hazell & Stuart, 2003).
  - Clonidine was more effective than placebo in reducing conduct symptoms but not hyperactivity.
  - Clonidine but not placebo also reduced stimulant side effects.
- Improvement of tics may be a benefit for patients with comorbid tic disorders.
  - May be more effective in ADHD with comorbid tic disorder.
- Guanfacine is better tolerated than clonidine.
  - Less sedation (21% vs. 35% for clonidine)
  - Fewer cardiovascular side effects
    - Low risk of hypotension
    - Less rebound hypertension on discontinuation
  - Longer duration of action
- Usual dose
  - Clonidine 4–5 µg/kg
  - Guanfacine 0.1 mg/kg, given bid or tid.
    - Start at 0.5 mg in morning.
    - Add 0.5 mg doses at noon and around 5 P.M.
    - Majority of dose can be given at bedtime because of half-life of 12 hours.
  - If clonidine is added to stimulant, start with 0.05 mg (half of a tablet).
    - Do not give > 0.3 mg/day.
- Lofexidine
  - In 44 medication-free children (mean age 10 years) with ADHD and comorbid tic disorders, lofexidine for 8 weeks produced 41% improvement in ADHD scores vs. 7% with placebo (Niederhofer, Staffen, & Mair, 2003).
    - Tic severity decreased by 27% with lofexidine versus 0 with placebo.

## Cholinesterase Inhibitors

- Cholinesterase inhibitors have had positive preliminary results in ADHD studies. (Spencer & Biederman, 2002).

## Iron Supplement

- Occasionally useful as adjunct
- 0.5 mg/kg/day
- Benefit uncertain

## Novel Treatments

- Sodium oxybate is approved for treatment of narcolepsy, based on double-blind placebo-controlled studies.
  - In 136 narcolepsy patients, improvement of cataplexy, daytime sleepiness, and nighttime awakenings were significantly more improved with 9 gm of sodium oxybate than with placebo (Anonymous, 2002).
  - A year-long open-label extension of a 4-week double-blind study in 118 patients with narcolepsy found that sodium oxybate 3–9 gm/night improved narcolepsy (Anonymous, 2003).
    - Improvement appeared at 4 weeks and was maximal after 8 weeks.
    - Significant decreases reported in cataplexy attacks and daytime sleepiness.
    - Significant improvement noted for nocturnal sleep quality, alertness, and ability to concentrate.
- Gamma hydroxybutyrate (GHB)
  - Schedule I drug
    - Medically formulated GHB may be moved to schedule III.
  - Useful for narcolepsy but is not patentable for this indication (Tunnicliff & Raess, 2002).

## Herbal Therapies

- Use of ephedra for ADHD is discussed on page 518.

Table 9.4 provides an overview of medications used to treat ADHD.

## Table 9.4  Medications for ADHD

| DRUG | BRAND NAME | DOSE FORMS (MG)* | DURATION OF ACTION (HOURS) | AVERAGE PEDIATRIC DOSE | AVERAGE COST/MONTH ($) |
|---|---|---|---|---|---|
| atomoxetine | Strattera | c: 10, 18, 25, 40, 60 | 8 | 1.2 mg/kg or 100 mg | 90 |
| dexmethylphenidate | Focalin | | 6 | 10 mg bid | 54.60 |
| dextroamphetamine | Dexedrine | t: 5, 10 | 4–6 | 10 mg bid or 5 mg tid | 48.80 |
| | Dexedrine Spansule | c: 5, 10, 15 | | | 64.80 |
| | DextroStat | t: 5 | | | |
| dextroamphetamine (long acting) | Generic | c: 5, 10, 15 | 6–8 | 20 mg q A.M. | 58.20 |
| dextroamphetamine + amphetamine | Generic | t: 5, 10, 20, 30 | 4–6 | 10 mg bid | 74.40 |
| | Adderall | | | | 84.00 |
| | Adderall-XR | t: 5, 7.5 c: 10, 20, 30 | 10–12 | 20 mg q A.M. | 73.20 |
| methylphenidate (immediate release) | Generic Ritalin | t: 5, 10, 20 | 3–5 | 10 mg tid or 20 mg bid | 37.20 54.00 |
| methylphenidate (intermediate acting) | Generic | | 3–8 | 40 mg q A.M. | 56.40 |
| | Metadate-ER | t: 10, 20 | | | 60.00 |
| | Methylin-ER | t: 5, 10, 20 | | | 62.40 |
| methylphenidate (long acting) | Metadate-CD | c: 20 | 8–12 | 40 mg q A.M. | 76.80 |
| | Ritalin-LA | c: 20, 30, 40 | | | 68.40 |
| | Ritalin-SR | | | | 68.40 |
| OROS methylphenidate | Concerta | t: 18, 27, 36, 54 | | 36–54 mg q A.M. | 74.70 |
| pemoline | Cylert | | 8–12 | 56.25–112.5 mg q A.M. | 101.70 |

* c = capsule; t = tablet

## CLINICAL INDICATIONS AND USE

### Childhood ADHD

- Greater likelihood of medication response in patients with signs and symptoms in several, rather than just one or two, settings.
  - 70% response rate to a single stimulant
  - Response rate to stimulants 85–90% with successive stimulant trials
  - Children with ADHD who take stimulants still have more behavioral problems than those who do not require medication.
- First choice is a short-acting stimulant.
  - A consensus panel recommended methylphenidate as initial treatment for children with ADHD because of high efficacy and safety (Greenhill, Beyer, et al., 2002).
    - Effective for inattention, hyperactivity, and impulsivity
    - If methylphenidate does not work, at least 25% chance that dextroamphetamine will be effective.
    - 75–90% of patients respond to one or the other medication.
  - Atomoxetine first choice for patients with risk of substance misuse, other concerns about using a stimulant, or if clinician prefers ease of prescription (not a controlled substance).
    - A randomized comparison of atomoxetine to methylphenidate in ADHD found similar improvement of inattention, hyperactivity, and impulsivity as well as similar tolerability and safety (Kratochvil et al., 2002).
    - Lack of placebo or blinding limits interpretation of results.
  - Sustained-release and other preparations are more expensive but can be taken less frequently.
    - Most useful when interdose withdrawal or decline in effect is a problem.
- Stimulant effect in ADHD
  - Appears within a few days
  - Decreased motor activity, impulsivity, irritability
  - Increased vigilance, attention, short-term memory, socially acceptable behavior
  - No tolerance over months–years
- Stimulants are highly effective for ADHD.
  - Effect size at least 1
  - Superior to placebo in 70–90%
    - 30% have marked improvement.

- 40–60% have moderate improvement.
- 10–30% are refractory to stimulants.
- Benefit is dose related.
  - Partial response may improve further with dosage increase.
  - However, single doses > 20 mg may reduce efficacy.
- Although stimulants can aggravate tics, most studies show no statistically significant increase in tics in patients with comorbid ADHD and tic disorders.
  - Randomized trial for 16 weeks in 136 children with ADHD and chronic tic disorder compared clonidine alone, methylphenidate alone, clonidine + methylphenidate, or placebo (Kurlan, 2002).
    - Greatest benefit of ADHD was with clonidine + methylphenidate.
    - Clonidine most helpful for hyperactivity and impulsivity; methylphenidate, for inattention.
    - Worsening of tics occurred in 22% on placebo, 20% on methylphenidate, and 26% on clonidine.
- Abnormal mood
  - Stimulants normally do not induce euphoria before puberty.
    - Euphoria is rare in ADHD children treated with stimulants.
  - Patients who develop elation, intense irritability, depression, mood swings, or psychosis at low doses should be reevaluated for possibility of unrecognized bipolar illness.
- In ADHD with comorbid conduct disorder, it is important to be sure that patient is not abusing drugs, especially nonprescription stimulants, or selling the medication.

## INITIATING AND MAINTAINING TREATMENT

### Before starting stimulants

- Document prior treatment, especially previous medications and psychosocial treatments.
- Perform a physical examination.
  - Obtain baseline blood pressure, pulse, height, and weight.
- Obtain baseline efficacy measures.

### Laboratory testing

- Methylphenidate occasionally decreases WBC count.
  - Obtain baseline white count and repeat every 3–6 months if clinical suspicion of neutropenia (e.g., fever).
- Pemoline can cause dangerous hepatotoxicity.
  - Monitor LFTs at baseline and every 3 months.

- Obtain LFTs immediately if evidence of hepatotoxicity (e.g., jaundice, abdominal pain).
- Monitor heart rate and blood pressure periodically, especially as dose is increased.
  - African American patients taking dextroamphetamine have higher risk of cardiac side effects.

Have parents and teachers rate symptoms and behavior at baseline and during treatment using Connors or similar validated rating scale.

Because of high placebo response rate
- It is desirable to determine whether active treatment is necessary.
- Have pharmacy prepare identical 1-week supplies of stimulant and placebo.
- Obtain daily rating scale scores on each treatment.
- If similar improvement with placebo and active drug, patient may not need stimulant.
- If similar lack of efficacy with both treatments, try a different medication.

Choosing between medications
- Immediate-release stimulants
  - Well studied
  - Clearly effective
  - Cheaper
  - Pemoline is effective but not an initial treatment because of risk of hepatotoxicity.
  - Start with 5 mg methylphenidate or 2.5 mg dextroamphetamine/amphetamines.
- Sustained-release stimulants
  - Less frequent dosing
  - Lower risk of interdose withdrawal
  - Fewer side effects
  - May be less effective than immediate-release stimulants.
  - More expensive
- Mixed amphetamine salts
  - May be better tolerated than standard stimulants.
  - Less frequent dosing
  - No more effective
  - More expensive
- Atomoxetine
  - Well tolerated

- Not a controlled substance
  - Can be refilled by telephone.
- Not as effective as stimulants
- Bupropion and venlafaxine
  - Not quite as effective as stimulants
  - Require divided dosing
  - Useful for ADHD with comorbid depression
- TCAs
  - Try stimulants, atomoxetine, bupropion, venlafaxine first.
  - Less frequent dosing
  - Not effective for childhood depression
  - Sudden death reported in prepubertal children taking desipramine.
- Alpha-2 agonists
  - Useful for hyperactivity but not inattention
  - Should usually be combined with other medications.
- Modafinil
  - May improve attention as well as alertness.
  - Consider as adjunct for partial response.
  - Should not be used for patients with left-ventricular hypertrophy, ischemic heart disease, or mitral valve prolapse because of a few reports of chest pain and ischemic EKG changes.
- Lithium
  - Useful for comorbid bipolar disorder
    - Can reduce inattention secondary to tangential thinking and distractibility in bipolar disorder.
  - May reduce impulsivity in ADHD with conduct disorder.
  - Can have cognitive side effects
- Carbamazepine may improve episode aggression and impulsivity.
  - Sometimes increases aggression in younger patients.

## MEDICATIONS TO AVOID

- Benzodiazepines
  - May cause paradoxical excitement and impair cognition.
- Antihistamines
  - May reduce hyperactivity but cause sedation and impair cognitive function.
- Antipsychotic drugs
  - Only useful for psychotic hyperactivity/inattention or severe agitation.
  - May be associated with state-dependent learning.

## Effect of Comorbid Conditions on Treatment Response

- ADHD + anxiety disorder
  - May have more side effects.
  - Probably no effect on treatment response.
- ADHD + major depression
  - Decreased ADHD symptoms may improve secondary depression.
  - If depression persists, antidepressant should be added.
    - However, bupropion and desipramine (second-line antidepressants in children) may treat both conditions.
- ADHD + Tourette's/tic disorder
  - Tics usually not increased by stimulant.
  - If tics do get worse, adding alpha-2 agonist may help.
- ADHD + conduct disorder
  - Antisocial behavior reduced by stimulant.
  - Adding lithium, divalproex, alpha-2 agonist, or atypical antipsychotic may reduce residual aggressive behavior.
- ADHD + bipolar disorder
  - Published data suggest no increase in mania if patient taking mood stabilizer.
  - Experience suggests risk of deterioration of mood with stimulant.
  - Cholinesterase inhibitor will not aggravate bipolar disorder.
- ADHD + pervasive developmental disorder (PDD)
  - PDD does not seem to impair response of ADHD to stimulants.

## Long-term Effects

- In randomized controlled trials lasting 24 months (Greenhill, Pliszka, et al., 2002)
  - Total methylphenidate dose 30–37.5 mg/day
  - No loss of efficacy over time

## Drug Holidays

- Many clinicians recommend drug holidays to address lack of weight gain or determine whether patient still needs medication.
- Schedule when patient is not in school or involved in important social activities.

### Adult ADHD

The majority of children with ADHD appear to continue to meet criteria for ADHD in adulthood. Hyperactivity tends to improve in adulthood, but inattention may persist in patients with onset of DSM-IV ADHD prior to age 7.

- Associated with poor work/academic performance, irritability, antisocial behavior, substance abuse.
- Most patients have comorbid mood, anxiety, substance use, or personality disorder.
  - Essential to obtain detailed substance use history and possibly toxicology screen.
  - Most important differential diagnosis is between adult ADHD and bipolar disorder.
    - Persistent hyperactivity suggests bipolar diagnosis.
  - History of positive response to stimulants does not confirm ADHD diagnosis.
    - Improvement of attention and psychomotor performance is a nonspecific effect of stimulants.
    - Bipolar disorder associated with paradoxical sedation with stimulants.
- Rating scales used for adults:
  - Conners Adult ADHD Rating Scale
  - Wender Utah Rating Scale
  - Brown Attention-Deficit Disorder Scale for Adults
- Stimulants (including mixed amphetamine salts) and atomoxetine appear to be effective.
  - Relative doses lower than children, for example:
    - 10 mg/day Adderall
    - 20–50 mg/day methylphenidate
  - Stimulant studies show 23–75% response rate.
  - Higher response rate seen with higher doses (e.g., 1 mg/kg methylphenidate).
- In two 10-week randomized double-blind placebo-controlled trials in a total of 536 adults with DSM-IV ADHD, atomoxetine was significantly better than placebo in reducing inattention, hyperactivity, and impulsivity (Michelson et al., 2003).
- Other medications reported to be effective for adult ADHD to consider when difficulty tolerating stimulants or risk of substance abuse are concerns:
  - Pemoline
  - Bupropion
  - Venlafaxine
  - Desipramine

- Fluoxetine
- Selegiline
- In four controlled and six open studies, desipramine, venlafaxine, atomoxetine, and bupropion were effective for adult ADHD, with most data supporting desipramine.
  - Atomoxetine appeared less effective than desipramine.

### Conduct Disorder

- Stimulants are sometimes useful for antisocial behavior.
  - Not correlated with level of ADHD symptomatology
- No long-term data
- Risk of stimulant abuse or selling medications is significant.

### Refractory Depression

- Stimulants are useful for depression in medically ill and geriatric patients.
  - When illness remits, depression often improves, making tolerance to antidepressant effect less of a concern.
- Stimulants also can be effective for depression in chronical illness (e.g., AIDS) when patients cannot tolerate antidepressants.
  - Bupropion also may be well tolerated by these patients.
- Stimulant augmentation in refractory depression may be most useful in older patients and patients who cannot tolerate therapeutic dose of antidepressant.

### Narcolepsy and Daytime Sleepiness/Sedation

- Of the REM phenomena in narcolepsy (hypnagogic hallucinations, sleep paralysis, cataplexy), only cataplexy is pathognomonic for narcolepsy.
- Stimulants are effective for sleep attacks and daytime sleepiness.
  - Total daily doses in published studies average 112.5 mg for methylphenidate and dextroamphetamine.
  - Pemoline is less effective at doses up to 312.5 mg.
  - Tolerance commonly develops.
  - Stimulants disrupt nighttime sleep.
    - Decreased sleep time
    - Decreased REM sleep

- Modafinil is approved for narcolepsy and excessive daytime sleepiness.
  - Benefit is similar to methylphenidate (decreased daytime sleepiness but sleep latency still decreased).
  - Does not affect cataplexy.
    - Adding venlafaxine may reduce cataplexy.
  - Improves but does not eliminate sleepiness.
  - In an 18 center 9-week randomized control trial in 283 patients with narcolepsy treated with 200 or 400 mg of modafinil or placebo (Fry, 1998), improvement in
    - 65% with 200 mg modafinil
    - 74% with 400 mg modafinil
    - 37% with placebo
  - In some studies, 400 mg more effective than 200 mg.
  - Also useful for medication-induced sedation.
  - Modafinil was used to treat residual hypersomnia in two patients with remitted bipolar depression (Fernandes & Petty, 2003).
    - Mania was not precipitated, but patients were not followed for extended periods of time.
- Gamma-hydroxybutyrate intensifies REM and non-REM sleep, possibly exhausting ability of sleep system to produce daytime sleepiness.
  - Very sedating
  - Short half-life
  - Taken at bedtime
  - Schedule I drug

### Restless Legs Syndrome

- Criteria for RLS
  - Desire to move limbs (including arms)
    - Associated with paresthesias or dysesthesias
  - Motor restlessness
  - Symptoms worse or only present at rest, with relief from activity.
  - Symptoms worse at night.
- May be secondary to renal disease, iron or folate deficiency, Charcot Marie Tooth disease, ADHD, vascular disease, neuropathy, pregnancy, caffeine use

Treatment
- Treat iron deficiency.
- Dopaminergic agents reduce RLS symptoms by 90–100%.

- Levodopa-carbidopa (Sinemet) 25/100 mg at bedtime is initially effective in 70% of patients.
  - Start at 20 mg levodopa, increase to 200 mg hs.
  - Rebound can result in escalating dose.
- Other dopaminergic agents also may be helpful, including
  - Pergolide ($D_1$, $D_2$ agonist)
  - Pramipexole ($D_3$ agonist)
    - Start with 0.125 mg.
    - Increase to maximum of 1.5 mg in two or three doses.
  - Ropinirole ($D_2$, $D_3$ agonist)
    - Start with 0.25 mg.
    - Increase to 3.0 mg in two or three doses.
  - Amantadine
  - Pergolide at dinner and 1 hour at bedtime
    - Start with 0.025 mg.
    - Increase by 0.05 mg q 3–7 days to maximum of 0.5 mg in two or three divided doses.
  - Bupropion sometimes effective.
  - Use of dopaminergic agents later in the day may cause insomnia and can destabilize mood in bipolar disorder.

### Anergia, Fatigue, and Depression in Chronically Debilitating Illnesses

- In addition to their antidepressant effect, stimulants may improve energy, interest, and motivation in patients with AIDS, cancer, and chronic fatigue syndrome.
  - Doses are lower than for ADHD.
    - For example, 15 mg/day methylphenidate
- No controlled studies, but stimulants effective for depression associated with stroke and other acute illnesses.
- Modafinil also may be helpful.
- Stimulants and modafinil can treat sedative side effects of medications used to treat medical illness.
- Primary adverse effect of concern in this population is appetite suppression.
- Misuse of stimulant a concern in patients who contracted AIDS through IV drug abuse.
- A number of medications should be considered first for chronic fatigue syndrome, including
  - Fluoxetine
    - Other SSRIs probably also effective.

- Bupropion
  - Improves energy as well as mood.
- TCAs (e.g., nortriptyline, imipramine, amitriptyline) have been reported to be effective, probably because of improvement in sleep, but are poorly tolerated and cause daytime sedation.
- Activating MAOIs (e.g., selegiline) may prove useful, but no studies.

## Obesity

- Commonly used medications (e.g., phentermine) produce modest weight loss that is often regained with time.
- A double-blind study randomly assigned 60 obese outpatients (BMI 30–45) with binge eating disorder (binge eating without purging) to placebo or 15 mg/day of sibutramine for 12 weeks (Appolinario et al., 2003).
  - Placebo patients gained 1.4 kg.
  - Sibutramine patients lost 7.4 kg ($p < 0.001$).
  - Sibutramine also decreased binge eating and depression scores.
- Zonesamide promotes weight loss in obese patients (see p. 63).

## SIDE EFFECTS

Adverse effects of stimulants involve
- Acute side effects
  - Usually begin within 2–3 weeks of starting medication.
  - Also develop when dose is escalated.
  - Moderate side effects occur in 4–10%.
  - Incidence of serious side effects is about 1/10,000.
- Withdrawal and rebound
  - May occur between doses with short-acting preparations.

### Cardiovascular Side Effects

HYPERTENSION

- Highly variable
  - Risk is highest in children of African ancestry.
- Reducing dose can ameliorate hypertension.
- If patient has excellent response but develops hypertension, it can be treated with an alpha-2 agonist or beta-blocker.

PALPITATIONS, TACHYCARDIA

- Usually benign
- May impair exercise tolerance.
- Dangerous for patients with ischemic heart disease

### Central Nervous System Side Effects

CHOREOATHETOID MOVEMENTS

- Most common with pemoline

CONFUSION

- Occasionally with higher doses of methylphenidate ($> 1$ mg/kg/day)

DIZZINESS

DYSPHORIA

- May be seen with all stimulants, especially methylphenidate, and associated with
  - Social withdrawal
  - Affective blunting
  - Hyperfocus
  - Perseveration
- Depression may occur in children.

EUPHORIA

- Seen primarily after puberty
- When marked at usual doses, often indicates treatment-emergent hypomania.

EXACERBATION OF TICS

- Not common, but can occur.

HEADACHE

- If severe, check patient's blood pressure.

INSOMNIA

- Usually difficulty falling asleep
- Dose related
- More likely to occur if medication is taken later in the day.

- Occurs in 30% of children on moderate or higher doses.
- Often develops early in treatment, before patient achieves therapeutic dose.
- Management:
  - Administer more of the medication earlier in the day.
  - Reduce dose.
  - Add trazodone.

## IRRITABILITY

- Ensure that patient is not developing treatment-emergent hypomania.
- Determine when irritability occurs.
  - If after dose, it may be caused by peak level.
    - Reduce dose.
  - If before dose or late in afternoon, it may be rebound.
    - Give medication more frequently.

## OBSESSIONS

- Rare
- Remit when medication discontinued

## OVERSTIMULATION

- Common with all stimulants
- If marked, consider emergence of hypomania.

## PSYCHOSIS

- Most common with amphetamines (dextroamphetamine, methamphetamine)
  - Especially with prolonged or IV use
- Dose related
  - Single dose of 300 mg amphetamine produces paranoia and hallucinations in normal subjects.
- Prominent signs and symptoms
  - Agitation
  - Paranoia > hallucinations
  - Tremor
  - Clear sensorium
  - Mimics paranoid schizophrenia
- May persist for months–years after medication discontinuation.
  - Prolonged amphetamine psychosis may represent schizophrenia precipitated by drug.

- Following the end of World War II, large quantities of methamphetamine that had been used to keep soldiers awake for long periods were released into the market by both the Japanese and the Allies.
  - Japanese factory workers took doses 50 times those used in children to work long hours during reconstruction.
  - A year later, the rate at which schizophrenia was diagnosed doubled.
    - Patients had good premorbid functioning and no family history of psychosis.
    - Negative symptoms persisted between exacerbations of psychosis.
  - During the following year, schizophrenia was diagnosed three times as frequently. The association with ready availability of methamphetamine was recognized and the drug was barred.
  - The rate of schizophrenia subsequently returned to baseline.
  - Most remissions of psychosis occurred during the first year after drug discontinuation.
    - The rate of remission decreased in each subsequent year.
  - However, it took 15% of patients with amphetamine-induced psychoses more than 5 years to recover, despite continued abstinence.

### Restlessness

- Move doses earlier in the day.
- Divide dosing more.
- Reduce dose.

### Stroke

- Cerebral infarction can be caused by hypertension or by vasospasm induced by stimulant.
- Chronic use of high doses of stimulants or cocaine may be associated with white matter hyperintensities and cognitive impairment.

### Tics

- Some children without tic disorders develop motor tics on stimulants.

## Endocrine and Sexual Side Effects

### Altered Libido

- Both increases and decreases have been reported.

### Erectile Dysfunction

- May occur with all stimulants.

GROWTH SUPPRESSION

- Appetite suppression may reduce rate of gain of weight.
- Risk of growth retardation on dextroamphetamine > methylphenidate > pemoline.
  - In 84 children with ADHD treated for 2 years with methylphenidate 10–80 mg/day, growth was significantly less in patients than in siblings who were not treated with the stimulant (Lisska & Rivkees, 2003).
- Compensatory rebound of growth occurs during drug holidays and when medication is discontinued.
- Child still may have low weight and short stature.

## Gastrointestinal Side Effects

ANOREXIA

- Decreased appetite occurs in 30% of children taking moderate or higher stimulant doses.
- Weight loss begins early in treatment.
  - Often remits.
  - Weight gain may follow with continuation of pemoline.
- Give stimulant with meals or snack.

DRY MOUTH

- Occurs primarily in adolescents.

HEPATOTOXICITY

- Reported in 1–3% of children taking pemoline
  - This is 17 times the incidence with other stimulants.
- Transaminases may increase during first few months of treatment with pemoline and return to baseline after drug discontinuation.

STOMACHACHE

- Common side effect
- Responds to lowering dose or changing timing of dosing.

COMMON SIDE EFFECTS OF MODAFINIL

- Anxiety
- Headache
- Nausea
- Rhinitis
- Insomnia

- Nervousness
- No clinically important effects on vital signs, EKG, or laboratory studies

## LESS FREQUENT BUT SEVERE SIDE EFFECTS OF MODAFINIL

- Amblyopia
- Amnesia
- Ataxia
- Cardiac arrhythmias
- Chills
- Confusion
- Fever
- Hyperglycemia
- Hypertension
- Hypotension
- Mental depression
- Pharyngitis
- Shortness of breath
- Urinary retention
- Vision changes

## COMMON SIDE EFFECTS OF ATOMOXETINE

- Abdominal pain
- Anorexia
- Constipation
- Cough
- Dry mouth
- Dysmenorrhea
- Fatigue
- Fever
- Nausea, vomiting
- Sexual dysfunction
- Urinary retention

## PREGNANCY AND LACTATION

### Teratogenicity

- Dextroamphetamine may cause cardiac anomalies and biliary atresia.
- Methylphenidate has not been linked to fetal malformations.

- There is usually no compelling reason to continue stimulants during pregnancy.

## Lactation

- Stimulants reduce prolactin release and inhibit lactation
  - Use not recommended for nursing mothers

### Direct Effects on Newborn

- Postnatal withdrawal from stimulants could cause anergia and irritability.
- Stimulants may aggravate preeclampsia.
- Stimulants are associated with premature delivery and low birth weight.

Table 9.5 summarizes interactions between stimulants and other drugs.

Table 9.6 presents the effects on laboratory tests.

## WITHDRAWAL

Stimulants can cause
- Psychological dependence
- Tolerance
- Physical dependence
- Modafinil does not cause withdrawal symptoms.
- Withdrawal manifested by
  - Increased appetite, weight gain
  - Increased sleep
  - Vivid dreams
  - Decreased energy, fatigue, anergia
  - Depression
  - Psychomotor retardation
  - Severe depression and suicidality with abrupt withdrawal
  - Occasional paranoia
  - EKG abnormalities
    - Myocardial ischemia
    - ST-T wave changes

**Table 9.5 Drug–Drug Interactions**

| DRUGS (X) INTERACT WITH: | DEXTRO-AMPHETAMINE (D) | COMMENTS |
|---|---|---|
| acidifying agents (e.g., ascorbic acid, fruit juice, glutamic acid) | D↓ ↓ | Decreases absorption of amphetamines. |
| acetazolamide (and some furosemides) | D↑ | Acetazolamide increases amphetamines. Monitor patients on acetazolamide or on other carbonic anhydrase inhibitors for excessive amphetamine levels. |
| alkalinizing agents (*see* sodium bicarbonate) | | |
| amantadine | X↑ | Increased amantadine effect with stimulation and agitation. |
| antihistamines | X↓ | Amphetamines reduce antihistamines' sedation. |
| antihypertensives | X↓ | Amphetamines may antagonize antihypertensives. |
| *antipsychotics:* chlorpromazine haloperidol | X↓ D↓ | Amphetamines inhibit antipsychotic actions, while neuroleptics block amphetamines' anorectic and stimulating effect. Antipsychotics effectively treat amphetamine overdose, but amphetamines should never treat an antipsychotic overdose. |
| ethosuximide | X↓ | Amphetamines delay absorption of anticonvulsant ethosuximide. |
| fluoxetine (*see* SSRIs) | | |
| fluvoxamine (*see* SSRIs) | | |
| furazolidone[†] | D↑ | Amphetamines induce hypertensive crises in patients given furazolidone, especially after 5 days. |
| guanethidine | X↓ D↑ | Amphetamines inhibit guanethidine's antihypertensive action. |
| haloperidol (*see* antipsychotics) | | |
| lithium | D↓ | Lithium slows weight reduction and stimulatory effects of amphetamines. No special precautions. |
| meperidine | X↑ | Amphetamines potentiate analgesic action. |
| MAOIs | X↑ | Hypertensive crisis. Most likely with tranylcypromine. |
| norepinephrine | X↑ | Amphetamine use may increase pressor response to norepinephrine. Combine with caution. |

*(continues)*

**Table 9.5  Continued**

| DRUGS (X) INTERACT WITH: | DEXTROAMPHETAMINE (A) | COMMENTS |
|---|---|---|
| phenobarbitol, phenytoin | X↓ | Amphetamines delay absorption. May also decrease seizure threshold. |
| Propoxyphene | X↑ D↑ | Can increase CNS symptoms in propoxyphene overdose, causing fatal convulsions. |
| opiates | X↑ | Amphetamines potentiate the analgesic and anorectic effect of opiates. |
| paroxetine (*see* SSRIs) | | |
| sedative hypnotics | X↓ | Reverses sedative and anxiolytic effects. |
| sertraline (*see* SSRIs) | | |
| sodium bicarbonate | D↑ | Sodium bicarbonate can increase amphetamines' effect; preferred by abusers. |
| SSRIs | X↑ D↑ | Increased agitation; may augment antidepressant effect. |
| TCAs | X↑ D↑ | Amphetamines may increase TCA effect; can also produce arrhythmias, agitation, and psychosis. TCAs (desipramine, protriptyline) increase amphetamine levels. |

| DRUGS (X) INTERACT WITH: | METHYLPHENIDATE (M) | COMMENTS |
|---|---|---|
| *anticonvulsants:* phenytoin diphenylhydantoin primidone | X↑ | Increases plasma levels; isolated cases of intoxication. |
| guanethidine | X↓ M↑ | Methylphenidate inhibits guanethidine's antihypertensive action. Try another antihypertensive. |
| MAOIs | X↑ | Methylphenidate poses less risk than amphetamines for hypertensive crisis, but methylphenidate should still be avoided with MAOIs. |
| TCAs | X↑ | Methylphenidate may facilitate TCAs' antidepressant and toxic effects and increase TCA levels. |
| warfarin | M↑ | Increases levels of methylphenidate; monitor closely. |

| DRUGS (X) INTERACT WITH: | PEMOLINE (P) | COMMENTS |
|---|---|---|
| sedative hypnotics | X↓ | Pemoline can interfere with anxiolytic and sedative effects. |
| anticonvulsants | X↓ | Pemoline may lower seizure threshold. |

↑ = increase, ↓ = decrease

**Table 9.6 Effects on Laboratory Tests**

| GENERIC NAMES | BLOOD/SERUM TESTS | URINE TESTS |
|---|---|---|
| dextroamphetamine | Corticosteroids[†] | Interferes with steroid determinations |
| methylphenidate | RBC ↓ r, WBC ↓ r | None |
| pemoline | LFT ↑ | None |

↑ Increases; ↓ Decreases; r = relative ? inconsistent; LFT are AST/SGOT, ALT/SGPT, LDH, alkaline phosphatase, and bilirubin.

- Bundle-branch block
- Left-ventricular hypertrophy
- Premature ventricular contractions
- Substance craving
- Drug misuse
  - ADHD is associated with increased risk of substance abuse and cigarette smoking.
  - Adolescents with ADHD have lower incidence of substance use disorders if they are treated with stimulants.
  - Greater abuse potential is associated with characteristics of dextroamphetamine, methamphetamine, methylphenidate:
    - High water solubility permits IV injection.
    - Stability at temperatures that produce a vapor facilitates smoking.
    - Stimulation of mesolimbic dopaminergic pathways.
  - Oral methylphenidate does not induce euphoria, but it can be injected.
    - Methylphenidate is mentioned 1/40th as frequently as cocaine in the Drug Abuse Warning Network.
  - A longitudinal study of 147 patients found that stimulant treatment of ADHD in childhood did not increase the risk of adolescent substance use (Fischer & Barkley, 2003).
  - Meta-analysis of seven studies found that stimulants for ADHD in childhood reduced risk for later substance use disorders by 50% (Faraone & Wilens, 2003).
  - Modafinil has low water solubility, is unstable at high temperatures, and does not act on dopaminergic systems, resulting in low abuse potential.
  - Risk of abuse in dextroamphetamine > methylphenidate > pemoline
  - Sustained-release preparations have lower abuse potential.
  - Gamma-hydroxybutyrate (GHB) was used during the 1980s in body-building and then became a "club drug."

- Approved for release at a single site in the United States as a treatment for narcolepsy.
- Can be neurotoxic.
- Acts at a specific receptor and at GABA$_B$ receptor.
- Abrupt discontinuation causes withdrawal.
- Multiple congeners have been synthesized.
- 1,4-butanediol, the most widely used, can be found in bodybuilding beverages and solvents, including printer cleaners.

Signs and symptoms of stimulant withdrawal:

- Dysphoria
- Depression
- Hypersomnia
- Increased appetite
- Lethargy
- Lasts 8 hours–2 weeks
- Often complicated by withdrawal from other substances used, such as alcohol and opiates.

Table 9.7 summarizes the drugs used to treat stimulant withdrawal.

Management of withdrawal from stimulants and cocaine:

- Observe patient closely.
- Institute suicide precautions.
- Treat depression.
    - Noradrenergic or dopaminergic agent preferred.
        - Bupropion may reduce craving.

**Table 9.7 Treatment of Stimulant Withdrawal**

| MEDICATION CLASS | EXAMPLES | COMMENT |
| --- | --- | --- |
| Direct dopamine agonists | Bromocriptine, pergolide | No efficacy |
| Indirect dopamine agonists | Methylphenidate | No effect on cocaine use, but lower dropout rate than placebo |
| | Amantadine | Better than placebo for cocaine-free urines at 1 month |
| Adrenergic antagonists | Propranolol | Reduced cocaine use and improved retention in one study |
| Antidepressants | Bupropion, desipramine | No efficacy |

Kosten & O'Connor (2003)

- Continued stimulant use may raise bupropion levels to range that increases seizure risk.
- Dopaminergic agents (e.g., bromocriptine, pergolide, pramipexole) may improve lethargy, depression, and substance craving.
- Patients with chronic anergia and depression after withdrawal from long-term stimulant use may be experiencing sequelae of reduced capacity to synthesize and release dopamine.
  - Dopaminergic antidepressant is best choice, for example:
    - Bupropion
    - Selegiline if patient can avoid more stimulant use
- Desipramine reduces craving and improves abstinence at 50–150 mg/day.
- 0.125 mg bromocriptine (dopamine agonist) every 6 hours reduces craving in early cocaine abstinence.
- Buprenorphine maintenance produces better reduction of cocaine use in opiate addicts than methadone.

## TOXICITY AND OVERDOSE

Despite a large therapeutic index, a 10-day supply of a stimulant may be toxic and occasionally lethal. Most severe overdoses involve illicit stimulants such as methamphetamine and cocaine

- Common signs and symptoms of stimulant overdose include
  - Agitation, anger
  - Suicidal ideation
  - Chest pain
  - Paranoia
  - Hallucinations (including haptic [somatic] hallucinations)
  - Confusion
  - Dysphoria
- Less common
  - Seizures
  - Hyperreflexia
  - Fever
  - Tremor
  - Rhabdomyolysis
  - Hypertension
  - Stroke
  - Palpitations
  - Headache

- Abdominal pain
- Leg pain
- Paresthesias
- Coma
- GHB intoxication produces
  - Delirium
  - Bradycardia
  - Hypothermia
  - Agitation
  - Myoclonus
  - Seizures
  - Coma
  - Apnea
  - Amnesia

Management of overdose:
- Nonspecific measures
  - Follow EKG and vital signs.
  - Obtain toxicology screening for other substances ingested.
  - Maintain circulation and airway.
  - Administer gastric lavage combined with endotracheal intubation to prevent aspiration if patient not conscious.
    - Most effective for ingestion within 4 hours
  - Administer activated charcoal 40–50 gm for adults or 20–25 gm for children po or through lavage tube.
- Specific measures
  - IV diazepam or short-acting barbiturate for seizures
  - Dopamine antagonist for psychosis
    - Haloperidol
    - Risperidone
    - Consider ziprasidone if injectable atypical antipsychotic is desired.
  - Isolate agitated or psychotic patient from environmental stimuli.
  - Use a hypothermia blanket for fever or increased intracranial pressure.
    - Administer mannitol if increased intracranial pressure is severe.
  - For hypertension
    - Hasten excretion by acidifying urine with ammonium chloride.
    - Administer phentolamine 4 mg IV.
  - Efficacy of dialysis not established.

## PRECAUTIONS

Contraindications to stimulants include
- Hypersensitivity to the medications
- Hyperthyroidism
- Severe stimulant abuse, especially with antisocial behavior or history of lying to physicians
- Agitation
- Uncontrolled hypertension
- Glaucoma
  - Stimulants can increase intraocular pressure.
- Hepatic disease (for pemoline)
- Active psychosis

Caution is necessary in the presence of
- Significant cardiovascular disease
- Tics
- History of stimulant abuse that may be self-treatment of ADHD and has not been associated with antisocial behavior
- History of abuse of other substances
- Tourette's disorder
- Seizure disorder
  - However, seizure frequency does not increase when methylphenidate is added.
- Ongoing treatment with MAO inhibitors
  - Stimulants can be cautiously combined with MAOIs for
    - Refractory depression
    - Management of MAOI-induced hypotension
- Growth retardation
  - Monitor child's growth regularly.

## ADVICE FOR CARETAKERS

Monitor the patient's
- Cardiovascular status
- Growth
- Blood sugar, if a diabetic patient has appetite suppression
- Use of the substance
  - Misuse is associated with escalating doses, lost prescriptions, running out of medication early, and use of the medication to get "high."

- If a suspicion arises that the patient is abusing, selling, or giving away medication, confront tactfully but firmly.

## NOTES FOR PATIENT AND FAMILY

Dosing recommendations
- Dextroamphetamine
  - Take on awakening or 30–60 minutes before breakfast.
  - Take other doses after meals to reduce risk of appetite suppression.
  - Take subsequent doses every 4–6 hours.
  - Do not take within 6 hours of bedtime.
  - If side effects are troublesome, switch to Adderall.
- Methylphenidate
  - Taking the first dose with breakfast may reduce stomachaches.
  - Do not take within 6 hours of bedtime.
  - Use a sustained-release form for
    - Significant side effects
    - Interdose withdrawal
    - Try Concerta before methylphenidate-SR
- Growth may be slowed initially, but patients eventually catch up with growth curve.
  - Growth may rebound with drug holidays.
  - Monitor height and weight every 6 months or so.
  - Growth retardation can be reduced by close attention to nutrition.
- If insomnia occurs, take medication earlier in the day.
- Do not stop stimulant abruptly.
  - May cause depression.
  - The stimulant itself may cause depression as a side effect.
- Monitor use of medication.
  - A 10-day supply can be dangerous.
- Avoid sodium bicarbonate.
  - Alkalinizes urine, reducing amphetamine excretion and prolonging its action.
- Excessive intake of vitamin C or citric acid may acidify urine, resulting in increased amphetamine excretion and reduced effect.
- If patient forgets a dose of an immediate-release stimulant, it can be taken up to 3 hours later.
  - Otherwise, wait for the next dose.
  - Do not double the dose.

- If patient forgets a dose of a sustained-release stimulant, wait until the next morning.
- Do not use stimulants for weight loss.
  - Any initial weight loss is usually reversed within a few months.

Be careful with caffeine.

# CHAPTER TEN

# Herbal, Complementary, and Hormonal Remedies and Treatments

A 1999 survey found that 10% of adults in the United States used an herbal medicine in the previous year, spending $5.1 billion on these preparations; one in six patients taking prescription medications also takes herbal remedies (de Smet, 2002; Straus, 2002).

- Most of these products are considered dietary supplements by the FDA.
    - They do not have to meet standards for medications.
    - They can be marketed without demonstration of their efficacy or safety.
    - The only requirement is that any claims made on the label must be truthful; but there is no standard for evidence of truthfulness of these claims.
- The amount of active substance varies considerably in herbal preparations and may not correspond to what is written on the container. For example, the amount of active ginsenosides and eleutherosides in ginseng products varies from 31–328% of the labeled amount (Straus, 2002).
- The common belief that herbal therapies are safe because they are "natural" is fallacious.
    - Many natural substances are toxic (e.g., radiation, arsenic, jimson weed)
    - Dangerous reactions can occur to herbal preparations (e.g., kava kava).
    - Many modern medications are derived from plants (e.g., digitalis).
    - Drug metabolizing systems evolved to eliminate xenobiotics (i.e., foreign plant material).
        - Herbal therapies may induce or inhibit these enzymes, resulting in important drug interactions.
- Manufacturers of herbal products are not required to demonstrate safety or efficacy prior to marketing; instead, the FDA must demonstrate that the product is not safe before its use can be modified.

The use of hormonal therapies in women has recently been reconsidered. These medications have traditionally been used to treat deficiency syndromes and as contraceptives in women, but clinicians also use them as adjunctive treatments for mood disorders—despite lack of compelling data on their efficacy and accumulating evidence that their use has medical risks. Antiandrogen treatment also is used to treat prostate cancer and paraphilias.

This chapter addresses some of the herbal therapies that are commonly used by psychiatric patients. A brief review of psychiatric applications of hormonal therapies is also included. Disorders considered include

- Depression (also discussed in Chapters 3 and 4)
- Bipolar disorder (also discussed in Chapters 5 and 6)
- Anxiety (also discussed in Chapters 3 and 7)
- Dementia (also discussed in Chapter 2)

Table 10.1 lists the substances discussed in this chapter.


## PHARMACOLOGY

Herbal and complementary therapies are produced in different ways and have diverse actions. For example:

- Ginkgo biloba is an extract of the leaves of the maidenhair tree (*Ginkgo biloba*). The active components of ginkgo include flavonoids (benzodiazepine receptor agonists), proanthocyanidins, and other agents that act as
  - Platelet activating factor inhibitors
  - Antioxidants
  - Free radical scavengers
  - Lipid peroxidation inhibitors
    - Lipid peroxidation contributes to neuronal loss.
- Kava kava, which is derived from the root of a South Pacific shrub (*Piper methysticum*), contains kava lactones and chalcones. It blocks voltage-dependent sodium and calcium channels, potentiates $GABA_A$ receptors, and reversibly inhibits MAO-B and cyclooxygenase, resulting in a number of actions:
  - Muscle relaxant
  - Analgesic
  - Anticoagulant
  - Antispasmodic

**Table 10.1  Herbal and Hormonal Therapies**

| NAME | GENUS | TRADE NAMES/ OTHER NAMES | DOSE FORMS |
|------|-------|--------------------------|------------|
| | | **HERBAL AND NATURAL SUBSTANCES** | |
| Ginkgo | *Ginkgo biloba* | Gincosan, Ginkai, Ginkoba, Ginkgo-gold, Ginkgo Power | c: 30, 40, 50, 60, 100, 120, 260, 400, 420, 440, 450, 500 mg<br>t: 30, 40, 60, 80, 120, 260 mg<br>l: 40 mg/5 mL<br>e: 50:1 |
| Kava kava | *Piper methysticum* | Kava Kava, Kava Kava Root, Kava Kava Power | c: 100, 125, 128, 150, 250, 390, 400, 425, 455, 500 mg<br>l: 1:1, 1:2 |
| Lemon balm | *Melissa officinalis* | Balm Sweet Mary, Honey Plant, Melissa | c: 395 mg |
| Ma-huang | *Ephedra sinica* | Ephedrine, Desert Herb | e: 1 gm/mL<br>t: 1:1, 1:4 |
| Melatonin | | Jarrow Melatonin<br>Source Naturals<br>Melaton<br>Country Life Melatonin | t: 1, 2, 3, 5 mg<br>s: 1, 2.5, 5 mg<br>l: 2, 4 oz |
| Omega-3 fatty acids | | Spectrum Essential Oil Omega-3<br>Spectrum Essential Ultra EFA Liquid<br>Omega 3 Twinlab<br>Natrol Omega-3<br>Enzymatic Therapy HF Eskimo-3 | c: 156, 300, 1000 mg<br>l: 2:1 Omega—3:6 |
| S-adenosyl methionine | | SAMe | |
| St. John's wort | *Hypericum perforatum* | St. John's Wort, Alterra, Mood Support, Hypericalm | c: (0.3% hypericin): 125, 150, 250, 300, 350, 370, 375, 400, 424, 434, 500, 510 mg<br>t: (0.3% hypericin): 100, 150, 300, 450 mg<br>er: (0.3% hypericin): 450, 900, 1000 mg<br>l: 300 mg/5 mL, 250 mg/5 mL<br>e: 1:1<br>i: 1%<br>ti: 1:10<br>td: 900 mg/24 hours |
| Valerian | *Valeriana officinalis* | Valerian Root, Nature's Root Nighttime, Quanterra Sleep, Valerian Power Time Release | c: 100, 250, 380, 400, 445, 475, 493, 500, 530, 550, 1000 mg<br>l: 1:1<br>t: 160, 550 mg |

*(continues)*

**Table 10.1 Continued**

| NAME | GENUS | TRADE NAMES/ OTHER NAMES | DOSE FORMS |
|---|---|---|---|
| Yohimbine | *Pausinystalia yohimbine* | Yocon, Actibine, Aphrobine, Testomar | c: 500 mg<br>t: 5.4 mg, 800 mg<br>l: 1000 mg/mL |

### HORMONAL AND RELATED PREPARATIONS

| NAME | GENUS | TRADE NAMES/ OTHER NAMES | DOSE FORMS |
|---|---|---|---|
| DHEA | | | c: 50 mg |
| Estrogen | Conjugated estrogen; esterified estrogen; estradiol | Activella<br>Conestin<br>Premarin<br>Premphase<br>Prempro<br>Estrase<br>Estratest<br>Estratest H.S.<br>Gyndiol<br>Menest<br>Vivelle | cr: 0.01%<br>t: 0.3, 0.625, 0.9, 1.25, 2.5 mg<br>td: 0.025, 0.0375, 0.05, 0.075, 0.1 mg/day |
| Testosterone | Testosterone enanthate and cypionate | | i: 200 mg/mL<br>t: 30 mg<br>td: 2.5, 5, 10 mg/day |
| Ketoconazole | | Nizoral | t: 200 mg |
| Leuprolide | Leuprolide acetate | Eligard<br>Lupron<br>Viadur | i: 1 mg/0.2 mL; 7.5, 22.5, 30 mg; 3.75, 7.5, 11.25, 22.5, 30 mg depot |

c = capsule; cr = cream; e = extract; er = extended-release capsule; i = injection; l = liquid; s = sublingual; t = tablet; td = transdermal; ti = tincture

- Ma-huang (ephedra), which is made from the branch of *Ephedra sinica,* contains 2-aminophenylpropane alkaloids, including ephedrine and pseudoephedrine, and has effects that include
  - Sympathomimetic
    - Direct and indirect alpha- and beta-adrenergic agonist
  - Bacteriostatic
- St. John's wort (SJW) is made from dried above-ground parts of the *Hypericum perforatum* plant. SJW has multiple constituents—hypericin, pseudohypericin, phloroglucinols, phenylpropanes, flavonol derivatives, biflavones, proanthocyanidins, xanthones, and amino acids—making it difficult to know which is the active agent. At least one of these components inhibits synaptic uptake of serotonin, dopamine, norepinephrine, GABA, L-glutamate, and melatonin.

- Flavonoids have antiinflammatory and antibacterial effects
- Hypericin does not inhibit MAO.
- Valerian root (*Valeriana officinalis*) contains iridoids, volatile oil, sesquiterpenes, pyridine alkaloids, and caffeic acid derivatives and glutamine. These substances
  - Inhibit GABA reuptake.
  - Increase GABA synthesis (glutamine crosses the blood–brain barrier and is converted to GABA).
- Commercial yohimbine is made from the dried bark of the *Pausinystalia yohimbine* tree, which contains indole alkaloids and tannins.
  - One of the indole alkaloids (rauwolscine) is a selective alpha-2 adrenergic antagonist.
    - Increases norepinephrine release.
    - Increases levels of the major CNS metabolite of NE, 3-methoxy-4-hydroxyphenylglycol (MHPG).
  - Clinical effects include
    - Sympathomimetic effect
    - Pressor agent
    - Decreased colonic tone
    - Analgesic
    - Improvement of sexual function
    - Increased salivary flow
- Lemon balm contains gycosides, caffeic acid derivatives, flavonoids, and triterpene acids. These substances have a number of actions:
  - Sedative
  - Antioxidant
  - Antiviral
  - Antibacterial
  - Spasmolytic
- S-adenosyl-L-methionine 1,4-butanedisulfonate (SAMe) is a methyl donor to biogenic amines, phospholipids, proteins, and nucleic acids.
- Essential amino acids (linoleic acid, γ-linolenic acid) must be consumed in the diet because humans cannot synthesize them.
  - Food sources: seeds, nuts, grains, legumes (flax, canola, soy), cold water fish
  - Linoleic acid and γ-linolenic acid are metabolized to long-chain polyunsaturated fatty acids that include
    - Omega-6 fatty acids (dihomo-γ-linolenic acid; arachidonic acid [AA]; arachidonic acid and docosahexaenoic acid, which account for half of total brain phospholipids; essential for synthesis of

cytokines that mediate inflammation, such as interleukins, TNF-α, interferon-γ)

- Omega-3 fatty acids (eicosapentaenoic acid [EPA]; docosahexaenoic acid [DHA]; decrease production of inflammatory cytokines; shift in ratio of omega-6/omega-3 fatty acids could lead to chronic inflammatory processes)

- Long-chain polyunsaturated fatty acids are needed for cell membrane functions, including receptor function, axon and dendrite growth, formation of new synapses, pruning of old synapses, actions of membrane-associated proteins, and cell signaling.

- Various factors can interfere with the synthesis of omega-6 and omega-3 fatty acids, for example:
  - Oxidative damage
  - Viral infection
  - Hormonal factors

- Omega-3 fatty acids inhibit protein kinase C activity and alter a number of other aspects of second messenger signaling.

- Gonadal steroids, including estrogens and androgens, are derived from dehydroepiandrosterone (DHEA), as indicated in Figure 10.1.

  - The most potent, naturally occurring estrogen is 17-β-estradiol, followed by estrone and estriol.

  - Progesterone has CNS-depressant and hypnotic properties.

  - Testosterone, the principal circulating androgen, has three fates:
    - Binding to androgen receptors
    - Conversion in certain tissues to dihydrotestosterone
    - Conversion to estradiol, which binds to estrogen receptors

  - Testosterone has important actions in the brain, skin, breast, cardiovascular system, prostate, and testes.

  - DHEA in its sulfated form (DHEA-S) is the most prevalent steroid in the body.
    - Influences neuronal excitability.
    - Enhances NMDA receptor activity.

- Analogues of gonadotrophin releasing hormone (GnRH) inhibit luteinizing hormone (LH) secretion and decrease testosterone synthesis.

- Mifepristone (RU-486) is a competitive antagonist of progesterone at low doses and of glucocorticoid receptors at higher doses.
  - Results in feedback inhibition from cortisol on ACTH secretion, resulting in increased cortisol and ACTH levels.

- Ketoconazole (Nizoral) is an antifungal drug.
  - At high doses (600–1200 mg/day) inhibits steroid hormone synthesis at multiple points.

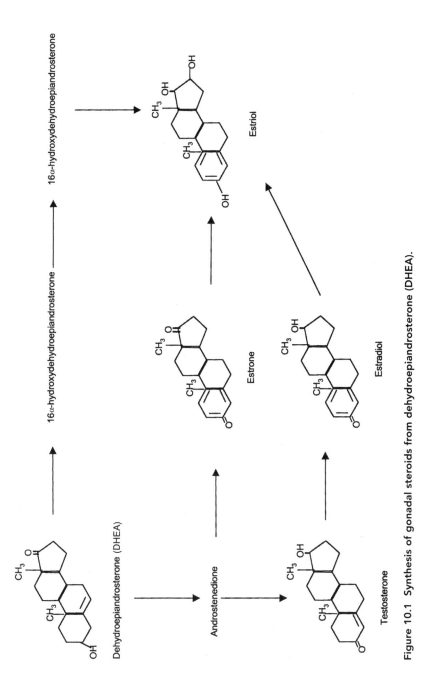

Figure 10.1 Synthesis of gonadal steroids from dehydroepiandrosterone (DHEA).

- Metyrapone is a selective inhibitor of 11-β-hydroxylase, which catalyzes synthesis of cortisol from 11-deoxycortisol.

## DOSES

Recommended doses of herbal therapies vary considerably, even within the same substance. In addition, because the FDA does not regulate these substances, the amount of active drug may differ substantially, not only between brands but even within the same brand. Table 10.2 provides guidelines for dosing.

**Table 10.2  Dosing Guidelines for Herbal Therapies**

| THERAPY | USUAL ADULT DOSE OF TABLETS/CAPSULES | DOSE OF RAW SUBSTANCE | SPECIAL CONSIDERATIONS |
|---|---|---|---|
| Ginkgo biloba | 40–80 mg tid | 3–6 gm of leaves/day as infusion | Protect from light and moisture |
| Kava kava | 150–300 mg bid | 30 drops of tincture tid, ½ cup of infusion bid | Take with food or liquid; do not use for > 3 months |
| Ma-huang (ephedra) | 120 mg/day | 1–4 gms in tea tid, 1–3 mL of extract tid, 6–8 mg of tincture tid | Protect from light |
| Melatonin | 1–3 mg hs | | Protect from light and moisture |
| Omega-3 fatty acids | 6.2 gm EPA/3.4 gm DHA | | Different doses for medical indications |
| SAMe | 400–1600 mg/day, 200–800 mg/day IV, 200–400 mg/day IM | | May augment TCAs |
| St. John's wort | 300 mg tid | 2–4 gms dried herb in boiling water or taken directly, 2–4 mL of liquid extract or tincture | Store at room temperature away from heat, moisture, and direct light |
| Valerian | 100–1800 mg/day | One cup infusion or tea 2–3 times per day, or ½–1 tsp tincture prn, 15 gm root powder, 400–900 mg extract hs | Store at room temperature in tightly closed, nonplastic container |
| Yohimbine | 5.4 mg tid; up to 30 mg/day if tolerated | | Dangerous in overdose |

## CLINICAL INDICATIONS AND USE

### Melatonin

Melatonin is usually used to treat insomnia and jet lag.

- Most studies find that doses around 1 mg are as effective as higher doses.
- Bioavailability varies from preparation to preparation.
- In a study in which 10 unmedicated patients with DSM-IV primary insomnia were randomly assigned to 0.3 mg melatonin, 1 mg melatonin, or placebo 60 minutes before bedtime (Montes, Uribe, Sotres, & Martin, 2003):
  - Each subject underwent each treatment for 7 days in a crossover design.
  - There were no significant differences between the two melatonin doses and placebo in amount or quality of sleep.

Bedtime melatonin can help to reset the sleep–wake cycle in patients with jet lag, especially when combined with morning bright light.

- In 9 of 10 controlled trials, melatonin taken close to the target bedtime at the destination decreased jet lag when crossing five or more time zones (Herxheimer & Petrie, 2002).
  - Doses of 0.5 and 5 mg were equally effective, except that sleep onset was sooner with 5 mg.
  - Doses > 5 mg are no more effective.
  - Slow-release melatonin was not as effective, suggesting that a short-lived high peak level is important.
  - The number needed to treat to produce meaningful benefit (NNT) in these trials was 2.

Melatonin has been used to improve the sleep disorder of dementia (see p. 432).

- A randomized double-blind crossover placebo-controlled trial in 44 demented patients found that 6 mg of melatonin did not affect time asleep, number of awakenings, or sleep efficiency (Serfaty, Kennell-Webb, Warner, Blizard, & Raven, 2002).

Demonstration of abnormality of melatonin release in recently abstinent alcoholics may imply that melatonin could be initial treatment of choice for insomnia in alcoholic patients.

### Ginkgo Biloba

- Ginkgo is most frequently used to treat dementia, peripheral vascular disease, and tinnitus. These applications are based on antagonism of platelet activating factor, scavenging of free radicals, antiinflammatory action, increased blood flow, inhibition of nitric oxide production with tissue damage, and antioxidant properties.

- In a year-long study of Alzheimer's disease and multiinfarct dementia, subjects taking 40 mg tid of ginkgo extract improved significantly more than subjects on placebo in cognitive function and daily behavior but not CGI (Le Bars et al., 1997).
  - Significantly more ginkgo- than placebo-treated patients had at least a 4-point improvement in cognitive function. The results suggested that six patients would have to be treated to obtain clinically meaningful improvement in one.
- A meta-analysis of 12–24-week randomized controlled trials in dementia found that ginkgo was significantly better than placebo in improving CGI scores, cognitive scores, activities of daily living, and emotional functioning.
  - Results of the better-designed studies were inconsistent (Birks, Grimley, Evans, & Van Dongen, 2002).
- A critical review of 9 double-blind, placebo controlled trials of ginkgo biloba in normal subjects found no consistent positive effect on any aspect of cognitive performance; any statistically significant changes were not noticeable by subjects (Canter & Ernst, 2002)
  - Such results may not apply to patients with dementia

Other uses of Ginkgo biloba
- Vertigo and/or dizziness caused by vascular or vestibular disorders
  - 80 mg BID reported to be effective in 65% of patients, similar to an antihistamine (Cesarini, Meloni, & Alpini, 1998)
- Peripheral artery occlusive disease
- Tinnitus
- Headache


## St. John's Wort

St. John's Wort (SJW) has been used widely to treat depression and anxiety.

- Response rates of mild-to-moderate depression to SJW were 23–55% higher than placebo response rates in early trials.
  - All of these were methodologically flawed (de Smet, 2002).
- A 6-week double-blind trial randomly assigned 375 patients with mild-to-moderate major depression (mean HRSD score 22) to SJW 300 mg tid (Lecrubier, Clerc, Didi, & Kieser, 2002).
  - Mean HRSD scores decreased by 9.9 points in the SJW group and 8.1 points in the placebo group.

- Although statistically significant, the difference between groups was not great, and differences between SJW and placebo groups in Montgomery–Asberg Depression Rating Scale scores were not statistically significant.
- In a placebo-controlled study, 300 mg of standardized hypericin extract taken three or four times/day produced a 27% response rate vs. 19% for placebo ($p$ = NS; Shelton et al., 2001).
- An 8-week study of moderately depressed outpatients compared 350 mg tid of SJW with just 100 mg/day of imipramine (Phillip, Kohnen, & Hiller, 2000).
  - Response rates were statistically significantly better for SJW (76%) than for imipramine (67%) or placebo (63%), but the difference was not clinically impressive.
- A multicenter double-blind trial randomly assigned 340 outpatients with moderate–major depression and mean HRSD scores of 22–23 to 900–1500 mg/day of hypericum, 50–100 mg/day of sertraline, or placebo (Group, 2002).
  - Responders at week 8 continued blinded treatment for another 18 weeks.
  - Reductions in total HRSD scores were
    - 9.2 for placebo
    - 8.7 for SJW
    - 10.5 for sertraline
    - Sertraline effect size was only 0.24 (effect size usually ~ 0.6; may reflect low antidepressant dose).
  - Sertraline but not SJW was more likely to improve CGI scores.
  - There were no differences in full response rates.
    - 32% for placebo
    - 24% for SJW
    - 25% for sertraline
  - The relatively low dose of sertraline makes this a poor comparator, although the study suggests that an active comparator as well as a placebo is necessary to determine whether or not a new antidepressant is effective.
- Based on these studies, there is no evidence that SJW is useful for more severe forms of major depression, but it may work as well as low doses of reference antidepressants for milder depression.

Other uses of SJW:
- Wound infections and eczema
  - SJW inhibits growth of gram positive bacteria.
- Skin inflammation

- Insect bites
- First-degree burns
- Chronic pain
- Malaria

### Kava Kava

- Kava has been found superior to placebo for nonpsychotic anxiety (Pittler & Ernst, 2000).
- Kava extract was compared to the benzodiazepines oxazepam and bromazepam in a double-blind study in 172 patients (Woelk, 1993)
  - Clinically significant decreases in anxiety were similar for kava and the two benzodiazepines.

Other uses of kava kava:
- Insomnia
- Agotatopm

Recent reports of severe hepatotoxicity may limit the usefulness of kava kava.

### Omega-3 Fatty Acids

In cross-national studies, higher intake of seafood is associated with lower rates of bipolar disorder and major depression.
- A 4-week controlled trial in unipolar depression found that 2 gm/day of EPA added to ongoing antidepressant treatment reduced HRSD scores by 12.4 points vs. 1.6 points with placebo (Nemets, Stahl, & Belmaker, 2002).
  - EPA reduced core depressive symptoms such as guilt, worthlessness, and insomnia.
- A 4-month study compared addition of 9.6 gm/day of a combination of EPA and DHA to olive oil placebo in 30 patients with bipolar disorder (Stoll, Severus, & Freeman, 1999).
  - Most patients were already taking mood stabilizers.
  - 8 patients were taking no other medication.
  - Omega-3 produced significantly better outcome than placebo.
    - Relapse rate 18% with active treatment vs. 40% with placebo.
- A randomized controlled trial in 231 prisoners found that those receiving an essential fatty acid supplement had 26% fewer disciplinary offenses than those receiving placebo (Gesch, Hammon, & Hamson, 2002).
- An 8-week randomized controlled study of ethyl-eicosapentaenoic acid (E-EPA) in women with borderline personality disorder and in women

with no current mood disorder assigned patients to 1000 mg of E-EPA (N = 20) or placebo (N = 10; Zanarini & Frankenburg, 2003).

- The E-EPA group had significantly greater reductions of mean scores on the Modified Overt Aggression Scale and the Montgomery–Asberg Depression Rating Scale.

Other uses of omega-3 fatty acids:

- Prevention of heart disease
- Arthritis
- Cyclosporine toxicity
- Dysmenorrhea
- Hypercholesterolemia
- Hypertriglyceridemia
- Hypertension
- Post MI
- Raynaud's syndrome
- Rheumatoid arthritis

## Ephedra

Compounds containing ephedrine alkaloids are usually used for weight loss or to enhance athletic performance.

- A careful literature review found 550 articles, 20 of which could not be located, that involved at least 8 weeks of follow-up for weight loss and no minimum for athletic performance (Shekelle et al., 2003).
  - Ephedra alone promoted weight loss of 0.6 kg/month > placebo.
  - Average weight loss at 4 months was 11%.
  - Only higher doses promoted weight loss.
  - Ephedra plus caffeine promoted weight loss of 0.4 kg/month > ephedrine alone.
  - Ephedra alone promoted weight loss of 0.8 kg > placebo.
  - Ephedra plus caffeine increased athletic performance by 20–30% vs. no change with either substance alone.
  - Risk of psychiatric, autonomic, GI, and cardiac effects was 2.2–3.6 times greater than that of placebo.
- A RAND report supported the finding of the FDA that "there is no safe dose of ephedra when taken without medical supervision" (Hollister & Kearns, 2003).
- The FDA has mandated removal of ephedra from the market.

Other uses of ephedra:

- Sedation, daytime sleepiness

- Mild broncospasm
- Bradycardia
- ADHD
    - Jiangqian granule for 3 months reduced ADHD symptoms in 93% of patients vs. 73% treated with methylphenidate (Chen, Chen, & Wang, 2002).
    - In a single-blind comparison, yizhidan improved "learning memory" in 46% and methylphenidate in 53% of patients.
        - Improvement in Conners scale scores was similar with both treatments.
        - Both substances increased cerebral monoamine concentrations to a similar extent.

### Lemon Balm

Lemon balm is sometimes used to treat anxiety and insomnia.

- In 71 elderly nursing home residents with dementia and clinically significant agitation, addition of 200 mg lemon balm oil (essential oil of *Melissa officinalis*) was significantly better than placebo (sunflower oil) in producing clinically meaningful decreases in agitation (60% with lemon balm vs. 14% with placebo), as well as quality of life and increased involvement with activities (Ballard, O'Brien, Reichelt, & Perry, 2002).

Other uses of lemon balm:

- Palpitations
- Headache

### Valerian

Valerian is usually used to treat insomnia:

- A multicenter controlled trial in 121 patients randomized to 600 mg valerian extract or placebo 1 hour before bedtime found that sleep was rated as good or very good after 28 days in 66% of valerian patients vs. 29% of placebo patients (Vorbach, Gortelmeyer, & Bruning, 1996).
    - Objective sleep laboratory measures were not obtained.
- Double-blind placebo-controlled crossover trial in nine healthy men and women of valerian 500 mg, valerian 1000 mg, triazolam 0.25 mg, or placebo (Hallam, Olver, McGrath, & Norman, 2003):
    - Triazolam caused significant impairment in cognitive tests.
    - Valerian had no effect on cognition or psychomotor performance.

Other uses of valerian:

- Anxiety
- Headache
- Menopausal symptoms
- Restlessness
- Irritable bowel syndrome

### Yohimbine

Yohimbine is primarily used to treat erectile dysfunction.

- Effective for antidepressant-induced sexual dysfunction.
- May improve anorgasmia in some patients.

Yohimbine is also used to increase salivary flow to treat medication-induced dry mouth.

### SAMe

Two multicenter trials comparing SAMe (S-adenosyl-L-methionine 1,4-butanedisulfonate) to imipramine found efficacy in major depression (Chiaie, Pancheri, & Scapicchio, 2002).

- One study involved 143 patients who received 400 mg oral SAMe and 138 who received 150 mg imipramine for 6 weeks.
- The other study assigned 147 patients to 400 mg IM SAMe and 148 patients to 150 mg imipramine for 4 weeks.
- In both studies, both SAMe and imipramine produced significant and equivalent reductions in HRSD scores.
- About two-thirds of patients responded to each treatment.
- SAMe was better tolerated than imipramine.

### Chromium Picolinate

Chromium picolinate has been used as an antidepressant.

- An 8-week placebo-controlled double-blind study of chromium picolate 600 mcg/day in 15 patients with major depression with atypical features reported that 80% of patients treated with it, vs. none on placebo, responded (Davidson, Abraham, Connor, & McLeod, 2003).

### Antiglucocorticoids

Reduced feedback inhibition of cortisol production at the level of the corticotrophin releasing factor (CRF) receptor appears to be a primary cause of hypothalamic–pituitary–adrenal cortical (HPA) hyperactivity in mood disorders. Short-term use of antagonists of cortisol production or cortisol receptors has been found to improve refractory depression, but potential long-term adverse effects on the HPA axis are significant.

- In an open-label study, up to 800 mg/day of ketoconazole (antifungal drug that inhibits cortisol synthesis) was added to ongoing treatment in patients with refractory bipolar depression (Brown, Bobadilla, & Rush, 2001).
  - Cortisol levels did not decrease, but depression was reduced in the three patients who received at least 400 mg/day.
- An 8-week trial in 20 patients with treatment-resistant major depression, whose previous medications had been discontinued, gave patients one of three drugs that block cortisol synthesis: aminoglutethimide, metyrapone, and ketoconazole (Murphy, Ghadirian, & Dhar, 1998).
  - All three drugs produced improvement of depression in 11 of 17 atients who completed the study.
  - ACTH levels increased with treatment, but cortisol levels did not change predictably.
- A double-blind study of 20 patients with refractory depression (eight of them with elevated cortisol levels) assigned patients to placebo or 400–800 mg/day of ketoconazole for 4 weeks (Wolkowitz et al., 1999).
  - Ketoconazole but not placebo improved depression in patients with, but not those without, hypercortisolemia.
- However, a 6-week double-blind placebo-controlled study of 16 adults with refractory major depressive disorder found that
  - Only two of eight patients randomly assigned to ketoconazole and none on placebo met criteria for response over 6 weeks of treatment (Malison et al., 1999).
  - Cortisol levels were not measured in this study.
- 5 patients with psychotic major depression were given 600 mg mifepristone (RU-486) in a 4-day double-blind placebo-controlled crossover study (Belanoff, Flores, Kalezhan, Sund, & Schatzberg, 2001).
  - All patients had significant improvement in HRSD scale scores, vs. no improvement with placebo.
  - An extension of this study involved 30 patients with psychotic major depression given open-label mifepristone 50, 600, or 1200 mg for 7 days (Belanoff et al., 2002). Of 19 patients who got 600 or 1200 mg of mifepristone
    - 12 had a 50% reduction of positive symptoms vs. 3 of 11 at the lower dose
    - 13 had at least a 30% reduction of overall BPRS scores, vs. 2 of 11 taking 50 mg, which served as a control because at that dose,

it is a progesterone receptor antagonist but not a glucocorticoid GR-1 receptor antagonist.

## Estrogen

Estrogen has unreliable effects on mood. Some studies suggest that estrogen may enhance mood in postmenopausal women.

- Estrogen increases sensitivity of dopamine D2 receptor.
  - Premenopausal women respond to lower antipsychotic doses and have more neurological side effects than menopausal women.
- Pregnant women (N = 29) who had a history of mania, hypomania, or schizoaffective disorder and were currently in remission started taking transdermal estradiol within 48 hours of delivery (Kumar et al., 2003).
  - There was no reduction in affective relapse rates in the 90 days following childbirth.
  - Patients who relapsed who were taking the highest estradiol dose (800 µg/day) required lower psychotropic doses and had briefer hospitalizations.

Contradictory findings have emerged in studies of estrogen for dementia.

- The Women's Health Initiative Memory Study assigned 4,532 postmenopausal women without probable dementia to 0.625 mg estrogen + 2.5 mg of medroxyprogesterone (i.e., hormone replacement therapy or HRT) or placebo for an average of 4.2 years (Shumaker et al., 2003).
  - OR for probable dementia was 2.05 with HRT.
    - Most cases of dementia were due to Alzheimer's disease.
  - There was no difference between groups in the risk of mild cognitive impairment.
- In the same study, women who did not develop dementia were more likely to have a clinically important decrease in MMSE scores ($\geq$ SDs, or $\geq$ 8 units) than patients on placebo (6.7% vs. 4.8%, $p = 0.008$).
  - HRT did not improve cognition significantly more than placebo (Rapp et al., 2003).

Conventional doses of estrogen (1 mg/day of 17β-estradiol or 0.625 mg/day of conjugated equine estrogen) reduce bone loss and decrease the risk of fracture in older women.

- A randomized double-blind placebo-controlled trial of just 0.25 mg/day of 17β-estradiol in 167 healthy women aged > 65 years found decreased bone turnover and increased bone mineral density of 2.6% in femur, 3.6% in hip, 2.8% in spine, and 1.2% in total body with low-dose estradiol vs. placebo (Prestwood, Kenny, Kleppinger, & Kulldorff, 2003).

### Androgens and AntiAndrogens

Testosterone has become a popular replacement therapy for signs and symptoms of hypogonadism in males, which include:

- Decreased libido
- Erectile dysfunction
- Reduced muscle mass and bone density
- Depression
- Anemia

  Affects 2–4 million men.
- Low bioavailable testosterone levels reported in 40% of men ages 60–69, 70% ages 70–79.

A testosterone patch has been used to improve antidepressant response rates in refractory depression. Testosterone also can improve libido in menopausal women.

- 15 men (mean age 61) with nonrefractory major depression who did not respond to a placebo run-in were randomly assigned to 100 mg/week or 200 mg/week of IM testosterone cypionate for 6 weeks (Perry et al., 2002).
    - Decreases in HRSD scores (from 19.8 to 9.3) were most notable in patients with onset of depression ≥ age 45.
    - No early-onset patients responded, vs. 60% of later-onset patients.
    - Testosterone therefore may be more helpful in late-onset depression in males.

GnRH hormone agonists, which reduce testosterone synthesis, have been used to treat paraphilias.

- An uncontrolled open study of 12 men with paraphilias followed for 6 months–6 years found that leuprolide acetate significantly suppressed self-reports of deviant sexual interests and behavior (Krueger & Kaplan, 2001).
- The response to 8–42 monthly injections of 3.75 mg triporelin, another GnRH agonist, was assessed in 30 men with long-standing paraphilias (mostly pedophilia; Rosler & Witztum, 1998).
    - All men had dramatic decreases in the number of deviant sexual fantasies and desires.
    - Serum testosterone concentrations decreased significantly.
- In open studies and case reports of 118 men treated with the luteinizing hormone releasing hormone agonists leuprolide and triptorelin, manifestations of various paraphilias (sadism, pedophilia, exhibitionism, voyeurism) were reduced.

- No relapses over follow-up lasting as long as 7 years if patients stayed on medications (Briken, Hill, & Berner, 2003).

## SIDE EFFECTS

Because of diverse actions of different herbal and hormonal therapies, this section considers side effects of each class of agents.

### Androgens and Androgen Antagonists

#### CARDIOVASCULAR SIDE EFFECTS

- No data supporting increased risk of cardiovascular disease.
- High testosterone levels may decrease risk of severe atherosclerosis and thrombosis.
- Fluid retention
- Hypertension (rare)

#### CENTRAL NERVOUS SYSTEM SIDE EFFECTS

- Exacerbation or new development of sleep apnea
  - Central effect rather than action on airway
- Aggression
- Psychosis

#### DERMATOLOGICAL SIDE EFFECTS

- Erythema, pruritus
  - More common with patch than with gel.
- Acne
- Increased body hair
- Oily skin

#### ENDOCRINE AND SEXUAL SIDE EFFECTS

- Bone demineralization
- Minimal effects on lipids and glucose metabolism
- Breast tenderness, gynecomastia
- Hot flashes
- Infertility
- Impotence
- Hypogonadism

### GASTROINTESTINAL SIDE EFFECTS

- Hepatic toxicity and both benign and malignant neoplasms have been reported with oral but not IM or transdermal preparations.

### HEMATOLOGIC SIDE EFFECTS

- Higher testosterone levels stimulate erythropoiesis.
  - Injection (44% risk) > transdermal (3–18% risk)
  - Increased hemoglobin levels
  - Increased hematocrit
    - Increased blood viscosity could aggravate vascular disorders.

### UROLOGICAL SIDE EFFECTS

- Increased prostate volume, especially during first 6 months.
- No significant impact on voiding.
- Could make prostate cancer more aggressive, but prospective studies demonstrate no increase in the risk of prostate cancer in patients receiving testosterone replacement (Rhoden & Morgentaler, 2004).
- Because of unknown risk that occult prostate cancer may be activated, biopsy prostate if PSA increases by 1.5 ng/mL in 2 years or by 2.0 in any period.
- Testicular atrophy

## Ephedra

The risk of adverse reactions to ephedra is greater than from all herbal therapies combined.

### CARDIOVASCULAR SIDE EFFECTS

- Arrhythmias
- Hypertension
- Myocardial infarction
- Tachycardia

### CENTRAL NERVOUS SYSTEM SIDE EFFECTS

- Drug dependence
- Headache
- Insomnia
- Irritability
- Restlessness

- Agitation
- Psychosis
- Stroke
- Tachyphylaxis

GASTROINTESTINAL SIDE EFFECTS

- Nausea and vomiting

### Estrogen

Estrogen increases bone mineral density. Concerns have been raised about increased risks of breast cancer, clotting disorders, and cardiovascular disease.

- The Women's Health Initiative found that estrogen 0.625 mg/day plus medroxyprogesterone acetate 2.5 mg/day had excess risk/10,000 person-years of (Investigators, 2002)
  - 7 more coronary events
  - 8 more pulmonary embolisms
  - 8 more strokes
  - 8 more invasive breast cancers
  - 6 fewer colorectal cancers
  - 5 fewer hip fractures
- A case control study of 155 consecutive patients with a first episode of venous thromboembolism found that oral but not transdermal estrogen increased the risk of venous thromboembolism three times (Scarabin, Oger, & Plu-Bureau, 2003).

### Ginkgo Biloba

ALLERGIC SIDE EFFECTS

- Anaphylaxis and phlebitis have been reported with IV use.
- Stevens–Johnson syndrome

CENTRAL NERVOUS SYSTEM SIDE EFFECTS

- Headache
- A few cases have been reported of cerebral or extracerebral hemorrhage with oral ginkgo.
- Seizures
- Spontaneous intracerebral hemorrhage

DERMATOLOGICAL SIDE EFFECTS

- Skin rash

GASTROINTESTINAL SIDE EFFECTS

- Nausea, GI distress, diarrhea

HEMATOLOGIC SIDE EFFECTS

- Increased bleeding time with chronic use

### Kava Kava

CARDIOVASCULAR SIDE EFFECTS

- Occasional palpitations and supraventricular arrhythmias

CENTRAL NERVOUS SYSTEM SIDE EFFECTS

- Choreoathetosis
- Decreased reflexes
- Dyskinesia
- Morning tiredness
- Suicide when taken by depressed patients

DERMATOLOGICAL SIDE EFFECTS

- Ichthyosis
- Seborrhea
- Yellowing of skin

EYES, EARS, NOSE, AND THROAT SIDE EFFECTS

- Eye irritation
- Impaired accommodation
- Mydriasis

GASTROINTESTINAL SIDE EFFECTS

- Hepatotoxicity
  - Increased GGT
  - The Centers for Disease Control (CDC) have reported 10 cases of fulminant hepatic toxicity requiring liver transplantation caused by kava (Centers for Disease Control, 2002).
    - Liver disease began 8 weeks–1 year after starting kava.
    - All patients had hepatic necrosis.

- A case of fulminant hepatitis and liver failure requiring transplantation was reported in a 14-year-old girl (Campo et al., 2002)
- Weight loss

## St John's Wort

### CARDIOVASCULAR SIDE EFFECTS

- Cardiovascular collapse during anesthesia

### CENTRAL NERVOUS SYSTEM SIDE EFFECTS

- Confusion
- Dizziness
- Fatigue (5%)
- Headache
- Insomnia
- Mania
- Relapse of schizophrenia
- Restlessness (0.3%)

### DERMATOLOGICAL SIDE EFFECTS

- Exanthema
- Photosensitization (dose related)
- Pruritis
- Skin rash

### ENDOCRINE AND SEXUAL SIDE EFFECTS

- Infertility
- Mutagenesis of sperm
- Serotonin syndrome
- Sexual dysfunction

### GASTROINTESTINAL SIDE EFFECTS (0.6%)

- Anorexia
- Diarrhea
- Dry mouth
- GI distress

- Nausea
- Stomachache

RENAL SIDE EFFECTS

- Urinary frequency

## Valerian

CARDIOVASCULAR SIDE EFFECTS

- Arrhythmias

CENTRAL NERVOUS SYSTEM SIDE EFFECTS

- Headache
- Insomnia
- Psychomotor impairment (impaired driving)
- Restlessness

## Yohimbine

CARDIOVASCULAR SIDE EFFECTS

- Hypertension
- Tachycardia

CENTRAL NERVOUS SYSTEM SIDE EFFECTS

- Anxiety
- Exacerbation of PTSD
- Insomnia
- Panic attacks in patients with panic disorder or Parkinson's disease
- Tremor

DERMATOLOGICAL SIDE EFFECTS

- Exanthema

GASTROINTESTINAL SIDE EFFECTS

- Nausea, vomiting
- Salivation

Table 10.3 lists common herbal preparations that are associated with adverse effects.

**Table 10.3  Adverse Effects Reported with Common Herbal Preparations**

| CARDIOTOXICITY | HEPATOTOXICITY | GASTROINTESTINAL PROBLEMS | WEIGHT GAIN | NEUROTOXICITY | RENAL DAMAGE | DECREASED GLYCEMIC CONTROL | MANIA | ANXIETY | HYPERTENSION |
|---|---|---|---|---|---|---|---|---|---|
| Aconite root tuber | Anthranoids | SAMe | Omega-3 fatty acids | Aconite root | β-Aescin | Essential fatty acids | Omega-3 fatty acids | SAMe | Omega-3 fatty acids |
| Colchicine | Chaparral leaf or stem | Omega-3 fatty acids | | Ascaridole | Cape aloe | | Flaxseed oil | | |
| Leigongteng | Germander | | | Colchicines | Cat's claw | | Fish oil | | |
| Licorice root | Green tea leaf | | | Ginkgo seed or leaf | Chaparral leaf/stem | | SAMe | | |
| Ma-huang | Protoberberine alkaloids | | | Kava rhizome | Chinese yew | | | | |
| Pokeweed root or leaf | Impila root | | | Ma-huang | Impila root | | | | |
| Scotch broom | Kava kava | | | Nux vomica | Jerring fruit | | | | |
| Squirting cucumber | Kombucha Ma-huang Pennyroyal oil Skullcap Soy phytoestrogen | | | Pennyroyal oil Star fruit Yellow jessamine | Pennyroyal oil Star fruit | | | | |

Information compiled from de Smet (2002) and Lake (2002).

## DRUG–DRUG INTERACTIONS

**Table 10.4  Interactions of Herbal Remedies and Hormones Used in Psychiatry with Other Medications/Substances**

| HERBAL OR HORMONE | MEDICATION | COMMENTS |
| --- | --- | --- |
| Ephedra | CNS stimulants | Additive stimulant effect |
| | MAOIs | Hypertensive crisis |
| Estrogen | Carbamazepine, oxcarbazepine, topiramate | Decreased oral contraceptive efficacy resulting from reduced estrogen concentration by CYP450 2C/3A induction by anticonvulsant |
| | Antidepressants | Increased antidepressant action at low estrogen doses due to displacement from binding protein; decreased antidepressant effect at high estrogen doses due to enzyme induction |
| Ginkgo biloba | Acetylsalicylic acid (ASA), rofecoxib, warfarin | Ginkgo has been associated with bleeding, both alone and in combination with ASA, rofecoxib and warfarin, and with intracerebral hemorrhage when taken along with thrombolytic drugs |
| | Trazodone | Coma reported in one patient with Alzheimer's disease treated with ginkgo plus trazodone |
| Omega-3 fatty acids | Aspirin | Additive antiplatelet effect increases risk of bleeding |
| | Dong quai, evening primrose, feverfew, ginkgo biloba, ginseng, heparin, licorice, NSAIDs | Additive anticoagulant effect increases risk of bleeding |
| | Oral hypoglycemics, insulin, metformin, sulfonylureas | Decreased efficacy of hypoglycemic agent; hyperglycemia |
| SAMe | MAOIs | Serotonin syndrome Hypertensive crisis |
| | SSRIs | Additive serotonergic effects |
| St. John's wort | Amitriptyline | SJW decreases amitriptyline and nortriptyline AUC |
| | Cyclosporine | SJW induces 3A4 and lowers cyclosporine levels; may result in transplanted organ rejection |
| | Digoxin | Reduced levels due to 3A4 induction |
| | Midazolam | |
| | MAOIs | Serotonin syndrome |

*(continues)*

**Table 10.4  Continued**

| HERBAL OR HORMONE | MEDICATION | COMMENTS |
|---|---|---|
| | Nefazodone, SSRIs, buspirone | Serotonin syndrome |
| | Narcotics | Prolonged CNS depression |
| | Oral contraceptives | Breakthrough bleeding |
| | Indinavir (protease inhibitor) | HIV treatment failure due to induction of 3A4 and 57% decrease in AUC |
| | Theophylline | Decreased levels |
| | Warfarin | Reduced anticoagulant effect |
| Asian ginseng | Phenelzine | Mania with ginseng alone and in combination with phenelzine |
| Kava kava | Alprazolam | Delirium and coma |
| | Alcohol, CNS depressants | Additive CNS depression |
| | Dopamine (e.g., L-dopa) | Interference with action of dopamine |
| Valerian | Benzodiazepines | Additive CNS depression |
| Yohimbine | Antihypertensives | Antagonism of antihypertensive action |
| | Ephedrine | Increased risk of hypertension |
| | Morphine | Enhanced analgesic effect |
| | Naltrexone | Potentiation of effects of yohimbine; increased anxiety |
| | TCAs | Increased autonomic and central effects (anxiety) of yohimbine |

Information compiled from de Smet, 2002.

## PREGNANCY AND LACTATION

Herbal preparations are not benign. Some preparations, in particular, should be avoided during pregnancy and lactation (see Table 10.5).

## TOXICITY AND OVERDOSE

Many herbal preparations are not dangerous, but some can cause severe toxicity in overdose.

### Kava Kava

Overdose can cause
- Abnormal movements

**Table 10.5 Herbs to Avoid During Pregnancy and Lactation**

| PREGNANCY (UTERINE CONTRACTION) | LACTATION (STIMULANT, LAXATIVE, TOXIC) |
|---|---|
| Black cohosh | Aloe supplement |
| Chamomile, roman | Black cohosh |
| Chaste tree berry | Cascara sagrada |
| Dong quai | Cocoa |
| Feverfew | Kava kava |
| Fresh horseradish | Ma-huang |
| Kava kava | Sage |
| Licorice | Senna |
| Pennyroyal | Wintergreen |
| Sage | |
| Senna | |
| St. John's wort | |
| Stinging nettle | |
| Aloe supplement | |
| > 1 gm fresh ginger root | |

- Fatigue
- Excessive sleep

Treatment is supportive.

### Ma-Huang

Lethal doses are 100 gm of ma-huang or 1–2 gm of L-ephedrine. Less severe overdoses produce

- Sweating
- Mydriasis
- Fever
- Muscle spasm
- Heart failure
- Asphyxiation
- Mania
- Stroke

Treatment of overdose involves

- Gastric lavage with potassium permanganate
- Activated charcoal
- Treat muscle spasm with diazepam.
- Administer sodium bicarbonate prophylactically to prevent acidosis.
- Intubation and ventilation may be necessary.

### Yohimbine

Overdose of yohimbine can cause

- Excessive salivation
- Mydriasis
- Hypotension
- Acidosis
- Arrhythmias
- Heart failure
- Shock
- Death

Treatment includes:

- Induction of vomiting
- Gastric lavage with potassium permanganate and sodium sulfate
- Activated charcoal
- Treat cardiac arrhythmias with lidocaine or physostigmine.
- Administer sodium bicarbonate for academia.
- Use volume expanders for shock.

## PRECAUTIONS

Biologically active herbs and hormonal treatments have the potential to produce significant toxicity and interactions.

- Patients should be made aware of the risk of hepatotoxicity with kava kava.
- Depressed people should not take kava kava because of the increased risk of suicide.
- Ma-huang and valerian should not be used during pregnancy or nursing.
- Anxious patients should not take yohimbine.
- The same precautions that apply to antidepressants should be observed with St. John's wort.
- In most cases, women with a past history of breast cancer should not take estrogen.

## ADVICE FOR CARETAKERS

Many people believe that because herbal therapies are "natural," they must be safe. However, many herbal treatments are produced in a factory, and many medications are derived from plants and metabolized by the same enzymes that eliminate plant products. In addition, "natural" elements such as arsenic, lead, ultraviolet radiation, and jimson weed are not necessarily safe.

- Patients should be informed about the potential risks of herbal therapies.
- Patients may not be inclined to report herbal treatments they are using because they do not consider them to be medicines or because they think that the physician will disapprove.

## NOTES FOR PATIENT AND FAMILY

Because the FDA does not regulate herbal and hormonal therapies, availability of active components can vary significantly from brand to brand and from batch to batch. The risk of interactions with psychiatric and other medications makes it important to tell the physician about any herbal therapies that are being taken and to incorporate them into the overall treatment plan.

- Be sure to tell health care providers about any herbal therapies being used.

# REFERENCES

Abrams RC (2002): Stimulus titration and ECT dosing. *Journal of ECT,* 18:3–9.

Adams CE, Eisenbruch M (2002): Depot fluphenazine for schizophrenia. *Cochrane Database of Systematic Reviews;* 2.

Afflelou S, Auriacombe M, Cazenave M, Chartres JP, Tignol J (1997): High dose levothyroxine for treatment of rapid cycling bipolar disorder: Review of the literature and application to 6 subjects. *Encephale,* 23:209–217.

Akhondzadeh S, Tavakolian R, Davari-Ashtiani R, Arabgol F, Amini H (2003): Selegiline in the treatment of attention deficit hyperactivity disorder in children: A double-blind and randomized trial. *Prog Neuro-Psychopharmacol & Biol Psychiatry,* 27:841–845.

Aldenkamp AP, Arends J, Bootsma HPR, et al (2002): Randomized double-blind parallel-group study comparing cognitive effects of a low dose lamotrigine with valproate and placebo in healthy volunteers. *Epilepsia,* 43:19–26.

Alderman CP, Seshadri P, Ben-Tovim DI (1996): Effects of serotonin reuptake inhibitors on hemostasis. *Ann Pharmacother,* 30:1232–1234.

Allison DB, Mentore JL, Heo M (1999): Antipsychotic-induced weight gain: A comprehensive research synthesis. *Am J Psychiatry,* 156:1686–1696.

Altshuler I, Suppes T, Black DW, et al (2003): Impact of antidepressant discontinuation after acute bipolar depression remission on rates of depressive relapse at 1-year follow-up. *Am J Psychiatry,* 160:1252–1262.

Altshuler LL, Post RM, Leverich GS, et al (1995): Antidepressant-induced mania and cycle acceleration: A controversy revisited. *Am J Psychiatry,* 152:1130–1138.

Amsterdam JD (2003): A double-blind, placebo-controlled trial of the safety and efficacy of selegiline transdermal system without dietary restrictions in patients with major depressive disorder. *J Clin Psychiatry,* 64:208–214.

Ananth J, Venkatesh R, Burgoyne K, Gunatilake S (2002): Atypical antipsychotic drug use and diabetes. *Psychotherapy and Psychosomatics,* 71:244–254.

Anderson GD, Yau MK, Gidal BE, et al (1996): Bidirectional interaction of valproate and lamotrigine in healthy subjects. *Clin Pharmacol Ther,* 60:145–156.

Andrade C, Kurinji S (2002): Continuation and maintenance ECT: A review of recent research. *Journal of ECT,* 18:149–158.

Andreoli V, Caillard V, Deo RS, Rybakowski JK, Versiani M (2002): Reboxetine, a new noradrenaline selective antidepressant, is at least as effective as fluoxetine in the treatment of depression. *J Clin Psychopharmacol,* 22:393–399.

Angst J, Hochstrasser B (1994): Recurrent brief depression: The Zurich Study. *J Clin Psychiatry,* 55(Suppl 4):3–9.

Anonymous (2002): A randomized, double-blind, placebo-controlled multicenter trial comparing the effects of three doses of orally administered sodium oxybate with placebo for the treatment of narcolepsy. *Sleep,* 25:42–49.

Anonymous (2003): A 12-month, open-label, multicenter extension trial of orally administered sodium oxybate for the treatment of narcolepsy. *Sleep,* 26:31–35.

Anton R, Swift RM (2003): Current pharmacotherapies of alcoholism: A U.S. perspective. *Am J Addictions,* 12(Suppl 1):S53–S68.

Appolinario JC, Bacaltchuk J, Sichieri R, et al (2003): A randomized, double-blind, placebo-controlled study of sibutramine in the treatment of binge-eating disorder. *Arch Gen Psychiatry,* 60:1109–1116.

Arango C, Summerfelt A, Buchanan RW (2003): Olanzapine effects on auditory sensory gating in schizophrenia. *Am J Psychiatry,* 160:2066–2068.

Areosa SA, Sheriff F (2003): Memantine for dementia. *Cochrane Database of Systematic Reviews;* 2.

Aronson TA, Shukla S, Gujavarty K, Hoff A, DiBuono M, Khan E (1988): Relapse in delusional depression: A retrospective study of the course of treatment. *Compr Psychiatry,* 29:12–21.

Bacaltchuk J, Hay P (2002): Antidepressants versus placebo for people with bulimia nervosa. *Cochrane Database of Systematic Reviews,* 4.

Baetz M, Bowen RC (1998): Efficacy of divalproex sodium in patients with panic disorder and mood instability who have not responded to conventional therapy. *Can J Psychiatry,* 43:73–77.

Baker R, Milton D, Stauffer VL, Gelenberg AJ, Tohen M (2003): Placebo-controlled trials do not find association of olanzapine with exacerbation of bipolar mania. *J Affect Disord,* 73:147–153.

Baldassano CF, Ballas C, Datto SM, et al (2003): Ziprasidone-associated mania: A case series and review of the mechanism. *Bipolar Disorders,* 5:72–75.

Baldessarini RJ, Tondo L, Faedda GL, et al (1996): Effects of the rate of discontinuing lithium maintenance treatment in bipolar disorders. *J Clin Psychiatry,* 57: 441–448.

Baldessarini RJ, Tondo L, Hennen J (2001): Treating the suicidal patient with bipolar disorder: Reducing suicide risk with lithium. *Ann N Y Acad Sci,* 932:24–38.

Ballantyne JC, Mao J (2003): Opioid therapy for chronic pain. *N Engl J Med,* 349:1943–1952.

Ballard C, O'Brien J, Reichelt K, Perry E (2002): Aromatherapy as a safe and effective treatment for the management of agitation in severe dementia: The results of a double-blind, placebo-controlled trial with *Melissa. J Clin Psychiatry,* 63:553–558.

Barbee JG, Jamhour NJ (2002): Lamotrigine as an augmentation agent in treatment-resistant depression. *J Clin Psychiatry,* 63:737–741.

Barbui C, Hotopf M, Freemantle N, et al (2003): Treatment discontinuation with selective serotonin reuptake inhibitors (SSRIs) versus tricyclic antidepressants (TCAs). *Cochrane Database of Systematic Reviews,* 1.

Barnett S, Kramer ML, Casat CD, Connor KM, Davidson J (2002): Efficacy of olanzapine in social anxiety disorder: A pilot study. *Journal of Psychopharmacology,* 16:365–368.

Basan A, Leucht S (2004): Valproate for schizophrenia. *Cochrane Database of Systematic Reviews,* 1.

Bauer J, Jarre A, Klingmuller D, Elger CE (2000): Polycystic ovary syndrome in patients with focal epilepsy: A study in 93 women. *Epilepsy Res,* 41:163–167.

Bauer MS, Whybrow PC (1990): Rapid cycling bipolar affective disorder. II. Treatment of refractory rapid cycling with high-dose levothyroxine: A preliminary study. *Arch Gen Psychiatry,* 47:435–440.

Bauer MS, Whybrow PC, Winokur A (1990): Rapid cycling bipolar affective disorder, I: Association with grade I hypothyroidism. *Arch Gen Psychiatry,* 47:427–432.

Belanoff J, Flores BH, Kalezhan M, Sund B, Schatzberg AF (2001): Rapid reversal of psychotic depression using mifepristone. *J Clin Psychopharmacol,* 21:516–521.

Belanoff J, Rothschild AJ, Cassidy F, et al (2002): An open label trial of C-1073 (mifepristone) for psychotic major depression. *Biol Psychiatry,* 52:386–389.

Berlant J, van Kammen DP (2002): Open-label topiramate as primary or adjunctive therapy in chronic civilian posttraumatic stress disorder: A preliminary report. *J Clin Psychiatry,* 63:15–20.

Beswick T, Best D, Bearn J, Gossop M, Rees S, Strang J (2003): The effectiveness of combined naloxone/lofexidine in opiate detoxification: Results from a double-blind randomized and placebo-controlled trial. *Am J Addictions,* 12:295–305.

Birks JS, Grimley Evans J, Van Dongen M (2002): Ginkgo biloba for cognitive impairment and dementia. *Cochrane Database of Systematic Reviews,* 4.

Birks JS, Melzer D, Beppu H (2002): Donepezil for mild and moderate Alzheimer's disease. *Cochrane Database of Systematic Reviews;* 2.

Bodkin JA, Amsterdam JD (2002): Transdermal selegiline in major depression: A double-blind, placebo-controlled, parallel-group study in outpatients. *Am J Psychiatry,* 159:1869–1875.

Bonnet U (2003): Moclobemide: Therapeutic use and clinical studies. *CNS Drug Reviews,* 9:97–140.

Bowden CL, Brugger AM, Swann AC (1994): Efficacy of divalproex vs lithium in the treatment of mania. *JAMA,* 271:918–924.

Bowden CL, Calabrese JR, McElroy SL, et al (2000): A randomized, placebo-controlled 12-month trial of divalproex and lithium in treatment of outpatients with bipolar I disorder: Divalproex Maintenance Study Group. *Arch Gen Psychiatry,* 57:481–489.

Bowden CL, Calabrese JR, Sachs G, et al (2003): A placebo-controlled 18-month trial of lamotrigine and lithium maintenance treatment in recently manic or hypomanic patients with bipolar I disorder. *Arch Gen Psychiatry,* 60:392–400.

Brady KT, Sonne SC, Anton R, Ballenger JC (1995): Valproate in the treatment of acute bipolar affective episodes complicated by substance abuse: A pilot study. *J Clin Psychiatry,* 56:118–121.

Brenner S, Wolf R, Landau M, Politi Y (1994): Psoriasiform eruption induced by anticonvulsants. *Isr J Med Sci,* 30:283–286.

Briken P, Hill A, Berner W (2003): Pharmacotherapy of paraphilias with long-acting agonists of luteinizing hormone-releasing hormone: A systematic review. *J Clin Psychiatry,* 64:890–897.

Brodaty H, Ames D, Snowdon J, et al (2003): A randomized placebo-controlled trial of risperidone for the treatment of aggression, agitation, and psychosis of dementia. *J Clin Psychiatry,* 64:134–143.

Broerse A, Crawford TJ, den Boer JA (2002): Differential effects of olanzapine and risperidone on cognition in schizophrenia? A saccadic eye movement study. *J Neuropsychiatry Clin Neurosci,* 14:454–460.

Brook S, Lucey JV, Gunn KP (2000): Intramuscular ziprasidone compared with intramuscular haloperidol in the treatment of acute psychosis. *J Clin Psychiatry,* 61:933–941.

Brown ES, Bobadilla L, Rush AJ (2001): Ketoconazole in bipolar patients with depressive symptoms: A case series and literature review. *Bipolar Disorders,* 3:23–29.

Buckley NA, McManus PR (2002): Fatal toxicity of serotoninergic and other antidepressant drugs: Analysis of United Kingdom mortality data. *BMJ,* 325:1332–1333.

Buckley PF (2001): Broad therapeutic uses of atypical antipsychotic medications. *Biol Psychiatry,* 50:912–924.

Burgess S, Geddes J, Hawton K, Townsend E, Jamison KR, Goodwin G (2002): Lithium for maintenance treatment of mood disorders. *Cochrane Database of Systematic Reviews;* 2.

Burke WJ, Gergel I, Bose A (2002): Fixed-dose trial of the single isomer SSRI escitalopram in depressed outpatients. *J Clin Psychiatry,* 63:331–336.

Byerly WG, Hartmann A, Foster DE, Tannenbaum AK (1991): Verapamil in the treatment of maternal paroxysmal supraventricular tachycardia. *Ann Emerg Med,* 20: 552–554.

Calabrese JR, Keck PE, McElroy SL, Shelton MD (2001): A pilot study of topiramate as monotherapy in the treatment of acute mania. *J Clin Psychopharmacol,* 21:340–342.

Calabrese JR, Sullivan JR, Bowden C, et al (2002): Rash in multicenter trials of lamotrigine in mood disorders: Clinical relevance and management. *J Clin Psychiatry,* 63:1012–1019.

Calabrese JR, Suppes T, Bowden CL, et al (2000): A double-blind, placebo-controlled, prophylaxis study of lamotrigine in rapid-cycling bipolar disorder: Lamictal 614 Study Group. *J Clin Psychiatry,* 61:841–850.

Callaghan N, Majeed T, O'Connell A, Oliveira DBG (1994): A comparative study of serum F protein and other liver function tests as an index of hepatocellular damage in epileptic patients. *Acta Neurol Scand,* 89:237–241.

Campo JV, McNabb J, Perel JM, Mazariegos GV, Hasegawa SL, Reyes J (2002): Kava-induced fulminant hepatic failure (letter to ed). *J Am Acad Child Adolesc Psychiatry,* 41:631–632.

Canter PH, Ernst E (2002): Ginkgo biloba: A smart drug? *Psychopharmacol Bull,* 36:108–123.

Capuron L, Hauser P, Hinze-Selch D, Miller AH, Neveu PJ (2002): Treatment of cytokine-induced depression. *Brain, Behavior and Immunity,* 16:575–580.

Caro J, Ward A, Levinton C, Robinson K (2002): The risk of diabetes during olanzapine use compared with risperidone use: A retrospective database analysis. *J Clin Psychiatry,* 63:1135–1139.

Carpenter LL, Friehs GM, Price LH (2003): Cervical vagus nerve stimulation for treatment-resistant depression. *Neurosurgery Clin North Am,* 14:275–282.

Carpenter LL, Yasmin S, Price LH (2002): A double-blind, placebo-controlled study of antidepressant augmentation with mirtazepine. *Biol Psychiatry,* 51:183–188.

Carvajal GP, Garcia D, Sanchez SA, Velasco MA, Rueda D, Lucena MI (2002): Hepatotoxicity associated with the new antidepressants. *J Clin Psychiatry,* 63:135–137.

Casper RC, Fleisher BE, Lee-Ancajas JC, Gaylor E, De Battista A, Hoyme HE (2003): Follow-up of children of depressed mothers exposed or not exposed to antidepressant drugs during pregnancy. *J Pediatr,* 142:402–408.

Cavallaro R, Brambilla P, Smeraldi E (1998): The sequential treatment approach to resistant schizophrenia with risperidone and clozapine: Results of an open study with follow-up. *Human Psychopharmacol,* 13:91–97.

Cavallaro R, Regazetti MG, Covelli G, Smeraldi E (1993). Tolerance and withdrawl with zolpidem. *Lancet,* 342:374–375.

Centers for Disease Control (2002): Hepatic toxicity possibly associated with kava-containing products—United States, Germany, and Switzerland, 1999–2002. *Morb Mortal Wkly Rep,* 51:1065–1067.

Cesarini A, Meloni F, Alpini D (1998): Ginkgo biloba (EGb 761) in the treatment of equilibrium disorders. *Adv Ther,* 15:291–304.

Chambers CD, Johnson KA, Dick LM, Felix RJ, Jones KL (1996): Birth outcomes in pregnant women taking fluoxetine. *N Engl J Med,* 335:1010–1015.

Chen B, Wang JF, Sun X, Young LT (2003): Regulation of GAP-43 expression by chronic desipramine treatment in rat-cultured hippocampal cells. *Biol Psychiatry,* 53:530–537.

Chen J, Chen Y, Wang X (2002): Clinical study on treatment of children with attention deficit hyperactivity disorder by jiangqian granule. *Chinese Journal of Integrated Traditional and Western Medicine,* 22:258–260.

Chengappa KN, Parepally H, Brar JS, Goldstein JM (2003): A random-assignment, double-blind, clinical trial of once-versus-twice-daily quetiapine fumarate in patients with schizophrenia or schioaffective disorder. *Can J Psychiatry,* 48:187–194.

Chiaie RD, Pancheri P, Scapicchio P (2002): Efficacy and tolerability of oral and intramuscular S-adenosyl-L-methionine 1,4-butanedisulfonate (SAMe) in the treatment of major depression: Comparison with imipramine in 2 multicenter studies. *Am J Clin Nutr,* 76(Suppl):1172S–1176S.

Chouinard G, Young SN, Annable L (1983): Antimanic effect of clonazepam. *Biol Psychiatry,* 18:451–466.

Clark N, Lintzeris N, Gijsbers A, et al (2002): LAAM maintenance vs methadone maintenance for heroin dependence. *Cochrane Database of Systematic Reviews;* 2.

Clark RD, Canive JM, Calais LA (1999): Divalproex in posttraumatic stress disorder: An open-label clinical trial. *Journal of Traumatic Stress,* 12:395–401.

Clayton AH, Pradko JF, Croft HA, et al (2002): Prevalence of sexual dysfunction among newer antidepressants. *J Clin Psychiatry,* 63:357–366.

Club AJ (1997): Fluoxetine worked as well as imipramine or desipramine for depression in primary care. *ACP Journal Club,* 126:16.

Club AJ (2000): Review: Newer and older antidepressants have similar efficacy and total discontinuation rates but different side effects. *ACP Journal Club,* 133:10.

Conley RR, Kelly DL (2001): Management of treatment resistance in schizophrenia. *Biol Psychiatry,* 50:898–911.

Corrigan MH, Denahan AQ, Wright CE, Ragual RJ, Evans DL (2000): Comparison of pramipexole, fluoxetine, and placebo in patients with major depression. *Depress Anxiety,* 11:58–65.

Corya SA, Andersen SW, Detke HC, et al (2003): Long-term antidepressant efficacy and safety of olanzapine/fluoxetine combination: A 76-week open-label study. *J Clin Psychiatry,* 64:1349–1356.

Da Costa CL, Younes RN, Lourenco MTC (2000): Stopping smoking: A prospective, randomized, double-blind study comparing nortriptyline to placebo. *Chest,* 122: 403–408.

Dalton SO, Johansen C, Mellemkjoer L, Norgard B, Sorensen HT, Olsen JH (2003): Use of selective serotonin reuptake inhibitors and risk of upper gastrointestinal tract bleeding: A population-based cohort study. *Arch Intern Med,* 163:59–64.

Dannon P, Dolberg O, Schreiber S (2002): Three and six-month outcome following courses of either ECT or rTMS in a population of severely depressed individuals: Preliminary report. *Biol Psychiatry,* 51:687–690.

Davidson JRT, Abraham K, Connor KM, McLeod MN (2003): Effectiveness of chromium in atypical depression: A placebo-controlled trial. *Biol Psychiatry,* 53:261–264.

Davis JM, Chen N, Glick ID (2003): A meta-analysis of the efficacy of second-generation antipsychotics. *Arch Gen Psychiatry* 60:553–564.

de Haan L, van Bruggen M, Lavalaye J, Booij J, Dingemans P, Linszen D (2003): Subjective experience and D2 receptor occupancy in patients with recent-onset schizophrenia treated with low-dose olanzapine or haloperidol: A randomized, double-blind study. *Am J Psychiatry,* 160:303–309.

DelBello MP, Schwiers ML, Rosenberg HL, Strakowski SM (2002): A double-blind, randomized, placebo-controlled study of quetiapine as adjunctive treatment for adolescent mania. *J Am Acad Child Adolesc Psychiatry,* 41:1216–1223.

Deshmukh R, Franco K (2003): Managing weight gain as a side effect of antidepressant therapy. *Cleveland Clinic J Med,* 70:614–623.

de Smet, PAGM (2002): Herbal remedies. *N Engl J Med,* 347:2046–2056.

Detke M, Lu Y, Goldstein DJ, Hayes JR, Demitrack MA (2002): Duloxetine, 60 mg once daily, for major depressive disorder: A randomized double-blind placebo-controlled trial. *J Clin Psychiatry,* 63:308–315.

Dirksen SJ, D'Imperio JM, Birdsall D, Hatch SJ (2002): A postmarketing clinical experience study of Metadate CD. *Current Medical Research & Opinion,* 18:371–380.

Dubovsky SL (1986): Using electroconvulsive therapy for patients with neurological disease. *Hosp Commun Psychiatry,* 37:819–825.

Dubovsky SL, Buzan RD (1997): Novel alternatives and supplements to lithium and anticonvulsants for bipolar affective disorder. *J Clin Psychiatry,* 58:224–242.

Dubovsky SL, Lee C, Christiano J (1991): Lithium decreases platelet intracellular calcium ion concentrations in bipolar patients. *Lithium,* 2:167–174.

Dubovsky SL, Thomas M (1992): Psychotic depression: Advances in conceptualization and treatment. *Hosp Commun Psychiatry,* 43:1189–1198.

Einarson A, Bonari L, Voyer-Lavigne S, Addis A, Johnson Y, Koren G (2003): A multicentre prospective controlled study to determine the safety of nefazodone use during pregnancy. *Can J Psychiatry,* 48:106–110.

Epperson N, Czarkowski KA, Ward-O'Brian D, et al (2001): Maternal sertraline treatment and serotonin transport in breast-feeding mother–infant pairs. *Am J Psychiatry,* 158:1631–1637.

Faraone SV, Wilens T (2003): Does stimulant treatment lead to substance use disorders? *J Clin Psychiatry*, 64(Suppl 11):9–13.

Fava M (2000): Weight gain and antidepressants. *J Clin Psychiatry*, 61(Suppl 11):37–41.

Felker BL, Sloan KL, Dominitz JA, Barnes RF (2003): The safety of valproic acid use for patients with hepatitis C infection. *Am J Psychiatry*, 160:174–178.

Fenton WS, Dickerson F, Boronow J (2001): A placebo-controlled trial of omega-3 fatty acid (ethyl eicosapentaenoic acid) supplementation for residual symptoms and cognitive impairment in schizophrenia. *Am J Psychiatry*, 158:2071–2073.

Fernandes PP, Petty F (2003): Modafinil for remitted bipolar depression with hypersomnia. *Ann Pharmacother*, 37:1807–1809.

Fischer M, Barkley RA (2003): Childhood stimulant treatment and risk for later substance abuse. *J Clin Psychiatry*, 64(Suppl 11):19–23.

Freedman R (2003): Schizophrenia. *N Engl J Med*, 349:1738–1749.

Friedman JL, Adler DN, Howanitz E, et al (2002): A double blind placebo controlled trial of donepezil adjunctive treatment to risperidone for the cognitive impairment of schizophrenia. *Biol Psychiatry*, 51:349–357.

Fry JM (1998): Treatment modalities for narcolepsy. *Neurology*, 50:S43–S48.

Frye MA, Ketter TA, Kimbrell TA, et al (2000): A placebo-controlled study of lamotrigine and gabapentin monotherapy in refractory mood disorders. *J Clin Psychopharmacol*, 20:607–614.

Fudala PJ, Bridge TP, Herbert S, et al (2003): Office-based treatment of opiate addiction with a sublingual-tablet formulation of buprenorphine and naloxone. *N Engl J Med*, 349:949–958.

Fuller MA, Shermock KM, Secic M, Grogg AL (2003): Comparative study of the development of diabetes mellitus in patients taking risperidone and olanzapine. *Pharmacotherapy*, 23:1037–1043.

Furukawa TA, Streiner D, Young LT (2002): Antidepressant and benzodiazepine for major depression. *Cochrane Database of Systematic Reviews*, 4.

Gadde KM, Franciscy DM, Wagner HR, Krishnan KRR (2003): Zonisamide for weight loss in obese adults. *JAMA*, 289:1820–1825.

Gagliardi JP, Krishnan KRR (2003): Evidence-based mental health use of anticonvulsants during pregnancy. *Psychopharmacol Bull*, 37:59–66.

Gelenberg AJ, Kane JM, Keller MB, et al (1989): Comparison of standard and low serum levels of lithium for maintenance treatment of bipolar disorder. *N Engl J Med*, 321:1489–1493.

Gershon AA, Dannon P, Grunhaus L (2003): Transcranial magnetic stimulation in the treatment of depression. *Am J Psychiatry*, 160:835–845.

Gesch CB, Hammon SM, Hamson SE (2002): Influence of supplementary vitamins, minerals and essential fatty acids on the antisocial behavior of young adult prisoners. *Br J Psychiatry*, 181:22–28.

Ghaemi SN, Ko JY, Katzow JJ (2002): Oxcarbazepine treatment of refractory bipolar disorder: A retrospective chart review. *Bipolar Disorders*, 4:70–74.

Ghaemi SN, Rosenquist KJ, Ko JK, Baldassano CF, Kontos NJ, Baldessarini RJ (2004): Antidepressant treatment in bipolar versus unipolar depression. *Am J Psychiatry*, 161:163–165.

Gianfrancesco FD, Grogg AL, Mahmoud RA, Wang R, Nasrallah HA (2002): Differential effects of risperidone, olanzapine, clozapine, and conventional antipsychotics on type 2 diabetes: Findings from a large health plan database. *J Clin Psychiatry,* 63:920–930.

Gill D, Hatcher S (2002): Antidepressants for depression in medical illness. *Cochrane Database of Systematic Reviews;* 2.

Gilmor ML, Owens MJ, Nemeroff CB (2002): Inhibition of norepinephrine uptake in patients with major depression treated with paroxetine. *Am J Psychiatry,* 159: 1702–1710.

Gitlin MJ, Suri R, Altshuler L, Zuckerbrow-Miller J, Fairbanks L (2002): Bupropion sustained release as a treatment for SSRI-induced sexual side effects. *J Sex Marital Ther,* 28:131–138.

Glassman A, Bigger JT (2001): Antipsychotic drugs: Prolonged QTc interval, torsades de pointes, and sudden death. *Am J Psychiatry,* 158:1774–1782.

Goodwin FK, Fireman B, Simons GE, Hunkeler EM, Lee J, Revicki D (2003): Suicide risk in bipolar disorder during treatment with lithium and divalproex. *JAMA,* 290: 1467–1473.

Gothelf D, Falk B, Singer P, et al (2002): Weight gain associated with increased food intake and low habitual activity levels in male adolescent schizophrenic inpatients treated with olanzapine. *Am J Psychiatry,* 159:1055–1057.

Gowing L, Ali R, White J (2002a): Buprenorphine for the management of opioid withdrawal. *Cochrane Database of Systematic Reviews,* 4.

Gowing L, Ali R, White J (2002b): Opioid antagonists under heavy sedation or anaesthesia for opioid withdrawal. *Cochrane Database of Systematic Reviews,* 2.

Grant JE, Kim SW (2002): An open-label study of naltrexone in the treatment of kelptomania. *J Clin Psychiatry,* 63:349–356.

Graudins A, Dowsett RP, Liddle C (2002): The toxicity of antidepressant poisoning: Is it changing? A comparative study of cyclic and newer serotonin-specific antidepressants. *Emergency Medicine,* 14:440–446.

Greenhill LL, Beyer DH, Finkleson J, et al (2002): Guidelines and algorithms for the use of methylphenidate in children with attention-deficit/hyperactivity disorder. *Journal of Attention Disorders,* 6(Suppl 1):S89–S100.

Greenhill LL, Pliszka S, Dulcan MK, AACAP (2002): Practice parameter for the use of stimulant medications in the treatment of children, adolescents, and adults. *J Am Acad Child Adolesc Psychiatry,* 41:26S–49S.

Greenwald MK, Schuh KJ, Hopper JA, Schuster CR, Johanson CE (2002): Effects of buprenorphine sublingual tablet maintenance on opioid drug-seeking behavior by humans. *Psychopharmacol,* 160:344–352.

Group HDTS (2002): Effect of *Hypericum perforatum* (St John's wort) in major depressive disorder. *JAMA,* 287:1807–1814.

Grunhaus L, Dolberg O, Polak D, Dannon P (2002): The antidepressant effects of transcranial magnetic stimulation: Comparison with electroconvulsive therapy. *Biol Psychiatry,* 51:123S–124S.

Grunze H, Langosch J, Born C, Schaub G, Walden J (2003): Levetiracetam in the treatment of acute mania: An open add-on study with an on–off–on design. *J Clin Psychiatry,* 64:781–784.

Grunze H, Normann C, Langosch J, et al (2001): Antimanic efficacy of topiramate in 11 patients in an open trial with an on–off–on design. *J Clin Psychiatry,* 62: 464–468.

Hallam KT, Olver JS, McGrath C, Norman TR (2003): Comparative cognitive and psychomotor effects of single doses of *Valeriana officinalis* and triazolam in healthy volunteers. *Human Psychopharmacol,* 18:619–625.

Hamner M, Faldowski R, Ulmer HG, Frueh BC, Huber MG, Arana GW (2003): Adjunctive risperidone treatment in posttraumatic stress disorder: A preliminary controlled trial of effects on comorbid psychotic symptoms. *Int Clin Psychopharmacol,* 18:1–8.

Hartong E, Moleman P, Hoogduin C, Broekman TG, Nolen W (2003): Prophylactic efficacy of lithium versus carbamazepine in treatment-naive bipolar patients. *J Clin Psychiatry,* 64:144–151.

Harvey BH, McEwen BS, Stein DJ (2003): Neurobiology of antidepressant withdrawal: Implications for the longitudinal outcome of depression. *Biol Psychiatry,* 54:1105–1117.

Hazell PL, Stuart JE (2003): A randomized controlled trial of clonidine added to psychostimulant medication for hyperactive and aggressive children. *J Am Acad Child Adolesc Psychiatry,* 42:886–894.

Heikkinen T, Ekblad U, Kero P, Ekblad S, Laine K (2002): Citalopram in pregnancy and lactation. *Clin Pharmacol Ther,* 72:184–191.

Heikkinen T, Ekblad U, Palo P, Laine K (2003): Prospective study of infant, maternal and breast milk levels in 11 women taking 20–40 mg fluoxetine. *Clin Pharmacol Ther,* 73:330–337.

Henderson DC, Cagliero E, Gray C, et al (2000): Clozapine, diabetes mellitus, weight gain, and lipid abnormalities: A five-year naturalistic study. *Am J Psychiatry,* 157:975–981.

Hendrick V, Smith LM, Suri R, Hwang S, Haynes D, Altshuler L (2003): Birth outcomes after prenatal exposure to antidepressant medication. *Am J Obstet Gynecol,* 188:812–815.

Hennessy S, Bilker WB, Knauss JS, et al (2002): Cardiac arrest and ventricular arrhythmia in patients taking antipsychotic drugs: Cohort study using administrative data. *BMJ,* 325:107–110.

Herxheimer A, Petrie K (2002): Melatonin for the prevention and treatment of jet lag. *Cochrane Database of Systematic Reviews;* 2.

Hirschfeld R (1999): Efficacy of SSRIs and newer antidepressants in severe depression: Comparison with TCAs. *J Clin Psychiatry,* 60:326–335.

Hoffman RE, Hawkins KA, Gueorguieva R, et al (2003): Transcranial magnetic stimulation of left temporoparietal cortex and medication-resistant auditory hallucinations. *Arch Gen Psychiatry,* 60:49–56.

Hollander E, Friedberg J, Wasserman S, Allen AJ, Birnbaum M, Koran LM (2003): Venlafaxine in treatment-resistant obsessive–compulsive disorder. *J Clin Psychiatry,* 64:546–550.

Hollister AS, Kearns GL (2003): American Society for Clinical Pharmacology and Therapeutics position statement on the public health risks of ephedra. *Clin Pharmacol Ther,* 74:403–405.

Hoopes SP, Reimherr FW, Hedges DW, et al (2003): Treatment of bulimia nervosa with topiramate in a randomzied, double-blind, placebo-controlled trial, part 1: Improvement in binge and purge measures. *J Clin Psychiatry,* 64:1335–1341.

Hu M, Wu H, Chao C (1997): Assisting effects of lithium on hypoglycemic treatment in patients with diabetes. *Biol Trace Elem Res,* 60:131–137.

Hummel B, Walden J, Stampfer R, et al (2002): Acute antimanic efficacy and safety of oxcarbazepine in an open trial with an on–off–on design. *Bipolar Disorders,* 4:412–417.

Iancu I, Rosen Y, Moshe K (2002): Antiepileptic drugs in posttraumatic stress disorder. *Clin Neuropharmacol,* 25:225–229.

Isojarvi JI, Laatikainen TJ, Pakarinen AJ, Juntunen KT, Myllyla VV (1993): Polycystic ovaries and hyperandrogenism in women taking valproate for epilepsy. *N Engl J Med,* 329:1383–1388.

Jacobsen NO, Mosekilde L, Myhre-Jensen EP, Wildenhoff KE (1967): Liver biopsies in epileptics during anticonvulsant therapy. *Acta Med Scand,* 199:345–348.

Janicak PG (1993): The relevance of clinical pharmacokinetics and therapeutic drug monitoring: Anticonvulsant mood stabilizers and antipsychotics. *J Clin Psychiatry,* 54:35–41.

Janicak PG, Keck PE, Davis JM, et al (2001): A double-blind, randomized, prospective evaluation of the efficacy and safety of risperidone versus haloperidol in the treatment of schizoaffective disorder. *J Clin Psychopharmacol,* 21:360–368.

Jerrell JM (2002): Cost-effectiveness of risperidone, olanzapine, and conventional antipsychotic medications. *Schizophrenia Bull,* 28:589–605.

Joffe RT, MacQueen GM, Marriott M, Robb J, Begin H, Young LT (2002): Induction of mania and cycle acceleration in bipolar disorder: Effect of different classes of antidepressants. *Acta Psychiatry Scand,* 105:427–430.

Kafantaris V, Coletti DJ, Dicker R, Padula G, Kane JM (2003): Lithium treatment of acute mania in adolescents: A large open trial. *J Am Acad Child Adolesc Psychiatry,* 42:1038–1045.

Kanba S, Yagi S, Kamijima K (1994): The first open study of zonisamide, a novel anticonvulsant, shows efficacy in mania. *Prog Neuro-Psychopharmacol Biol Psychiatry,* 18:707–715.

Kane JM, Eerdekens M, Lindenmayer JP, Keith SJ, Lesem MD, Karcher K (2003): Long-acting injectable risperidone: Efficacy and safety of the first long-acting atypical antipsychotic. *Am J Psychiatry,* 160:1125–1132.

Kapstan A, Yaroslavsky Y, Applebaum J, Belmaker RH, Grisaru N (2003): Right prefrontal TMS versus sham treatment of mania: A controlled study. *Bipolar Disorders,* 5:36–39.

Karpa KD, Cavanaugh JE, Lakoski JM (2002): Duloxetine pharmacology: Profile of a dual monoamine modulator. *CNS Drug Reviews,* 8:361–376.

Keck PE, Ice K (2000): A 3-week, double-blind, randomized trial of ziprasidone in the acute treatment of mania. *40th Annual NCDEU Meeting.* Boca Raton, Fl.

Keck PE, Versiani M, Potkin SG, West SA, Giller EL, Ice K (2003): Ziprasidone in the treatment of acute bipolar mania: A three-week, placebo-controlled, double-blind, randomized trial. *Am J Psychiatry,* 160:741–748.

Kemner C, Willemsen-Swinkels SHN, de Jonge M, Tuynman-Qua M, van Engeland H (2002): Open-label study of olanzapine in children with pervasive developmental disorder. *J Clin Psychopharmacol,* 22:455–460.

Kennedy R, Mittal D, O'Jile J (2003): Electroconvulsive therapy in movement disorders: An update. *J Neuropsychiatry Clin Neurosci,* 15:407–421.

Kiefer F, Holger J, Tarnaske T, et al (2003): Comparing and combining naltrexone and acamprosate in relapse prevention of alcoholism. *Arch Gen Psychiatry,* 60:92–99.

Kirby D, Harrigan S, Ames D (2002): Hyponatremia in elderly psychiatric patients treated with selective serotonin reuptake inhibitors and venlafaxine: A retrospective study in an inpatient unit. *Int J Geriatr Psychiatry,* 17:231–237.

Kirchmayer U, Davoli M, Verster A (2002): Naltrexone maintenance treatment for opioid dependence. *Cochrane Database of Systematic Reviews;* 2.

Kirsch I, Moore TJ, Scoboria A, Nicholls SS (2002): The emperor's new drugs: An analysis of antidepressant medication data submitted to the U. S. Food and Drug Administration. *Prevention and Treatment,* 5: article 23.

Koenigsberg HW, Reynolds D, Goodman M, et al (2003): Risperidone in the treatment of schizotypal personality disorder. *J Clin Psychiatry,* 64:628–634.

Koller EA, Doraiswamy PM (2002): Olanzapine-associated diabetes mellitus. *Pharmacotherapy,* 22:841–852.

Kontkanen O, Toronen P, Lakso M, Wong G, Castren E (2002): Antipsychotic drug treatment induces differential gene expression in the rat cortex. *Journal of Neurochemistry,* 83:1043–1053.

Koro CE, Fedder DO, L'Italien GJ, et al (2002a): Assessment of independent effect of olanzapine and risperidone on risk of diabetes among patients with schizophrenia: Population based nested case-control study. *BMJ,* 325:243–245.

Koro CE, Fedder DO, L'Italien GJ, et al (2002b): An assessment of the independent effects of olanzapine and risperidone exposure on the risk of hyperlipidemia in schizophrenic patients. *Arch Gen Psychiatry,* 59:1021–1026.

Kosten TR, O'Connor PG (2003): Management of drug and alcohol withdrawal. *N Engl J Med,* 348:1786–1795.

Kowatch RA, Carmody TJ, Suppes T, et al (2000): Acute and continuation pharmacological treatment of children and adolescents with bipolar disorders: A summary of two previous studies. *Acta Neuropsychiatrica,* 12:145–149.

Kozel FA, George MS (2002): Meta-analysis of left prefrontal repetitive transcranial magnetic stimulation (rTMS) to treat depression. *J Psychiatr Res,* 8:270–275.

Kratochvil C, Heiligenstein JH, Dittmann R, et al (2002): Atomoxetine and methylphenidate treatment in children with ADHD: A prospective, randomized, open-label trial. *J Am Acad Child Adolesc Psychiatry,* 41:776–784.

Krishnan KRR, Charles HC, Doraiswamy PM, et al (2003): Randomized, placebo-controlled trial of the effects of donepezil on neuronal markers and hippocampal volumes in Alzheimer's disease. *Am J Psychiatry,* 160:2003–2011.

Krueger RB, Kaplan MS (2001): Depot-leuprolide acetate for treatment of paraphilias: A report of twelve cases. *Archives of Sexual Behavior,* 30:409–422.

Krystal JH, Cramer JA, Krol WE, Kirk GE, Rosenheck R (2001): Naltrexone in the treatment of alcohol dependence. *N Engl J Med,* 345:1734–1739.

Kumar C, McIvor R, Davies T, et al (2003): Estrogen administration does not reduce the rate of recurrence of affective psychosis after childbirth. *J Clin Psychiatry,* 64:112–118.

Kurdyak PA, Gnam WH, Streiner D (2002): Antidepressants and the risk of breast cancer. *Can J Psychiatry,* 47:966–970.

Kurlan R (2002): Treatment of ADHD in children with tics: A randomized controlled trial. *Neurology,* 58:527–536.

Kurz A (2002): Non-cognitive benefits of galantamine treatment in vascular dementia. *Acta Neurol Scand,* 106:19.

Lake JT (2002): Omega-3 fatty acids: theory, clinical trials and safety issues. *Psychiatric Times,* 19:1–16.

Lake MB, Birmaher B, Wassick S, Mathos K, Yelovich AK (2000): Bleeding and selective serotonin reuptake inhibitors in childhood and adolescence. *J Child Adolesc Psychopharmacol,* 10:35–38.

Lam RWA, Wan DDC, Cohen NL, Kennedy S (2002): Combining antidepressants for treatment-resistant depression: A review. *J Clin Psychiatry,* 63:685–693.

Landi F, Cesari M, Russo A, Onder G, Sgadari A, Bernabei R (2002): Benzodiazepines and the risk of urinary incontinence in frail older persons living in the community. *Clin Pharmacol Ther,* 72:729–734.

Lattanzi L, Dell'Osso L, Cassano P, et al (2002): Pramipexole in treatment-resistant depression: A 16-week naturalistic study. *Bipolar Disorders,* 4:307–314.

Le Bars PL, Katz MM, Berman N, Itil TM, Freedman AM, Schatzberg AF (1997): A placebo-controlled, double-blind, randomized trial of an extract of Ginkgo biloba for dementia: North American EGb Study Group. *JAMA,* 278:1327–1332.

Lecrubier Y, Clerc G, Didi R, Kieser M (2002): Efficacy of St. John's wort extract WS 5570 in major depression: A double-blind, placebo-controlled trial. *Am J Psychiatry,* 159:1361–1366.

Lerer B, Shapira B, Calev A, et al (1995): Antidepressant and cognitive effects of twice- versus three-times-weekly ECT. *Am J Psychiatry,* 152:564–570.

Lesem MD, Zajecka J, Swift RH, Reeves KR, Harrigan EP (2001): Intramuscular ziprasidone 2 mg versus 10 mg in the short-term management of agitated psychotic patients. *J Clin Psychiatry,* 62:12–18.

Levin ED, Rezvani AH (2002): Nicotinic treatment for cognitive dysfunction. *Current Drug Targets: CNS and Neurological Disorders,* 1:423–431.

Lewis J (2002): Mirtazepine for PTSD. *Am J Psychiatry,* 159:1948–1949.

Liebowitz MR, DeMartinis NA, Weihs K, et al (2003): Efficacy of sertraline in severe generalized social disorder: Results of double-blind, placebo-controlled study. *J Clin Psychiatry,* 64:785–792.

Liebowitz MR, Turner SM, Piancentini J, et al (2002): Fluoxetine in children and adolescents with OCD: A placebo-controlled trial. *J Am Acad Child Adolesc Psychiatry,* 41:1431–1438.

Lima AR, Soares-Weiser K, Bacaltchuk J, Barnes TR (2002a): Benzodiazepines for neuroleptic-induced acute akathisia. *Cochrane Database of Systematic Reviews,* 4.

Lima AR, Weiser KV, Bacaltchuk J, Barnes TR (2002b): Anticholinergics for neuroleptic-induced acute akathisia. *Cochrane Database Systematic Reviews,* 2.

Lindenmayer JP, Czobor P, Volkan K, et al (2003): Changes in glucose and cholesterol levels in patients with schizophrenia treated with typical or atypical antipsychotics. *Am J Psychiatry,* 160:290–296.

Lisanby SH (2002): Update on magnetic seizure therapy: A novel form of convulsive therapy. *Journal of ECT,* 18:182–188.

Lisska MC, Rivkees SA (2003): Daily methylphenidate use slows the growth of children: A community based study. *J Pediatr Endocrin Metabolism,* 16:711–718.

Lopez-Arrieta A, Birks JS (2002): Nimodipine for primary degenerative, mixed and vascular dementia. *Cochrane Database of Systematic Reviews;* 4.

Luef GJ, Abraham I, Trinka E, et al (2002): Hyperandrogenism, postprandial hyperinsulinism and the risk of PCOS in a cross sectional study of women with epilepsy treated with valproate. *Epilepsy Res,* 48:91–102.

MacIntyre RS, Mancini DA, McCann S, Srinivasan J, Kennedy S (2003): Valproate, bipolar disorder and polycystic ovarian syndrome. *Bipolar Disorders,* 5:28–35.

Maina G, Albert U, Ziero S, Bogetto F (2003): Antipsychotic augmentation for treatment resistant obsessive–compulsive disorder: What if antipsychotic is discontinued? *Int Clin Psychopharmacol,* 18:23–38.

Maj M, Pirozzi R, Bartoli L, Magliano L (2002): Long-term outcome of lithium prophylaxis in bipolar disorder with mood-incongruent psychotic features: A prospective study. *J Affect Disord,* 71:195–198.

Makela E, Cutlip WD, Stevenson JM, et al (2003): Branded versus generic clozapine for treatment of schizophrenia. *Annals of Pharmacotherapy,* 37:350–353.

Malison RT, Anand A, Pelton GH, et al (1999): Limited efficacy of ketoconazole in treatment-refractory major depression. *J Clin Psychopharmacol,* 19:466–470.

Manna V (1991): *Disturbi affectivi bipolari e ruolo del calcio intraneuronale. Effetti terapeutici del trattamento con cali di litio e/o calcio antagonista in pazienti con rapida inversione di polarita.* [Bipolar affective disorders and intraneuronal calcium. Therapeutic effects of treatment with lithium and/or a calcium antagonist in patients with rapid cycling] *Minerva Medica,* 82:757–763.

Marangell L, Rush AJ, George MS, et al (2002): Vagus nerve stimulation (VNS) for major depressive episodes: One year outcomes. *Biol Psychiatry,* 51:280–287.

Marco MCG, Hofer H, Gekle W, et al (2002): Risperidone, 2 mg/day vs. 4 mg/day, in first-episode, acutely psychotic patients: Treatment efficacy and effects on fine motor functioning. *J Clin Psychiatry,* 63:885–891.

Marder SR, Essock SM, Miller AL, et al (2002): The Mount Sinai conference on the pharmacotherapy of schizophrenia. *Schizophrenia Bull,* 28:5–16.

Matthews JD, Bottonari KA, Polania LM, et al (2002): An open study of olanzapine and fluoxetine for psychotic major depressive disorder: Interim analyses. *J Clin Psychiatry,* 63:1164–1170.

McCall WV, Reboussin DM, Weiner RD (2000): Titrated moderately suprathreshold vs fixed high-dose right-unilateral electroconvulsive therapy. *Arch Gen Psychiatry,* 57:438–444.

McCracken J, McGough J, Shah B, et al (2002): Risperidone in children with autism and serious behavioral problems. *N Engl J Med,* 347:314–321.

McDougle CJ, Kem DL, Posey D (2002): Case series: Use of ziprasidone for maladaptive symptoms in youths with autism. *J Am Acad Child Adolesc Psychiatry,* 41:921–927.

McElroy SL, Arnold LM, Shapira NA, et al (2003): Topiramate in the treatment of binge eating disorder associated with obesity: A randomized, placebo-controlled trial. *Am J Psychiatry,* 160:255–261.

McElroy SL, Keck PE (2000): Pharmacologic agents for the treatment of acute bipolar mania. *Biol Psychiatry,* 48:539–557.

McGrath JJ, Soares JC (2002): Benzodiazepines for neuroleptic-induced tardive dyskinesia. *Cochrane Database of Systematic Reviews;* 4.

McGrath JJ, Soares-Weiser K (2002): Miscellaneous treatments for neuroleptic-induced tardive dyskinesia. *Cochrane Database of Systematic Reviews;* 4.

McIntyre RS, Mancini DA, McCann S, Srinivasan J, Sagman D, Kennedy S (2002): Topiramate versus bupropion SR when added to mood stabilizer therapy for the depressive phase of bipolar disorder: A preliminary single-blind study. *Bipolar Disorders,* 4:207–213.

McIntyre R, Trakas K, Lin D, Hwang P, Robinson K, Eggleston A (2003): Risk of weight gain associated with antipsychotic treatment: Results of the Canadian National Outcomes Measurement Study in Schizophrenia. *Can J Psychiatry,* 48: 689–694.

Meatherall R, Younes J (2002): Fatality from olanzapine-induced hyperglycemia. *J Forensic Sci,* 47:893–896.

Meehan K, Zhang F, David SR, et al (2001): A double-blind, randomized comparison of the efficacy and safety of intramuscular injections of olanzapine, lorazepam, or placebo in treating acutely agitated patients diagnosed with bipolar mania. *J Clin Psychopharmacol,* 21:389–397.

Meltzer HY, Alphs L, Green AI, et al (2003): Clozapine treatment for suicidality in schizophrenia: International suicide prevention trial. *Arch Gen Psychiatry,* 60:82–91.

Meltzer HY, McGurk S (1999): The effect of clozapine, risperidone and olanzapine in cognitive function in schizophrenia. *Schizophrenia Bull,* 25:233–256.

Mendell JR, Sahenk Z (2003): Painful sensory neuropathy. *N Engl J Med,* 348:1243–1255.

Mendelson WB (1996): The use of sedative/hypnotic medication and its correlation with falling down in the hospital. *Sleep,* 19:698–701.

Merello M, Nouzeilles MI, Cammarota A, Leiguarda R (1999): Effect of memantine (NMDA antagonist) on Parkinson's disease: A double-blind crossover randomized study. *Clin Neuropharmacol,* 22:273–276.

Meyer JM (2001): Effects of atypical antipsychotics on weight and serum lipid levels. *J Clin Psychiatry,* 62(Suppl 27):27–34.

Michelson D, Adler LA, Spencer T, et al (2003): Atomoxetine in adults with ADHD: Two randomized placebo-controlled trials. *Biol Psychiatry,* 53:112–120.

Michelson D, Allen AJ, Busner J, et al (2002): Once-daily atomoxetine treatment for children and adolescents with attention deficit hyperactivity disorder: A randomized, placebo-controlled study. *Am J Psychiatry,* 159:1896–1901.

Mintzer JE, Kershaw P (2003): The efficacy of galantamine in the treatment of Alzheimer's disease: Comparison of patients previously treated with acetylcholinesterase inhibitors to patients with no prior exposure. *Int J Geriatr Psychiatry,* 18:292–297.

Moncrieff J (2003): Clozapine v. conventional antipsychotic drugs for treatment-resistant schizophrenia: A re-examination. *Br J Psychiatry,* 183:161–166.

Montes LG, Uribe MP, Sotres JC, Martin GH (2003): Treatment of primary insomnia with melatonin: A double-blind, placebo-controlled, crossover study. *J Psychiatry Neurosci,* 28:191–196.

Montgomery DB, Roberts A, Green M, Bullock T, Baldwin D, Montgomery SA (1994): Lack of efficacy of fluoxetine in recurrent brief depression and suicidal attempts. *Eur Arch Psychiatry Clin Neurosci,* 244:211–215.

Montgomery SA, Mahe V, Haudiquet V, Hackett D (2002): Effectiveness of venlafaxine, extended-release formulation, in the short-term and long-term treatment of generalized anxiety disorder: Results of a survival analysis. *J Clin Psychopharmacol,* 22:561–567.

Moore CM, Demopulos CM, Henry ME (2002): Brain-to-serum lithium ratio and age: An in vivo magnetic resonance spectroscopy study. *Am J Psychiatry,* 159:1240–1242.

Morello CM, Leckband SG, Stoner CP (1999): Randomized dougle-blind study comparing the efficacy of gabapentin with amitriptyline on diabetic peripheral neuropathy pain. *Arch Intern Med,* 159:1931–1937.

Morihisa JM, Rosse RB, Cross CD (1994): Laboratory and other diagnostic tests in psychiatry. In Hales RE, Frances AJ (eds), *American Psychiatric Press Textbook of Psychiatry,* 3 ed. Washington, DC: American Psychiatric Press, pp. 277–310.

Mortimer AM, Martin M, Wheeler JA, Tyson PJ (2003): Conventional antipsychotic prescription in unipolar depression, II: Withdrawing conventional antipsychotics in unipolar, nonpsychotic patients. *J Clin Psychiatry,* 64:668–672.

Movig KKL, Leufkens HGM, Lendernik AW, et al (2002): Association between antidepressant drug use and hyponatremia: A case-control study. *Br J Clin Pharmacol,* 53:363–369.

Muller N, Riedel M, Scheppach C, et al (2002): Beneficial antipsychotic effects of celecoxib add-on therapy compared to risperidone alone in schizophrenia. *Am J Psychiatry,* 159:1029–1034.

Mulsant B, Sweet R, Rosen J, et al (2001): A double-blind randomized comparison of nortriptyline plus perphenazine versus nortriptyline plus placebo in the treatment of psychotic depression in late life. *J Clin Psychiatry,* 62:597–604.

Murphy BE, Ghadirian AM, Dhar V (1998): Neuroendocrine responses to inhibitors of steroid biosynthesis in patients with major depression resistant to antidepressant therapy. *Can J Psychiatry,* 43:279–286.

Nahas Z, Kozel FA, Li X, Anderson B, George MS (2003): Left prefrontal transcranial magnetic stimulation (TMS) treatment of depression in bipolar affective disorder: A pilot study of acute safety and efficacy. *Bipolar Disorders,* 5:40–47.

Nemeroff CB (2003): Safety of available agents used to treat bipolar disorder: Focus on weight gain. *J Clin Psychiatry,* 64:532–539.

Nemets B, Stahl Z, Belmaker RH (2002): Addition of omega-3 fatty acid to maintenance medication treatment for recurrent unipolar depressive disorder. *Am J Psychiatry,* 159:477–479.

Neutel I (1998): Benzodiazepine-related traffic accidents in young and elderly drivers. *Human Psychopharmacol,* 13(Suppl 2):S115–S123.

Niederhofer H, Staffen W, Mair A (2003): A placebo-controlled study of lofexidine in the treatment of children with tic disorders and attention deficit hyperactivity disorder. *J Psychopharmacol,* 17:113–119.

Normann C, Hummel B, Scharer LO, Horn M, Grunze H, Walden J (2002): Lamotrigine as adjunct to paroxetine in acute depression: A placebo-controlled, double-blind study. *J Clin Psychiatry,* 63:337–344.

Nulman I, Rovet J, Stewart DE, et al (1997): Neurodevelopment of children exposed in utero to antidepressant drugs. *N Engl J Med,* 336:258–262.

Nurnberg HG, Gelenberg AJ, Hargreave TR, Harrison W, Siegel RL, Smith MD (2001): Efficacy of sildenafil citrate for the treatment of erectile dysfunction in men taking serotonin reuptake inhibitors. *Am J Psychiatry,* 158:1926–1928.

Obrocea GV, Dunn R, Frye MA, et al (2002): Clinical predictors of response to lamotrigine and gabapentin monotherapy in refractory affective disorders. *Biol Psychiatry,* 51:253–260.

O'Donovan C, Kusumaker V, Graves GR, Bird DC (2002): Menstrual abnormalities and polycystic ovary syndrome in women taking valproate for bipolar mood disorder. *J Clin Psychiatry,* 63:322–330.

Okuma T (1983): Therapeutic and prophylactic effects of carbamazepine in bipolar disorders. *Psychiatr Clin North Am,* 6:157–174.

Okuma T (1993): Effects of carbamazepine and lithium on affective disorders. *Neuropsychobiology,* 27:138–145.

Olin J, Schneider L (2002): Galantamine for Alzheimer's disease. *Cochrane Database of Systematic Reviews;* 2.

Pande AC, Crockatt JG, Feltner DE, et al (2003): Pregabalin in generalized anxiety disorder: A placebo-controlled trial. *Am J Psychiatry,* 160:533–540.

Pande AC, Crockatt JG, Janney CA, Werth JL, Tsaroucha G (2000): Gabapentin in bipolar disorder: A placebo-controlled trial of adjunctive therapy—Gabapentin Bipolar Disorder Study Group. *Bipolar Disorders,* 2(3 Pt 2):249–255.

Pande AC, Davidson J, Jefferson JW, et al (1999): Treatment of social phobia with gabapentin: A placebo-controlled study. *J Clin Psychopharmacol,* 19:341–348.

Pande AC, Pollack MH, Crockatt JG, et al (2000): Placebo-controlled study of gabapentin treatment of panic disorder. *J Clin Psychopharmacol,* 20:467–471.

Park Y, Zhu S, Palaniappan L, Heshka S, Carnethon MR, Heymsfield SB (2003): The metabolic syndrome: Prevalence and associated risk factor findings in the U. S. population from the Third National Health and Nutrition Examination Survey, 1988–1994. *JAMA,* 163:427–436.

Patton WW, Misri S, Corral MR, Perry KF, Kuan AJ (2002): Antipsychotic medication during pregnancy and lactation in women with schizophrenia: Evaluating the risk. *Can J Psychiatry,* 47:959–965.

Pazzaglia PJ, Post RM, Ketter TA, George MS, Marangell LB (1993): Preliminary controlled trial of nimodipine in ultra-rapid cycling affective dysregulation. *Psychiatry Res,* 49:257–272.

Pellock JM, Willmore LJ (1991): A rational guide to routine blood monitoring in patients receiving antiepileptic drugs. *Neurology,* 41:961–964.

Perry PJ (2001): Therapeutic drug monitoring of antipsychotics. *Psychopharmacol Bull,* 35:19–29.

Perry PJ, Yates WR, Williams RD, et al (2002): Testosterone therapy in late-life major depression in males. *J Clin Psychiatry,* 63:1096–1101.

Perugi G, Toni C, Frare F, et al (2002): Effectiveness of adjunctive gabapentin in resistant bipolar disorder: Is it due to anxious-alcohol abuse comorbidity? *J Clin Psychopharmacol,* 22:584–591.

Perugi G, Toni C, Ruffolo G, Frare F, Akiskal HS (2001): Adjunctive dopamine agonists in treatment-resistant bipolar II depression: An open case series. *Pharmacopsychiatry,* 34:137–141.

Phillip M, Kohnen R, Hiller KO (2000): Hypericum extract versus imipramine or placebo in patients with moderate depression: Randomised multi-centre study of treatment for eight weeks. *BMJ,* 319:1534–1538.

Piccinelli M, Pini S, Bellantuono C, Wilkinson G (1995): Efficacy of drug treatment in obsessive–compulsive disorder: A meta-analytic review. *Br J Psychiatry,* 166:424–443.

Pittler MH, Ernst E (2000): Efficacy of kava extract for treating anxiety: Systematic review and meta-analysis. *J Clin Psychopharmacol,* 20:84–89.

Pope HG, Cohane GH, Kanayama G, Siegel AJ, Hudson JI (2003): Testosterone gel supplementation for men with refractory depression: a randomized, placebo-controlled trial. *Am J Psychiatry,* 160:105–111.

Poyurovsky M, Isaacs I, Fuchs C, et al (2003): Attenuation of olanzapine-induced weight-gain with reboxetine in patients with schizophrenia: A double-blind, placebo-controlled study. *Am J Psychiatry*, 160:297–302.

Poyurovsky M, Pashinian A, Gil-Ad I, et al (2002): Olanzapine-induced weight gain in patients with first-episode schizophrenia: A double-blind, placebo-controlled study of fluoxetine addition. *Am J Psychiatry*, 159:1058–1060.

Preskhorn SH, Burke MJ, Fast GA (1993): Therapeutic drug monitoring: Principles and practice. *Psychiatr Clin North Am*, 16:611–640.

Prestwood KM, Kenny AM, Kleppinger A, Kulldorff M (2003): Ultralow-dose micronized 17B-estradiol and bone density and bone metabolism in older women. *JAMA*, 290:1042–1048.

Purdon SE, Jones BDW, Stip E (2000): Neuropsychological changes in early phase schizophrenia during 12 months of treatment with olanzapine, risperidone or haloperidol. *Arch Gen Psychiatry*, 57:553–559.

Quitkin F, Petkova E, McGrath PJ, et al (2003): When should a trial of fluoxetine for major depression be declared failed? *Am J Psychiatry*, 160:734–740.

Quraishi S, David A (2002): Depot haloperidol decanoate for schizophrenia. *Cochrane Database of Systematic Reviews;* 2.

Rabey JM, Nissipeanu P, Korczyn AD (1992): Efficacy of memantine, an NMDA receptor antagonist, in the treatment of Parkinson's disease. *J Neural Transm Park Dis Dement Sect,* 4:277–282.

Rapp SR, Espeland MA, Shumaker SA, et al (2003): Effect of estrogen plus progestin on global cognitive function in postmenopausal women. *JAMA*, 289:2663–2672.

Raskin J, Goldstein DJ, Mallinckrodt CH, Ferguson MB (2003): Duloxetine in the long-term treatment of major depressive disorder. *J Clin Psychiatry*, 64:1237–1244.

Reilly J, Ayis SA, Ferrier IN, Jones SJ, Thomas SHL (2002): Thioridazine and sudden unexplained death in psychiatric in-patients. *Br J Psychiatry*, 180:515–522.

Reisberg B, Doody RS, Stoffler A, Schmitt F, Ferris SH, Mobius HJ (2003): Memantine in moderate-to-severe Alzheimer's disease. *N Engl J Med*, 348:1333–1341.

Rengo F, Carbonin P, Pahor M, et al (1996): A controlled trial of verapamil in patients after acute myocardial infarction: Results of the calcium antagonist reinfarction Italian study (CRIS). *Am J Cardiol*, 77:365–369.

Rhoden EL, Morgentaler A (2004): Risks of testosterone-replacement therapy and recommendations for monitoring. *N Engl J Med*, 350:482–492.

Richardson MA, Bevans ML, Read LL, et al (2003): Efficacy of the branched-chain amino acids in the treatment of tardive dyskinesia in men. *Am J Psychiatry*, 160: 1117–1124.

Rickels K, Downing R, Schweizer E, Hassman H (1993): Antidepressants for the treatment of generalized anxiety disorder: A placebo-controlled comparison of imipramine, trazodone and diazepam. *Arch Gen Psychiatry*, 50:884–895.

Rickels K, Zaninelli R, McCafferty J, Bellew K, Iyengar M, Sheehan DV (2003): Paroxetine treatment of generalized anxiety disorder: A double-blind, placebo-controlled study. *Am J Psychiatry*, 160:749–756.

Rinne T, Van den Brink W, Wouters L, van Dyck R (2002): SSRI treatment of borderline personality disorder: A randomized, placebo-controlled clinical trial for female patients with borderline personality disorder. *Am J Psychiatry*, 159:2048–2054.

Rosenheck R, Davis JM, Evans DL, Herz A (2003): Olanzapine versus haloperidol in schizophrenia. *JAMA,* 290:2693–2702.

Rosler A, Witztum E (1998): Treatment of men with paraphilia with a long-acting analogue of gonadotropin-releasing hormone. *N Engl J Med,* 338:416–422.

Rossouw JE, Anderson GL, Prentice RL, et al. (2002): Risks and benefits of estrogen plus progestin in healthy postmenopausal women: Principal results from the Women's Health Initiative randomized controlled trial. *JAMA,* 288(3):321–333.

Rothschild AJ, Duval SE (2003): How long should patients with psychotic depression stay on the antipsychotic medication? *J Clin Psychiatry,* 64:390–396.

Rothschild AJ, Samson JA, Bessette MP, Carter-Campbell JT (1993a): Efficacy of the combination of fluoxetine and perphenazine in the treatment of psychotic depression. *J Clin Psychiatry,* 54:338–342.

Rothschild AJ, Samson JA, Bessette MP, Carter-Campbell JT (1993b): Efficacy of the combination of fluoxetine and perphenazine in the treatment of psychotic depression. *J Clin Psychiatry,* 54:338–342.

Rudolph RL (2002): Achieving remission from depression with venlafaxine and venlafaxine extended release: A literature review of comparative studies with selective serotonin reuptake inhibitors. *Acta Psychiatr Scand,* 106:24–30.

Rull J, Quibrera R, Gonzalez-Millan H, Lozano Castenada O (1969): Symptomatic treatment of peripheral diabetic neuropathy with carbamazepine (Tegretol): Double blind crossover trial. *Diabetologia,* 5:215–218.

Rush AJ, George MS, Sackeim HA, et al (2000): Vagus nerve stimulation (VNS) for treatment-resistant depression: A multicenter study. *Biol Psychiatry,* 47:276–286.

Ryan MCM, Collins P, Thakore JH (2003): Impaired fasting glucose tolerance in first-episode, drug-naive patients with schizophrenia. *Am J Psychiatry,* 160:284–289.

Sachs G, Rosenbaum JF, Jones L (1990): Adjunctive clonazepam for maintenance treatment of bipolar affective disorder. *J Clin Psychopharmacol,* 10:42–47.

Sackeim HA, Prudic J, Devanand DP (2000): A prospective, randomized, double-blind comparison of bilateral and right unilateral electroconvulsive therapy at different stimulus intensities. *Arch Gen Psychiatry,* 57:425–434.

Sackeim HA, Rush AJ, George MS, et al (2001): Vagus nerve stimulation (VNS) for treatment-resistant depression: Efficacy, side effects, and predictors of outcome. *Neuropsychopharmacol,* 25:713–728.

Sanger T, Grundy SL, Gibson P, Namjoshi M, Greaney MG, Tohen M (2001): Long-term olanzapine therapy in the treatment of bipolar I disorder: An open-label continuation study. *J Clin Psychiatry,* 62:273–281.

Sanger T, Tohen M, Vieta E, et al (2003): Olanzapine in the acute treatment of bipolar I disorder with a history of rapid cycling. *J Affect Disord,* 73:155–161.

Santarelli L, Saxe M, Gross C, et al (2003): Requirement of hippocampal neurogenesis for the behavioral effects of antidepressants. *Science,* 301:805–809.

Sarchiapone M, Amore M, De Risio S, et al (2003): Mirtazepine in the treatment of panic disorder: An open-label trial. *Int Clin Psychopharmacol,* 18:35–38.

Sasaki H, Hashimoto K, Inada T, Fukui S, Iyo M (1995): Suppression of oro-facial movements by rolipram, a cAMP phosphodiesterase inhibitor, in rats chronically treated with haloperidol. *Eur J Pharmacol,* 282:71–76.

Sasaki Y, Matsuyama T, Inoue S, et al (2003): A prospective, open-label, flexible-dose study of quetiapine in the treatment of delirium. *J Clin Psychiatry,* 64:1316–1321.

Sassi R, Nicoletti M, Brambilla P, et al (2002): Increased gray matter volume in lithium-treated bipolar disorder patients. *Neuroscience Letters,* 329:243.

Sato Y, Kondo I, Ishida S, et al (2001): Decreased bone mass and increased bone turnover with valproate therapy in adults with epilepsy. *Neurol,* 57:445–449.

Scarabin PY, Oger E, Plu-Bureau G (2003): Differential association of oral and transdermal oestrogen-replacement therapy with venous thromboembolism risk. *Lancet,* 362:428–432.

Schacter SC (2002): Vagus nerve stimulation: Where are we? *Current Opinion Neurol,* 15:201–206.

Schneider LS, Small GW (2002): The increasing power of placebos in trials of antidepressants [letter]. *JAMA,* 288:450.

Schoeneberger RA, Tanasijevic MJ, Jha A, Bates DW (1995): Appropriateness of antiepileptic drug level monitoring. *JAMA,* 274:1622–1626.

Schwartz TL (2002): The use of tiagabine augmentation for treatment-resistant anxiety disorders: A case series. *Psychopharmacol Bull,* 36:53–57.

Schwartz TL, Beale M (2003): Psychotropic drug-induced weight gain alleviated with orlistat: A case series. *Psychopharmacol Bull,* 37:5–9.

Segal J, Berk M, Brook S (1998): Risperidone compared with both lithium and haloperidol in mania: A double-blind randomized controlled trial. *Clin Neuropharmacol,* 21:176–180.

Segraves RT (2003): Pharmacologic management of sexual dysfunction: Benefits and limitations. *CNS Spectrums,* 8:225–229.

Segraves RT, Saran A, Segraves K, Maguire E (1993): Clomipramine versus placebo in the treatment of premature ejaculation: A pilot study. *J Sex Marital Ther,* 19: 198–200.

Seidman S, Pesce VC, Roose SP (2003): High-dose sildenafil citrate for selective serotonin reuptake inhibitor-associated ejaculatory delay: Open clinical trial. *J Clin Psychiatry,* 64:721–725.

Semenchuk MR, Sherman S, Davis B (2001): Double-blind, randomized trial of bupropion SR for the treatment of neuropathic pain. *Neurology,* 57:1383–1388.

Serfaty M, Kennell-Webb S, Warner J, Blizard R, Raven P (2002): Double blind randomised placebo controlled trial of low dose melatonin for sleep disorders in dementia. *Int J Geriatr Psychiatry,* 17:1120–1127.

Sernyak MJ, Godleski LS, Griffin RA, Mazure CM, Woods SW (1997): Chronic neuroleptic exposure in bipolar outpatients. *J Clin Psychiatry,* 58:193–195.

Shekelle PG, Hardy ML, Morton SC, et al (2003): Efficacy and safety of ephedra and ephedrine for weight loss and athletic performance. *JAMA,* 289:1537–1545.

Shelton RC, Keller MB, Gelenberg AJ, et al (2001): Effectiveness of St. John's wort in major depression: A randomized controlled trial. *JAMA,* 285:1978–1986.

Shumaker SA, Legault C, Rapp SR, et al (2003): Estrogen plus progestin and the incidence of dementia and mild cognitive impairment in postmenopausal women. *JAMA,* 289:2651–2662.

Simon GE, Cunningham ML, Davis RL (2002): Outcomes of prenatal antidepressant exposure. *Am J Psychiatry,* 159:2055–2061.

Simpson DM, Olney R, McArthur JC, Khan A, Godbold J, Ebel-Frommer K (2000): A placebo-controlled trial of lamotrigine for painful HIV-associated peripheral neuropathy. *Neurol,* 54:2115–2119.

Simpson DM, Perry CM (2003): Atomoxetine. *Paediatric Drugs,* 5:407–415.

Simpson GM, El Sheshai A, Rady A, Kingsbury SJ, Fayek M (2003): Sertraline as monotherapy in the treatment of psychotic and nonpsychotic depression. *J Clin Psychiatry,* 64:959–965.

Sjogren MJC, Hellstrom PTO, Jonsson MAG, Runnerstam M, Silander HC, Ben-Menachem E (2002): Cognition-enhancing effect of vagus nerve stimulation in patients with Alzheimer's disease: A pilot study. *J Clin Psychiatry,* 63:972–980.

Smith D, Dempster C, Glanville J, Freemantle N, Anderson IM (2002): Efficacy and tolerability of venlafaxine compared with selective serotonin reuptake inhibitors and other antidepressants: A meta-analysis. *Br J Psychiatry,* 180:396–404.

Smith D, Wesson DR (1999): Benzodiazepines and other sedative-hypnotics. In Galanter M, Kleber HD (eds), *American Psychiatric Press Textbook of Substance Abuse Treatment,* 2nd ed. Washington, DC: American Psychiatric Press, pp. 239–250.

Smith DL, Angst MS, Brock-Utne JG, DeBattista C (2003): Seizure duration with remifentanil/methohexital vs. methohexital alone in middle-aged patients undergoing electroconvulsive therapy. *Acta Anaesthesiol Scand,* 47:1064–1066.

Smith WT, Londborg PD, Glaudin V, Painter JR (2002): Is extended clonazepam cotherapy of fluoxetine effective for outpatients with major depression? *J Affect Disord,* 70:251–259.

Soares KV, McGrath JJ (2001): Vitamin E for neuroleptic-induced tardive dyskinesia. *Cochrane Database Systematic Reviews;* 2.

Soumerai SB, Simoni-Wastila L, Singer C, et al (2003): Lack of relationship between long-term use of benzodiazepines and escalation to high doses. *Psychiatric Services,* 54:1006–1011.

Spencer T, Biederman J (2002): Non-stimulant treatment for attention-deficit/ hyperactivity disorder. *J Attention Disord,* 6(Suppl 1):S109–S119.

Sproule B (2002): Lithium in bipolar disorder: Can drug concentrations predict therapeutic effect? *Clin Pharmacokinet,* 41:639–660.

Srisurapanont M, Jarusuraisin N (2002): Opioid antagonists for alcohol dependence. *Cochrane Database of Systematic Reviews;* 2.

Stahl S, Entusah R, Rudolph RL (2002): Comparative efficacy between venlafaxine and SSRIs: A pooled analysis of patients with depression. *Biol Psychiatry,* 52: 1166–1174.

Stahl S, Gergel I, Li D (2003): Escitalopram in the treatment of panic disorder: A randomized, double-blind, placebo-controlled trial. *Am J Psychiatry,* 64:1322–1327.

Stassen HH, Delrur-Stula A, Angst J (1993): Behandlung von angst-patienten. *Z Allgemeinmed,* 10:271–277.

Stearns V, Beebe KL, Iyengar M, Dube E (2003): Paroxetine controlled release in the treatment of menopausal hot flashes: A randomized controlled trial. *JAMA,* 289: 2827–2834.

Stein DJ, Versiani M, Hair T, Kumar R (2002): Efficacy of paroxetine for relapse prevention in social anxiety disorder. *Arch Gen Psychiatry,* 59:1111–1118.

Stein MB, Kline NA, Matloff JL (2002): Adjunctive olanzapine for SSRI-resistant combat-related PTSD: A double-blind, placebo-controlled study. *Am J Psychiatry,* 159:1777–1779.

Steiner H, Petersen ML, Saxena K, Ford S, Matthews Z (2003): Divalproex sodium for the treatment of conduct disorder: A randomized controlled clinical trial. *J Clin Psychiatry,* 64:1183–1191.

Sternbach H (2003): Are antidepressants carcinogenic? A review of preclinical and clinical studies. *J Clin Psychiatry,* 64:1153–1162.

Stoler JM (2001): Maternal antiepileptic drug use and effects on fetal development. *Current Opinion Pediatr,* 13:566–571.

Stoll AL, Severus E, Freeman MP (1999): Omega-3 fatty acids in bipolar disorder: A preliminary double-blind, placebo-controlled trial. *Arch Gen Psychiatry,* 56: 407–412.

Straus S (2002): Herbal medicines: What's in the bottle? *N Engl J Med,* 347:1997–1998.

Strous RD, Maayan R, Lapidus R, et al (2003): Dehydroepiandrosterone augmentation in the management of negative, depressive, and anxiety symptoms in schizophrenia. *Arch Gen Psychiatry,* 60:133–141.

Suppes T (2002): Review of the use of topiramate for treatment of bipolar disorders. *J Clin Psychopharmacol,* 22:599–609.

Suppes T, Chisholm K, Dhavale D, et al (2002): Tiagabine in treatment refractory bipolar disorder: A clinical case series. *Bipolar Disorders,* 4:283–289.

Suppes T, Webb A, Paul B, Carmody T, Kraemer HC, Rush AJ (1999): Clinical outcome in a randomized 1-year trial of clozapine versus treatment as usual for patients with treatment-resistant illness and a history of mania. *Am J Psychiatry,* 156: 1164–1169.

Suri R, Stowe ZN, Hendrick V, Hostetter AM, Widawski M, Altschuler LL (2002): Estimates of nursing infant daily dose of fluoxetine through breast milk. *Biol Psychiatry,* 52:446–451.

Swanson J (2003): Development of a new once-a-day formulation of methylphenidate for the treatment of attention-deficit/hyperactivity disorder. *Arch Gen Psychiatry,* 60:204–211.

Tammenmaa IA, McGrath JJ, Sailas E, Soares-Weiser K (2002): Cholinergic medications for neuroleptic-induced tardive dyskinesia. *Cochrane Database Systematic Reviews;* 3.

Tasmuth T, Hartel B, Kalso E (2002): Venlafaxine in neuropathic pain following treatment of breast cancer. *Eur J Pain,* 6:17–24.

Tew JD, Mulsant B, Haskett RF, Dolata D, Hixson L, Mann J (2002): A randomized comparison of high-charge right unilateral electroconvulsive therapy in older depressed patients who failed to respond to 5 to 8 moderate-charge right unilateral treatments. *J Clin Psychiatry,* 63:1102–1105.

Thambi L, Kapcala LP, Chambers WJ, et al (2001): Topiramate-associated secondary angle-closure glaucoma: A case series. *Arch Ophthalmol,* 119:1210–1211.

Tharyan P, Adams CE (2002): Electroconvulsive therapy for schizophrenia. *Cochrane Database Systematic Reviews;* 2.

Tiihonen J, Hallikainen T, Ryynanen O-P, et al (2003): Lamotrigine in treatment-resistant schizophrenia: A randomized placebo-controlled cross-over trial. *Biol Psychiatry,* 54:1241–1248

Tohen M, Baker R, Altshuler L, Zarate CA, Suppes T, Ketter TA (2002a): Olanzapine versus divalproex in the treatment of acute mania. *Am J Psychiatry,* 159: 1011–1017.

Tohen M, Chengappa KN, Suppes T, Zarate CA, Calabrese JR, Bowden C (2002b): Efficacy of olanzapine in combination with valproate or lithium in the treatment of mania in patients partially nonresponsive to valproate or lithium monotherapy. *Arch Gen Psychiatry,* 59:62–69.

Tohen M, Chengappa KN, Suppes T, et al (2002c): Efficacy of olanzapine in combination with valproate or lithium in the treatment of mania in patients partially responsive to valproate or lithium monotherapy. *Arch Gen Psychiatry*, 59:62–69.

Tohen M, Jacobs TG, Grundy SL, et al (2000): Efficacy of olanzapine in acute bipolar mania: A double-blind, placebo-controlled study—The Olanzapine HGGW Study Group. *Arch Gen Psychiatry*, 57:841–849.

Tohen M, Sanger TM, McElroy SL, et al (1999): Olanzapine versus placebo in the treatment of acute mania. *Am J Psychiatry*, 156:702–709.

Tohen M, Vieta E, Calabrese JR, et al (2003): Efficacy of olanzapine and olanzapine–fluoxetine combination in the treatment of bipolar I depression. *Arch Gen Psychiatry*, 60:1079–1088.

Tondo L, Baldessarini RJ, Floris G, Rudas N (1997): Effectiveness of restarting lithium treatment after its discontinuation in bipolar I and bipolar II disorders. *Am J Psychiatry*, 154:548–550.

Tondo L, Baldessarini RJ, Hennen J, Floris G, Silvetti F, Tohen M (1998): Lithium treatment and risk of suicidal behavior in bipolar disorder patients. *J Clin Psychiatry*, 59:405–414.

Tran PV, Bymaster FP, McNamara RK, Potter WZ (2003): Dual monoamine modulation for improved treatment of major depressive disorder. *J Clin Psychopharmacol*, 23:78–86.

Trinh N, Hoblyn J, Mohanty S, Yaffe K (2003): Efficacy of cholinesterase inhibitors in the treatment of neuropsychiatric symptoms and functional impairment in Alzheimer's disease. *JAMA*, 289:210–216.

Trivedi MH, Rush AJ, Carmody T, et al (2001): Do bupropion SR and sertraline differ in their effects on anxiety in depressed patients? *J Clin Psychiatry*, 62:776–781.

Tunnicliff G, Raess BU (2002): Gamma-hydroxybutyrate. *Current Opinion in Investigational Drugs*, 3:278–283.

Vaage-Nilsen M, Hansen JF, Hagerup L, Sigurd B, Steinmetz E (1995): Effect of verapamil on the prognosis of patients with early postinfarction electrical or mechanical complications: The Danish Verapamil Infarction Trial II (DAVIT II). *Int J Cardiol*, 48:255–258.

Van Ameringen M, Mancini C, Pipe B, Campbell M, Oakman J (2002): Topiramate treatment for SSRI-induced weight gain in anxiety disorders. *J Clin Psychiatry*, 63:981–984.

van Minnen A, Hoogduin KAL, Keijsers GPJ, Hellenbrand I, Hendriks G-J (2003): Treatment of trichotillomania with behavioral therapy or fluoxetine: A randomized, waiting-list controlled study. *Arch Gen Psychiatry*, 60:517–522.

Verma NP, Haidukewych D (1993): Differential but infrequent alterations of hepatic enzyme levels and thyroid hormone levels by anticonvulsant drugs. *Arch Neurol*, 2:319–323.

Verster JC, Volkerts E, Verbaten N (2002): Effects of alprazolam on driving ability, memory functioning and psychomotor performance: A randomized, placebo-controlled study. *Neuropsychopharmacol*, 27:260–269.

Vestergaard P, Schou M (1987): Does long-term lithium treatment induce diabetes mellitus? *Neuropsychobiol*, 17:130–132.

Vieta E, Goikolea J, Corbella B (2001): Group for the Study of Risperidone in Affective Disorders (GSRAD): Risperidone safety and efficacy in the treatment of bipolar and schizoaffective disorders—results from a 6-month, multicenter, open study. *J Clin Psychiatry,* 62:818–825.

Vieta E, Parramon G, Padrell E, et al (2002): Quetiapine in the treatment of rapid cycling bipolar disorder. *Bipolar Disorders,* 4:335–340.

Vieta E, Torrent C, Garcia-Ribas G, Gilabert A (2002): Use of topiramate in treatment-resistant bipolar spectrum disorders. *J Clin Psychopharmacol,* 22:431–435.

Viola J, Ditzler T, Batzer W (1997): Pharmacological management of posttraumatic stress disorder: Clinical summary of a five-year restrospective study 1990–1995. *Military Med,* 162:616–619.

Vorbach EU, Gortelmeyer R, Bruning J (1996): *Therapie von insomnien. Wirksamkeit und vertraeglichkeit eine baldrianpraeparats.* [*Treatment of insomnia*] *Psychopharmakotherapie,* 3:109–115.

Vorona R, Catesby WJ (2000): Update on nonapnea sleep disorders. *Current Opinion in Pulmonary Med,* 6:507–511.

Wagner KD, Ambrosini PJ, Rynn MA, et al (2003): Efficacy of sertraline in the treatment of children and adolescents with major depressive disorder: Two randomized controlled trials. *JAMA,* 290:1033–1041.

Wagner KD, Weller EB, Carlson G, et al (2002): An open-label trial of divalproex in children and adolescents with bipolar disorder. *J Am Acad Child Adolesc Psychiatry,* 41:1224–1230.

Wahlbeck K, Cheine MV, Essali A, Adams CE (1999): Evidence of clozapine's effectiveness in schizophrenia: A systematic review and meta-analysis of randomized trials. *Am J Psychiatry,* 156:990–999.

Walden J, Schaerer L, Schloesser S, Grunze H (2000): An open longitudinal study of patients with bipolar rapid cycling treated with lithium or lamotrigine for mood stabilization. *Bipolar Disorders,* 2:336–339.

Wall M, Baird-Lambert J, Buchanan N, Farrell G (1992): Liver function tests in persons receiving anticonvulsant medications. *Seizure,* 1:187–190.

Walsh BT, Seidman SN, Sysko R, Gould M (2002): Placebo response in studies of major depression: Variable, substantial, and growing. *JAMA,* 287:1840–1847.

Wang PW, Santosa C, Schumacher M, Winsberg ME, Strong CM, Ketter TA (2002): Gabapentin augmentation therapy in bipolar depression. *Bipolar Disorders,* 4:296–301.

Wang SJ, Sihra TS, Gean PW (2001): Lamotrigine inhibition of glutamate release from isolated cerebrocortical nerve terminals (synaptosomes) by suppression of voltage-activated calcium channel activity. *Neuroreport,* 12:2255–2258.

Wecker L, James S, Copeland N, Pacheco MA (2003): Transdermal selegiline: Targeted effects on monoamine oxidases in the brain. *Biol Psychiatry,* 54:1099–1104.

Wheeler V, Jason A, Mortimer AM, Tyson PJ (2000): Somatic treatment of psychotic depression: Review and recommendations for practice. *J Clin Psychopharmacol,* 20:509–514.

Whitehead C, Moss S, Cardno A, Lewis G (2002): Antidepressants for people with both schizophrenia and depression. *Cochrane Database of Systematic Reviews;* 2.

Wilens T, Pelham W, Stein MB, et al (2003): ADHD treatment with once-daily OROS methylphenidate: Interim 12-month results from a long-term open-label study. *J Am Acad Child Adolesc Psychiatry,* 42:424–433.

Wilkinson D, Holmes C, Woolford J, Stammers S (2002): Prophylactic therapy with lithium in elderly patients with unipolar major depression. *Int J Geriatr Psychiatry,* 17:619–622.

Wimo A, Winblad B, Stoffler A, Wirth Y, Mobius HJ (2003): Resource utilization and cost analysis of memantine in patients with moderate to severe Alzheimer's disease. *Pharmacoeconomics,* 21:327–340.

Wirshing DA, Boyd JA, Meng LR, Ballon JS, Marder SR, Wirshing WC (2002): The effects of novel antipsychotics on glucose and lipid levels. *J Clin Psychiatry,* 63:856–865.

Wisner KL, Peindl KS, Perel JM, Hanusa BH, Piontek CM, Baab S (2002): Verapamil treatment for women with bipolar disorder. *Biol Psychiatry,* 51:745–752.

Wolkowitz OD, Reus VI, Chan T, et al (1999): Antiglucocorticoid treatment of depression: Double-blind ketoconazole. *Biol Psychiatry,* 45:1070–1074.

Woods SW (2003): Chlorpromazine equivalent doses for the newer atypical antipsychotics. *J Clin Psychiatry,* 64:663–667.

Worthington JJ, Simon NM, Korbly NB, Perlis RH, Pollack MH (2002): Ropinirole for antidepressant-induced sexual dysfunction. *Int Clin Psychopharmacol,* 17: 307–310.

Yatham LN, Grossman F, Augustyns I, Vieta E, Ravindran A (2003): Mood stabilisers plus risperidone or placebo in the treatment of acute mania: International double-blind, randomised controlled trial. *Br J Psychiatry,* 182:141–147.

Yatham LN, Kusumaker V, Calabrese JR, Rao R, Scarrow G, Kroeker G (2002): Third generation anticonvulsants in bipolar disorder: A review of efficacy and summary of clinical recommendations. *J Clin Psychiatry,* 63:275–283.

Yingling DR, Utter G, Vengalil S, Mason BJ (2002): Calcium channel blocker, nimodipine, for the treatment of bipolar disorder during pregnancy. *Am J Obstet Gynecol,* 187:1711–1712.

Zajecka J, Weisler RH, Sachs G, Swann AC, Wozniak PJ, Sommerville KW (2002): A comparison of the efficacy, safety and tolerability of divalproex sodium and olanzapine in the treatment of bipolar disorder. *J Clin Psychiatry,* 63:1148–1155.

Zanardi R, Franchini L, Gasperini M, Perez J, Smeraldi E (1996): Double-blind controlled trial of sertraline versus paroxetine in the treatment of delusional depression. *Am J Psychiatry,* 153:1631–1633.

Zanarini MC, Frankenburg FR (2003): Omega-3 fatty acid treatment of women with borderline personality disorder: A double-blind, placbo-controlled pilot study. *Am J Psychiatry,* 160:167–169.

Zarate CA, Tohen M (2004): Double-blind comparison of the continued use of antipsychotic treatment versus its discontinuation in remitted manic patients. *Am J Psychiatry,* 161:169–171.

Zerjav-Lacombe S, Tabarsi E (2001): Lamotrigine: A review of clinical studies in bipolar disorders. *Can J Psychiatry,* 46:328–333.

Zohar J, Keegstra H, Barrelet L (2003): Fluvoxamine as effective as clomipramine against symptoms of severe depression: Results from a multicentre, double-blind study. *Human Psychopharmacol,* 18:113–119.

Zornberg GL, Jick H (2000): Antipsychotic drug use and risk of first-time idiopathic venous thromboembolism: A case-control study. *Lancet,* 356:1219–1223.

# INDEX

Page numbers in *italics* refer to figures or tables.